(73)

Art 2.

Apt. E-9

Lakeland Drive 15

Optic Foramen – Post. boundary of Ant. Cranial fossa

3538207

Shearer's

Manual of

HUMAN DISSECTION

Shearer's

Manual of

HUMAN DISSECTION

Edited by

CHARLES E. TOBIN, Ph.D.

Associate Professor of Anatomy, The University
of Rochester School of Medicine and Dentistry

FOURTH EDITION

THE BLAKISTON DIVISION

McGraw-Hill Book Company, Inc., New York, Toronto, London

Fourth Edition

Shearer's MANUAL OF HUMAN DISSECTION

Preface ·

As originally conceived, this manual was intended to supply the inexperienced dissector with concise, specific directions for dissection procedures. Because of the decreased amount of time allotted to gross anatomy and the increased number of students, it was hoped such a manual would facilitate and enhance instruction in the laboratory. The need for this fourth edition substantiates the original concept.

In answer to the requests of numerous instructors, however, additional dissection procedures for the brain, eyeball, oral cavity, middle ear, and fascial spaces of the head and neck have been added, but in accord with the basic plan all directions have been kept concise and clear. Terminology has been modernized, and most of the newer, more descriptive terms from the *Nomina Anatomica* (Paris, 1955) have been adopted. Wherever a new term is introduced, however, the old (BNA) term is also given so that the student may be familiar with both terminologies.

An endeavor has been made to achieve a workable balance between the amount of procedure for dissection and the descriptive text. The manual is, therefore, a compromise between the classical, lengthy manuals and the very brief guides for dissection. It is adaptable to various plans or sequences of dissection without overburdening the dissector with detailed instructions or, on the other hand, neglecting to indicate and correlate the parts of the human body. Certain structures, notably, the lymphatic system and some of the articulations, purposely have been given only minor consideration, since the medical student usually does not have the time to dissect them adequately. In the author's opinion, knowledge of these parts, which is essential to further progress in medical education, can be best gained from lectures, reading, or demonstrations.

The sequential presentation of regional dissections in this manual is based on the traditional order of dissection, although it may be changed to suit the plans or preferences of the staff teaching the course. At the author's school, in order to achieve correlation in the anatomy courses, the order of dissection is so arranged that the students dissect the gross structures prior to or at the same time as these structures are being studied in embryology, histology, or neuroanatomy.

Since the manual is designed as an autonomous unit, it does not have to be used in conjunction with, or with reference to, any specific descriptive text on human anatomy. *The dissector should use this book in view of the purpose for which it has been written— a guide for human dissection. If he is to obtain a thorough understanding of human anatomy, the student should supplement the information gained from the dissection and from the brief descriptions and illustrations in this manual with collateral reading in one of the standard descriptive texts.* Frequent reference to one of the standard medical dictionaries will also help to familiarize the dissector with the meaning, origin, and pronunciation of the numerous terms he will encounter. Many interesting sidelights on the development of medical science will be brought out by this means.

Most of the illustrations are the original ones made by Dr. Shearer for the first edition of this manual. They have been changed only where additional guide lines or labels and slight changes in the legends would enhance the usefulness of the illustrations. The reader must be cognizant of the fact that many of these illustrations are not exact portrayals of the dissections, since the dissection procedures have been altered considerably from those given by Dr. Shearer when the original drawings were made. To enhance visualization of the material presented, the size of some of the original illustrations has been enlarged. Other illustrations have been added for the new chapters.

References to original papers have been cited only where descriptions in this manual differ radically from those in the standard descriptive texts.

I am greatly indebted to the many students, staff members, publishers, and reviewers who have made suggestions to help improve the usefulness of this manual.

CHARLES E. TOBIN

Introduction ·

The right to dissect the human body has been won with difficulty after centuries of struggle against the prejudice of the unenlightened. The medical student of the present day is apt to forget that having legally at his disposal, without effort on his own part, a well-preserved body for dissection is a privilege for which the anatomist of 300 years ago would have given much. The body on the dissecting table is all the corporeal remains of what was once a human being, and it should be regarded with respect.

The early anatomist was frequently confronted with the necessity for secrecy and stealth, if he was so fortunate as to procure a body at all; and, in addition to this, his work had to be done hurriedly because of the rapidity of decay. With modern methods of embalming and preservation, decay has ceased to be a factor, and the only responsibility of the dissector for the preservation of the body in the dissecting room is to see that it does not become too dry. To avoid drying, the body should always be kept wrapped in damp cloths when not in use.

The technique of human dissection is something that can be acquired only by practice. Fortunately, however, an adequate technique is usually acquired with relatively little practice. It differs from the technique of dissection with which the student may already be familiar from studies of comparative anatomy chiefly because of the vastly larger size of the body. For this reason, it is less difficult than the technique of the comparative anatomist, often requiring patience rather than great skill.

The essential instruments for the dissection of the human body are a strong pair of blunt pointed forceps and a sharp scalpel with a broad blade of medium to large size. Since proper results cannot be achieved with a dull scalpel, a stone for sharpening the blade should always be at hand. A flexible probe and a pair of scissors of medium size with one rounded and one pointed end are occasionally needed. Small, sharp, pointed forceps; narrow bladed, sharp-pointed knives; and various elaborate surgical instruments are quite useless for dissecting. The number and kind of instruments do not necessarily have to conform to this list. They may vary with the ones selected to suit the needs and plan of study in various medical schools.

The method followed in dissecting the body is the regional method, in which the design is to see everything that is to be seen in a single region of the body at one time, as opposed to the systematic method more commonly followed in studies of comparative anatomy. In approaching any region of the body, the first procedure is to identify the surface landmarks (bones, muscles, vessels, etc.) which can be palpated through the skin and then the reflection of the skin which covers it. Skin should be reflected from a region only when that region is to be studied, as skin is the best protection against drying of the underlying parts. The actual technique of skin reflection is best learned by practice, but it is well to remember that the incisions which mark out a flap of skin for reflection must be made completely through the skin and along its entire length before reflection is begun and that the skin must always be reflected cleanly from the underlying fascia.

The structures which it is desired to expose and study after the skin is reflected are embedded in the various types of connective tissue which come under the generic term *fascia*.

Before the fascia is removed, its form, extent, and connections should be studied. This tissue not only forms the framework for and encloses the various structures, but it is also important in limiting and directing the spread of infections. The further dissection of the body consists, to a very great extent, in the removal of this fascia without injury to the structures it contains. This removal of fascia is known as the cleaning of the embedded muscles, nerves, arteries, etc. It is a tedious business, and the dissector will often be tempted to leave it incomplete and pass on to other things when he has sufficiently cleaned the particular muscle or nerve he is seeking only in order to see that it actually exists. This, however, is a bad practice not only because careless work is, in itself, detrimental to proper observation but also because it is cumulative in its effect on the dissection as a whole. The more thoroughly a particular region is cleaned, the more easily and satisfactorily can ensuing and deeper regions be cleaned and observed.

When all the structures in a particular region have been cleaned, time should be taken for review and study of these structures as they appear in the body. A definite plan of study should be followed for each structure dissected. This plan should include: the plane or part of the body in which it is located; the form, size, and shape of the structure; its origin, course, and distribution; and its function. Although the function of the structures dissected will be studied in more detail in future courses, gross anatomy can be made more dynamic and interesting for the dissector if he has some knowledge, however brief, of the function of the structure he is dissecting.

Too often there is a tendency on the part of the dissector merely to go through the motions of dissection in the dissecting room and to do his actual anatomical study elsewhere from textbooks. The purpose of dissection is not, however, to provide a mild gymnastic exercise but to afford the opportunity for observation and study of the actual structure of the body itself.

Since human anatomy is the introductory course in the medical career of the dissector, he should early form the habit of accurate observation and concise expression of the knowledge gained in this as well as future courses. If at any time the dissector wishes to test the knowledge which he has obtained of any structure or region, this can be done by drawing or diagraming with labels, describing to his fellow dissectors, or writing in exact terms a brief description of the part or parts of the body being studied.

An occasional source of pardonable distress to the inexperienced dissector is the reflection that from a regional study he is expected to acquire a systematic knowledge of human anatomy. The only consolation that can be offered is that here is an opportunity for exercise of the mild integrative intellectual powers that one who embarks on the study of anatomy may be assumed to possess. Though it is a practical necessity to prosecute the dissection as a series of separate regions, it is by no means a necessity to keep the observations so made in separate regional compartments of the mind. As the dissection proceeds, the knowledge acquired region by region should be associated in the mind of the dissector so that he will eventually see the body as a whole and be able to reproduce his knowledge in systematic form, even though, for example, he may never actually have seen the entire arterial system or the entire nervous system at one time.

Contents ·

Pectoral Region ·

Before starting the dissection of the **pectoral region,** identify the bony points which may be felt through the skin. In the midline at the base of the neck is the **jugular notch,** which marks the superior border of the manubrium sterni. At each side of the jugular notch the prominent medial end of the **clavicle** may be felt; it takes part in the sternoclavicular articulation. The clavicle may be felt along its entire length. At its lateral end it articulates with the **acromion process** of the scapula, which also is subcutaneous, and which forms the bony prominence of the shoulder. The **sternum** may be felt through the skin in the midline along the entire length of the **manubrium** and **corpus sterni.** At the lower end of the corpus sterni is a depression in the anterior body wall corresponding to the **xiphoid process** of the sternum. About 1½ in. below the jugular notch is a marked transverse bony ridge. This is the **sternal angle,** which marks the junction of the manubrium and corpus sterni; it is of importance in that it indicates the level at which the second rib joins the sternum and may be used as a starting point for counting the ribs on the surface of the body.

Observe the position of the **nipple.** It usually corresponds to the fourth intercostal space, about 4 in. from the sternum. In the female it is at the summit of a rounded elevation formed by the superficial fascia which contains the mammary gland.

Abduct the arms and observe the **axillary folds.** These are folds of skin, fascia, and muscle which bound the **axilla** or armpit. The anterior fold is caused by the lower border of the pectoralis major muscle. The posterior fold, which extends farther inferiorly, is caused principally by the latissimus dorsi. Between the two folds the skin, here covered with hair, is indented to form the arched floor of the axilla.

For the dissection of the pectoral region and axilla, the arms should be abducted and tied in this position to a long board placed under the shoulders and extending outward on each side. This abduction should only be about 12 in. from the side of the body when beginning this dissection. Full abduction will tear the muscles. During subsequent dissection periods, gradually abduct the arms until the axilla is fully exposed. With the body so placed, the following skin incisions should be made: (1) in the midline from the jugular notch to the middle of the xiphoid process; (2) from the upper end of the first incision, one laterally on each side along the full length of the clavicle to the tip of the acromion; (3) from the lower end of the first incision, one laterally and somewhat inferiorly across the thoracic wall to the posterior axillary fold; (4) from the lower end of the first incision, one upward and laterally to the nipple, which it should encircle, then upward and laterally along the line of the anterior axillary fold and down the front of the arm for about 6 in. Transverse incisions should then be made across the front of the arm for about 2 in. The large flaps of skin thus marked out on each side should be reflected laterally. Some difficulty may be met in reflecting the skin of the axilla, since this skin, which is quite thin, is rather firmly attached to strands of axillary fascia.

When the skin flaps are reflected, the **superficial fascia** of the pectoral and axillary regions are exposed. In the male subject, the superficial fascia of this region has no specific characteristics, except that in its uppermost part will be found the fibers of origin of the

1

platysma, a superficial muscle of the neck. In the female, however, it contains the mammary gland, which should now be studied. Dissect the vessels and nerves within the superficial fascia, paying particular attention to those related to the mammary gland in the female. Consult one of the standard descriptive texts for the **lymphatic drainage of the mammary gland.**

The **mammary gland** does not have a distinct capsule of connective tissue. Its essential glandular portion, the **corpus mammae,** is embedded in the general subcutaneous fatty tissue, which is here increased in amount. The corpus mammae consists of from 15 to 20 **lobes,** each of which has a single **excretory duct** opening separately into a depression on the nipple. Pass a bristle into one of these openings and attempt by dissection to demonstrate the **lactiferous duct** whose termination it is. Look also for the **sinus lactiferus,** a dilation of the lactiferous duct just internal to its opening. Internal to the sinus each duct breaks up into smaller and smaller branches within the substance of the gland. These cannot ordinarily be demonstrated in gross dissection.

The pectoralis major muscle should now be cleaned. On one side, remove the superficial fascia (including the mammary gland and nipple) and the deep fascia covering the muscle. Cut through the fascia (until the red muscle fibers are exposed) in a transverse line running from the lower border of the medial end of the clavicle outward to the anterior aspect of the arm and in a vertical line along the lateral part of the anterior aspect of the sternum. This will mark out a triangular flap of fascia which can then be reflected laterally and downward to expose the sternocostal portion of the muscle. In cutting the strands of fascia from the surface of the muscle, the blade of the scalpel should be moved in the direction in which the muscle fibers run. When the lower border of the muscle, corresponding to the anterior axillary fold, is reached, the

flap of fascia removed from its surface may be cut away and discarded. Next remove the fascia from the upper or clavicular portion of the muscle in the same manner by reflecting it upward and laterally.

On the other side, leave the mammary gland as a landmark and for observation of its blood supply from vessels supplying the pectoral muscles in a later stage of the dissection. The pectoralis major muscle on this side can be cleaned by cutting and reflecting the fascia from the peripheral borders of the mammary gland.

The **pectoralis major** is a large triangular muscle consisting of a smaller **clavicular portion** and a larger, inferior **sternocostal portion.** The clavicular portion arises from the anterior surface of the medial half of the clavicle. The superficial fibers of the sternocostal portion arise from the lateral part of the entire length of the anterior surface of the manubrium and corpus sterni. Its deeper fibers arise from the anterior surfaces of the second to sixth costal cartilages, but this cannot be demonstrated until the muscle is reflected. Laterally, the fibers of both parts converge to be inserted together into the outer lip of the **intertubercular sulcus** of the humerus, which is now under cover of the deltoid muscle.

Attempt to demonstrate some of the small anterior **cutaneous nerves** and **vessels** which pierce the pectoralis major in longitudinal series slightly lateral to the sternum. These are the terminal portions of the upper intercostal nerves and vessels, and they supply the skin over the anterior part of the chest.

Identify and clean the **cephalic vein.** This is a superficial vein of the arm, usually large but sometimes reduced in size or lacking, which will be found in the present area of dissection in the groove between the upper border of the pectoralis major and the deltoid. It disappears from view behind the clavicle in the **deltopectoral triangle.** This is a small triangular depression bounded by the anterior border of the deltoid, the upper border of the pectoralis major, and the lower border of the middle portion of the clavicle. Remove the fat which it contains and look for the small **deltopectoral lymph glands** which are often present. Emerging through the fat of the delto-pectoral triangle will also be found the **deltoid branch** of the **thoracoacromial artery,** which accompanies the cephalic vein laterally and supplies the anterior border of the deltoid.

The anterior wall of the axilla is formed principally by the pectoralis major. To prepare the axilla for dissection this muscle should now be reflected. *Before the pectoralis major (or any other muscle) is reflected, it is advisable to insert a finger beneath the muscle and, by palpation, ascertain its bony attachments, re-lationships to other structures, and nerve and blood supply.* This procedure will avoid the error of cutting through not only the muscle being dissected but also the adjacent structures, since the thickness of the muscle to be reflected cannot be fully appreciated until it is palpated. On one side dissect the fat and fascia from the axilla (follow procedure given on p. 4) before reflecting the pectoralis major. Then, detach the clavicular portion from its origin, and cut through the sternocostal portion by an incision running parallel and about 1 in. lateral to its medial border. The detached lateral segment of muscle can then be turned laterally toward its insertion. As this is done, the subjacent pec-toralis minor muscle will be exposed and the nerves and vessels which supply the pectoralis major will be seen entering its deep surface. The nerves and arteries should be cleaned. The nerves are branches of the **medial** and **lateral anterior thoracic (pectoral) nerves.** These nerves are derived in the axilla from the brachial plexus, to which origin they will later be traced. The lateral pectoral nerve reaches the deep surface of the pectoralis major by winding around the medial border of the pectoralis minor. The medial pectoral nerve usually pieces the pectoralis minor but may

appear at its lateral border. The arteries enter-ing the deep surface of the pectoralis major are the **pectoral branches** of the **thoracoacromial artery;** they also appear at the medial border of the pectoralis minor. The pectoralis major cannot usually be properly reflected without dissecting these vessels and nerves free from the undersurface of the pectoralis major. Then cut them so that sufficiently long pieces will be retained to later identify and trace them to their origins (Fig. 1).

Clean and study the **pectoralis minor. It** arises from the anterior surfaces of the **second to fifth ribs** near their cartilages; the fibers run upward and converge to a tendinous insertion on the **coracoid process** of the scapula.

Observe the **clavipectoral fascia.** This sheet of fascia occupies the triangular gap between the medial border of the pectoralis minor, the lower border of the clavicle, and the anterior thoracic wall. It is pierced by the cephalic vein, the lateral pectoral nerve, and the deltoid and pectoral branches of the thoracoacromial artery. Together with the pectoralis minor, it aids the pectoralis major in forming the an-terior wall of the axilla. Superiorly it splits to enclose the subclavius muscle. Cut through the clavipectoral fascia just below the clavicle to expose this muscle. The **subclavius** is a small **muscle** which arises from the **first rib** and its cartilage near their junction and runs upward and laterally to be inserted into a groove on the under surface of the middle third of the **clav-icle.** The axilla may now be completely opened from the front by removal of the clavipectoral fascia and reflection of the pectoralis minor. Detach the pectoralis minor from its origin on the ribs and turn it upward to its insertion. As this is done, the **medial pectoral nerve,** whose terminal portion has already been seen entering the pectoralis major, will be found entering the deep surface of the pectoralis minor, which it also supplies. This nerve should be preserved for future reference.

The **axilla** is a potential space, roughly pyramidal in shape, lying between the upper part of the arm and the upper lateral thoracic wall. Its anterior wall has already been studied and removed; its remaining boundaries will be exposed as the dissection proceeds. The medial wall of the axilla is formed by the upper ribs and intercostal muscles, covered externally for the most part by the **serratus anterior muscle.** Its narrow lateral wall is formed by the medial surface of the upper part of the humerus, covered by the **coracobrachialis muscle.** Its posterior wall, which extends farther inferiorly than does the anterior wall, is formed from above downward and laterally by the **subscapularis, teres major,** and **latissimus dorsi muscles.** The apex of the axilla is a triangular gap bounded by the first rib, the upper border of the scapula, and the posterior border of the clavicle and is known as the **cervicoaxillary canal,** through which the axilla communicates with the posterior triangle of the neck. The base or floor of the axilla is formed by the **axillary fascia** and skin.

The dissection of the axilla consists in the removal of the axillary fascia and fat without injury to the structures embedded in it. As the fat is removed, numerous lymph vessels and glands will also be found within it. Their form, position, and the areas which they drain should be noted, but they need not be retained. Those parts of the latissimus dorsi, teres major, and subscapularis muscles, forming the posterior wall of the axilla, should also be cleaned at this time to aid in the identification of their nerve and blood supply. The ventral part of the latissimus dorsi muscle should be freed from the chest wall and retracted laterally. The lateral cutaneous branches of the intercostal nerves in this area should also be cleaned and studied.

The nerves and vessels entering the arm

from the lateral part of the axilla should first be exposed. Start by removing the deep fascia from the upper part of the arm, where it forms the lateral wall of the axilla. This will expose the **coracobrachialis muscle** and the **short head of** the **biceps brachii,** which arise together from the coracoid process of the scapula. Descending along the medial border of the coracobrachialis, the large **median nerve** will be found. Medial to this nerve the distal part of the **axillary artery** should be exposed and cleaned. Medial to the artery is the **ulnar nerve.** This latter nerve may be overlapped by the **axillary vein,** whose general position is medial and somewhat anterior to the artery. Also medial to the axillary artery and closely related to the axillary vein will be found the **medial cutaneous nerve of** the **forearm** (medial antibrachial cutaneous nerve) and the **medial cutaneous nerve of** the **arm** (medial brachial cutaneous nerve). The latter usually· communicates by a branch with another small nerve, the **intercostobrachial.** This nerve will be found in the fascia near the floor of the axilla. It is usually the lateral cutaneous branch of the second intercostal nerve, which emerges from the second intercostal space and crosses the axilla to reach the medial aspect of the arm. Now push the coracobrachialis laterally and expose the **musculocutaneous nerve.** This nerve lies lateral to the median nerve in the upper part of the arm and disappears from view by entering the substance of the coracobrachialis. Trace the median nerve proximad and observe that it is formed at about the level of the outer margin of the pectoralis minor by the junction of two smaller nerve trunks. These are known as the **lateral** and **medial heads of** the **median nerve.** The medial head crosses in front of the axillary artery. If the distal part of the axillary artery is now drawn forward and medially, a very large nerve which lies immediately behind it in the lateral part of the axilla may be exposed. This is the **radial nerve.**

The various nerves which have been exposed are the terminal branches of the brachial plexus. Their distribution cannot be studied until the arm is dissected, but they may be traced back to their origins in the more medial parts of the axilla. Before doing this, however, it is well to have a general idea of the

The three trunks enter the upper medial part of the axilla through the cervicoaxillary canal, and each breaks up into an **anterior** and a **posterior branch** (division), which are recombined to form the **cords** of the plexus. The **lateral cord** is formed by the anterior branches of the upper and middle trunks, the **medial cord** is a direct continuation of the anterior branch of the lower trunk, and the **posterior cord** is formed by the junction of all three

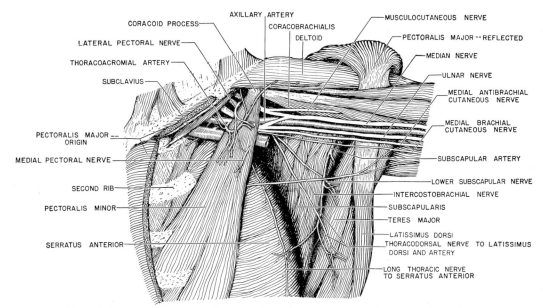

FIG. 1. The axilla, opened from the front by reflection of the pectoralis major.

plan of the brachial plexus and its relation to the axillary artery.

The **brachial plexus** is derived from the anterior primary divisions of the fifth, sixth, seventh, and eighth cervical and the first thoracic nerves. These nerves, which are known as the **roots** of the plexus, are situated in the posterior triangle of the neck. Here they combine to form the **trunks** of the plexus as follows: the **fifth** and **sixth** cervical roots form the **upper trunk,** the **seventh** cervical alone forms the **middle trunk,** and the **eighth** cervical and **first thoracic,** the **lower trunk.**

posterior branches. The three cords are grouped about the middle portion of the axillary artery in positions corresponding to their names. The nerves already exposed in the lateral part of the axilla are derived from these three cords. Before tracing them back to the various cords, the axillary vessels should be studied.

The **axillary vein,** while usually described as a single channel, is often found to consist of two or more parallel anastomosing vessels. Its tributaries, in so far as they are constant, correspond to and accompany the branches of the axillary artery. Having once observed the important fact that throughout its course the axillary vein lies medial and somewhat anterior to the artery, *the dissector is advised to cut the veins (and in future dissections other veins) away whenever by so doing he may facilitate the cleaning and study of the arteries and nerves.*

Clean and study the **axillary artery** and its branches. The axillary artery is an arbitrary anatomical subdivision of the great arterial channel which supplies the superior extremity. It begins at the outer border of the **first rib** as a direct continuation of the **subclavian artery** and ends at the outer border of the **teres major muscle** (which corresponds roughly to the lateral part of the posterior axillary fold), beyond which point its continuation is known as the **brachial artery.** It is further arbitrarily divided for descriptive purposes into **three parts.** Of these, the **first** is **medial** to the pectoralis minor and, consequently, posterior to the clavipectoral fascia, the **second** lies **behind** the pectoralis minor, and the **third** and longest part is **lateral to** the **pectoralis minor.** Observe that the distal half of the third part, where it extends beyond the lower border of the pectoralis major, is quite superficial, being covered only by the fascia and skin.

The branches of the axillary artery are subject to some variation, but in the majority of cases are as follows. From the **first part** arises a small branch, the **supreme thoracic,** distributed to the upper part of the thoracic wall. From the **second part,** near its beginning, arises the **thoracoacromial artery.** This is a short, thick trunk, some of whose branches have already been met, which runs forward into the costocoracoid membrane to break up into a group of radiating branches, which are described from the regions they supply as **deltoid, pectoral, acromial,** and **clavicular.** The **lateral thoracic artery** arises from the middle of the **second part** of the axillary and runs downward

under cover of the pectoralis minor to be distributed to the lateral thoracic wall and the pectoral muscles.

The **third part** of the axillary artery has three branches which all arise close together at about the middle of its course. The **anterior humeral circumflex artery** is a small branch which arises from the anterolateral aspect of the axillary and runs laterally across the front of the arm to disappear behind the coracobrachialis muscle. The **posterior humeral circumflex** is considerably larger. It arises from the posterior aspect of the axillary and runs backward and downward to disappear almost at once into a groove in the posterior wall of the axilla. Accompanying the artery into this groove, which lies between the adjacent borders of the subscapularis and teres major muscles, will be found a large nerve, not previously uncovered. This is the **axillary nerve.** Running downward from the axillary artery in close relation to the posterior wall of the axilla is the **subscapular artery.** About 1 in. below its origin it ends by dividing into the **thoracodorsal** and **scapular circumflex arteries.** The scapular circumflex leaves the axilla by passing backward into the groove between the subscapularis and the teres major. The thoracodorsal continues its descent on the posterior wall of the axilla and is distributed chiefly to the latissimus dorsi and teres major muscles. In cleaning it, secure the nerve of supply to the latissimus dorsi. This is the **thoracodorsal nerve,** which runs downward and laterally in the fat on the posterior wall of the axilla to be distributed to the latissimus dorsi in company with branches of the thoracodorsal artery (Fig. 2).

Now complete the study of those parts of the brachial plexus which lie in the axilla. Begin with the **lateral cord.** This lies lateral to the second part of the axillary artery and may be identified by tracing proximally the **musculocutaneous nerve** and the **lateral head of** the

median nerve, which are its terminal branches. Its only other branch is the **lateral pectoral nerve,** which was previously identified and should now be traced to its origin. Trace the lateral cord proximad and identify the anterior branches of the upper and middle trunks, which join to form it.

The **medial cord** lies medial to the second part of the axillary artery. Its terminal branches are the **ulnar nerve** and the **medial head of** the

minal branches, the **axillary** and **radial nerves,** have been identified and may now be traced back to their origins. Its other branches are three smaller nerves, the upper and lower subscapular nerves and the **thoracodorsal.** The latter has already been seen as the nerve of supply to the latissimus dorsi. The subscapular nerves will be found by dissecting in the fat close to the posterior wall of the axilla. The **upper subscapular,** often represented by two

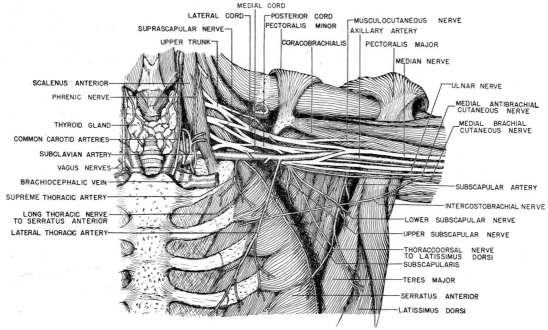

FIG. 2. Complete dissection of the brachial plexus. The medial end of the clavicle has been removed and both pectoral muscles reflected.

median nerve, which crosses in front of the third part of the axillary artery. Proximal to its termination the medial cord gives rise to the **medial cutaneous nerve of** the **forearm,** the **medial cutaneous nerve of** the **arm,** and the **medial pectoral nerve,** all of which have already been identified. As the medial cord is traced proximad, it will be found to be a direct continuation of the anterior branch of the lower trunk.

The **posterior cord** lies behind the second part of the axillary artery. Its two large ter-

branches, supplies the subscapularis; the **lower subscapular,** the teres major. The two subscapular nerves and the thoracodorsal often arise from the posterior cord by a common trunk and sometimes appear to arise from the axillary nerve rather than directly from the posterior cord. Trace the posterior cord proximad and observe that it is formed by the union of the posterior branches of all three trunks.

As the final step in the dissection of the axilla, clear away the fascia from its medial wall to expose the **serratus anterior muscle** and **long thoracic nerve (to serratus anterior).** The serratus anterior is a large flat muscle which arises by a series of pointed slips from the outer surfaces of the **first eight ribs** about 1 in. lateral to their junction with their cartilages. Its fibers run posteriorly around the thoracic wall to be inserted into the inner aspect of the **vertebral border of** the **scapula** along its entire length. It is supplied by the long thoracic nerve. This nerve will be found running downward over the external surface of the muscle in about the midaxillary line. It is derived in the posterior triangle of the neck from the fifth, sixth, and seventh cervical nerves.

Triangles of Neck ··············

The anterior and posterior triangles of the neck are regions which depend for their anatomical recognition principally upon the position of the **sternomastoid muscle.** The **anterior triangle,** of which the apex is directed inferiorly, lies in front of the sternomastoid, whose anterior border forms the posterolateral boundary of the triangle; its superior boundary is formed by the lower border of the mandible, and its medial boundary is formed arbitrarily by the median line of the neck from the mandibular symphysis to the jugular notch of the sternum. It is only by this line that the anterior triangles of the two sides are separated from each other. The **posterior triangle,** of which the apex is directed superiorly, lies behind the sternomastoid, whose posterior border forms its anterior boundary; its inferior boundary is formed by the middle third of the clavicle; its posterior boundary is formed by the anterior border of the trapezius muscle (Fig. 3).

The skin should now be reflected in a single flap from the surface of both triangles and the sternomastoid muscle. For this purpose three skin incisions should be made: (1) a median incision running from the mental protuberance downward to the jugular notch; (2) from the upper end of the first incision, one backward and laterally along the inferior border of the mandible to the angle, and then backward and somewhat upward, to pass below the ear, across the mastoid process, and for about 1 in. along the superior nuchal line; (3) from the lower end of the first incision, one laterally along the clavicle to the acromion. The skin should then be reflected backward and laterally from the front and side of the neck. As this is done, be extremely careful to reflect the skin cleanly away from the underlying fascia, particularly as the posterior portion of the area is reached, since if the skin is carelessly reflected in this region, the anterior border of the **trapezius** is liable to injury or even to reflection with the skin. The superficial fascia which is exposed by the reflection of the skin shows no particular characteristics differentiating it from the same layer in other regions, except that it is extremely thin and contains the platysma muscle.

Clean the **platysma** by the removal of that part of the superficial fascia which covers it. This thin, sheetlike muscle belongs to the general group of the muscles of facial expression and is often poorly developed. Do not mistake the fibers of the sternomastoid for those of the platysma; this confusion can be avoided by observation of the direction in which the fibers run. The **platysma** arises from the skin and

cervical IV of facial to
platysma m ?

superficial fascia covering the upper portion of the pectoralis major; from here its fibers pass upward and medially across the clavicle in a broad, flat sheet which covers the lower anterior part of the posterior triangle, the lower two-thirds of the sternomastoid, and the superolateral part of the anterior triangle; it is inserted into the inferior border of the mandible

muscle should be rolled up from its caudal end and left attached to the facial muscles. This must be done with care to avoid injury to the nerves and vessels which lie immediately subjacent to the platysma. As the angle of the mandible is approached, attempt to secure the **cervical branch of the facial nerve,** which emerges from behind the lower part of the

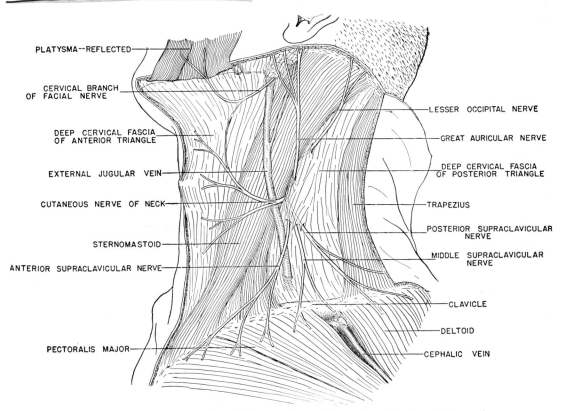

FIG. 3. Superficial dissection of the anterior and posterior triangles of the neck.

and the skin of the lower part of the cheek and the angle of the mouth. This latter part of its insertion cannot be seen at present. Locate the branches of the **supraclavicular nerves** within the superficial fascia at the caudal edge of the platysma muscle, separating the lower fibers of this muscle, if necessary, to identify these nerves. When the platysma has been cleaned and observed, it should be reflected from the clavicle upward and medially to the lower border of the mandible. The platysma

parotid gland to enter the deep surface of the platysma, which it supplies. Observe that the lower tip of the **parotid gland** fills in the narrow interval between the posterior border of the ramus of the mandible and the anterior border of the sternomastoid. The main body of the parotid is still covered by the skin of the face.

Now clean the sternomastoid muscle, cleaning at the same time and retaining in position the structures which cross its external surface.

These are the **external jugular vein** and four nerves. These nerves are **cutaneous branches of the cervical plexus;** they become superficial by piercing the deep fascia of the posterior triangle close to the posterior border of the sternomastoid and turning forward across that muscle. The **lesser occipital nerve** crosses the upper posterior part of the sternomastoid to be distributed to the skin of the lower lateral part of the scalp. The **great auricular nerve** runs upward and slightly forward over the upper half of the sternomastoid to supply the skin of this part of the neck, a small part of the skin of the face in the region of the angle of the mandible, and the posterior part of the auricle. The **cervical cutaneous nerve** crosses the sternomastoid transversely at about its middle to supply the skin over the anterior triangle. The **anterior supraclavicular nerve** crosses the lower lateral portion of the sternomastoid to be distributed to the skin in the region of the sternoclavicular articulation (Fig. 3).

The **external jugular vein** is somewhat variable in size and occasionally entirely missing. Typically, it is formed on the sternomastoid below and behind the angle of the mandible by the junction of the **posterior auricular vein** with a branch of the **posterior facial (retromandibular).** It descends across the sternomastoid and pierces the deep fascia of the lower anterior part of the posterior triangle to terminate in the **subclavian vein.**

The **sternomastoid muscle** (m. sternocleidomastoideus) arises by two heads, a medial one from the front of the **manubrium sterni** and a more lateral one from the upper border of the medial third of the **clavicle.** It is inserted on the outer surface of the **mastoid process** and the lateral half of the **superior nuchal line.**

Posterior Triangle

When the sternomastoid and the structures crossing it have been cleaned and studied, proceed to the dissection of the posterior triangle. For this dissection, the shoulder should be depressed and the head turned as far as possible to the opposite side.

The **trapezius** muscle cannot be studied as a whole until the back is dissected. Its upper anterior border should now be cleaned, however, in order to define completely the boundaries of the posterior triangle. This border runs downward and laterally from about the middle of the superior nuchal line to the upper border of the clavicle at about the junction of its middle and lateral thirds. The superficial boundary or roof of the posterior triangle is formed by a layer of the **deep cervical fascia** which stretches between the sternomastoid and the trapezius and is limited inferiorly by the clavicle. This fascia is pierced by the structures which have already been seen to cross the sternomastoid and by the remaining supraclavicular nerves, which should now be identified. The **supraclavicular nerves** are all derived, as will be apparent later, from a single trunk that arises from the lowest loop of the cervical plexus. They usually pierce the deep fascia of the posterior triangle as three separate trunks, **anterior, middle,** and **posterior,** supply the skin over the lower part of the posterior triangle, and descend across the clavicle to supply the skin covering the upper part of the pectoralis major and the region of the acromion. Posterior supraclavicular branches cross the trapezius superficially (Fig. 3).

The deep boundary or floor of the posterior triangle is formed by the external surfaces of several of the deeper muscles of the neck. The actual extent of the triangle is the potential space, much deeper below than above, which intervenes between this muscular floor and the fascial roof. The further dissection of the posterior triangle consists in the cleaning of the structures contained within it and the muscles which make up its floor by the careful removal of the fascia and fat. It should be noted that inferiorly the posterior triangle is directly continuous with the axilla by means of a triangular aperture known as the **cervico-axillary canal;** this canal is bounded by the clavicle, the upper border of the scapula, and the first rib. The muscles which form the floor of the triangle are, from above down, the **splenius capitis,** the **levator scapulae,** and the **scalenus medius** and **posterior.** Only a portion of each of these muscles appears in the triangle, but they should be identified as the dissection proceeds. The scalenus anterior sometimes appears in the lower anterior corner of the triangle but is usually completely covered by the sternomastoid.

The **cutaneous nerves** which have already been displayed should now be traced back to the points at which they emerge from under cover of the posterior border of the sternomastoid. The cervical plexus, from which all these nerves arise, is under cover of the sternomastoid and will be displayed later, when that muscle is reflected. Next identify and clean the **accessory nerve.** This is the eleventh cranial nerve; it emerges from under cover of the sternomastoid in close relation to the **lesser occipital nerve** and runs downward and posteriorly on the levator scapulae to disappear under cover of the trapezius, which it supplies. Somewhat lower one or two smaller nerve twigs will be found following a similar course through the triangle; these are **muscular branches of** the **cervical plexus,** for the additional supply of the trapezius (Fig. 4).

Clean the **posterior belly of** the **omohyoid muscle** and locate its nerve supply. This muscle subdivides the posterior triangle into an upper **occipital** and a lower **subclavian triangle,** as it courses from behind the sternomastoid and in front of the anterior scalene toward its attachment to the superior border of the scapula. On a slightly deeper plane, the **transverse cervical artery** may be exposed and cleaned. This vessel is usually a branch of the **thyrocervical trunk of** the **subclavian artery;**

emerging from behind the sternomastoid, it crosses the posterior triangle about ½ in. above, and roughly parallel to, the clavicle, to divide into two branches. The **ascending (superficial) branch** passes laterally under cover of the trapezius. The **descending (deep) branch** enters the floor of the triangle in the interval between the scalenus medius and the levator scapulae. The origin and course of these arteries is variable, and a superficial branch, the **superficial cervical artery,** may replace part of the transverse cervical artery.

Attention should next be directed to the roots and trunks of the **brachial plexus,** which lie deeply in the lower anterior part of the posterior triangle. The **roots** of the plexus are the anterior primary divisions of the fifth, sixth, seventh, and eighth cervical and the first thoracic nerves. They pass downward and laterally into the triangle from the interval behind the scalenus anterior and in front of the scalenus medius and combine to form the upper, middle, and lower trunks of the plexus. The **trunks** continue their course downward and laterally, resting against the scalenus medius, to enter the axilla through the cervicoaxillary canal.

Clean first the **upper trunk.** This is formed by the junction of the anterior primary divisions of the fifth and sixth cervical nerves and gives rise to two branches in the posterior triangle. These are the **suprascapular nerve** and the **nerve to** the **subclavius.** The latter is a small twig which passes downward and forward through the areolar tissue of the lower part of the triangle and behind the clavicle to supply the subclavius muscle. The suprascapular nerve is a much larger branch which passes laterally toward the upper border of the scapula. The **middle trunk** of the plexus lies below the upper trunk and is a direct continuation of the anterior primary division of the seventh cervical nerve; it has no branches in the posterior triangle. The **lower trunk** is formed by the junction of the anterior rami of the eighth cervical and first thoracic nerves; its course in the posterior triangle is very short, and it also is devoid of branches in this area.

Identify and clean the **dorsal scapular** and the **long thoracic (nerve to serratus anterior)**. These are both derived from the upper roots

transverse cervical artery. The **nerve to serratus anterior** takes a more nearly vertical course and passes behind the trunks of the plexus into the axilla (Fig. 4).

Clean the portions of the **subclavian vein** and the **subclavian artery** which are at present available for study. The subclavian vein lies

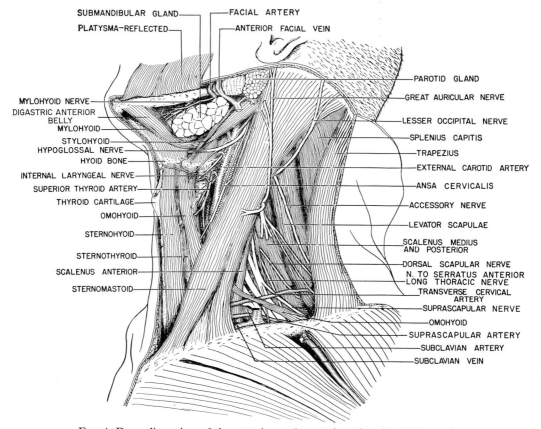

FIG. 4. Deep dissection of the anterior and posterior triangles of the neck.

of the plexus, but their origin is too far medial to be seen at present. They will be found to enter the triangle through the substance of the scalenus medius and pass downward on the surface of that muscle, inclining somewhat posteriorly. The **dorsal scapular nerve** is the higher of the two; it leaves the triangle by entering its floor in the interval between the scalenus medius and the levator scapulae in close relation to the descending branch of the

immediately behind the clavicle in the lower anterior corner of the posterior triangle and passes medially behind the sternomastoid and in front of the scalenus anterior. It receives in this region the termination of the external jugular vein. Behind the subclavian vein, the **suprascapular artery** will be found emerging from in front of the scalenus anterior to cross the lowest part of the posterior triangle and join the **suprascapular nerve** close to the upper border of the scapula. The second part of the subclavian artery lies behind the scalenus anterior, which separates it from the vein. The third part extends from the outer border of the scalenus anterior to the outer border of the first rib and should now be cleaned. It rests on the upper surface of the first rib and lies below and in front of the lower trunk of the brachial plexus; at the outer border of the first rib, it becomes the axillary artery. It typically has no branches, but occasionally either the transverse cervical or the suprascapular artery, or both, may arise from it.

Anterior Triangle

The **anterior triangle** is also roofed by a layer of **deep cervical fascia.** This fascia stretches from the anterior border of the sternomastoid muscle of one side to that of the other. Superiorly it is attached to the lower border of the mandible and more posteriorly blends with the fascia forming the sheath of the parotid gland. It is firmly attached to the body of the hyoid bone, whose position should be determined by palpation. Inferiorly, the fascia splits into anterior and posterior layers which are attached to the anterior and posterior borders, respectively, of the jugular notch of the sternum and enclose between them a potential space filled with areolar tissue known as the **suprasternal space.** On the external surface of this fascia is the **anterior jugular vein.** This vein is formed by several small veins in the region of the mental protuberance and descends just lateral to the median line to enter the suprasternal space. Just above the manubrium, it turns laterally behind the sternomastoid to terminate in the external jugular or the subclavian vein. It shows variable communications with other veins and is apt to be particularly large if the external jugular is small.

The layer of deep cervical fascia which forms the roof of the anterior triangle must be carefully removed. The layers of the deep cervical fascia should be reviewed from the diagrams and descriptions in the standard descriptive texts. Clean first the **digastric muscle.** The two bellies of this muscle have the form of a wide V. The **anterior belly** arises from the **digastric fossa** of the mandible; the **posterior belly** arises from the **mastoid notch** of the temporal bone. The latter attachment is at present hidden by the mastoid process and the sternomastoid muscle. The two bellies narrow to an **intermediate tendon** which lies just above the lateral part of the body of the **hyoid bone,** to which it is bound by a slip of the deep cervical fascia. In close relation to the posterior belly will be found the **stylohyoid muscle.** This slender muscle arises from the base of the **styloid process** and is inserted on the **hyoid bone** near the junction of the body and the greater cornu; it is usually pierced near its insertion by the intermediate tendon of the digastric. Crossing the posterior belly of the digastric and the stylohyoid externally will be found the **common facial vein,** which should be preserved.

Identify the position of the **thyroid cartilage.** This cartilage, which forms the prominence of the larynx commonly known as the Adam's apple, lies a short distance below the hyoid bone, to which it is connected by the thyrohyoid membrane. Both cartilage and membrane are at present largely covered by the **infrahyoid muscles,** which should now be cleaned. The **sternohyoid** arises from the inner surfaces of the **manubrium sterni** and the capsule of the sternoclavicular joint; its fibers run almost vertically upward to be inserted on the lower border of the **hyoid bone** just lateral to the median line. The **posterior belly of** the **omohyoid** has already been seen in the posterior triangle, where it takes origin from the **upper border of** the **scapula.** The intermediate tendon lies behind the sternomastoid. The **anterior belly** runs upward and forward through the anterior triangle to be inserted on the **hyoid bone** just lateral to the insertion of the sternohyoid. The sternothyroid and thyrohyoid muscles are partially covered externally by the two muscles just described. The **sternothyroid** arises from the inner surface of the **manubrium,** below the origin of the sternohyoid, and is inserted on an oblique line on the lamina of the **thyroid cartilage.** The **thyrohyoid** arises from this same line on the **thyroid cartilage** and is inserted on the lower border of the **hyoid bone** under cover of the insertions of the sternohyoid and the omohyoid.

Identify the branches of the **ansa cervicalis** supplying the sternohyoid, sternothyroid, and omohyoid muscles. These nerves enter the sternohyoid and sternothyroid at their caudolateral borders. The branch to the posterior belly of the omohyoid should have been identified in the previous dissection. That to the anterior belly of the omohyoid enters its lateral border. Later these nerves can be traced back to their sources, but it is advisable to identify them now, since the ansa cervicalis may be variable and hard to identify in the subsequent dissection of the neck.

Observe that by means of the **digastric** and the **omohyoid muscles** the anterior triangle of the neck is divided into three subsidiary triangular spaces, which are known as the digastric, the carotid, and the muscular triangles. The **muscular triangle** is bounded by the midline of the neck below the hyoid bone, the posterior border of the anterior belly of the omohyoid, and the anterior border of the lower half of the sternomastoid; its principal contents are the infrahyoid muscles, which have already been cleaned. The **carotid triangle** is bounded by the posterior border of the omohyoid, the anterior border of the upper half of the sternomastoid, and the lower border of the posterior belly of the digastric. The **digastric triangle,** to which attention will next be directed, is bounded by the two bellies of

the digastric and the lower border of the mandible. Bounded by the anterior bellies of the digastric muscles of the two sides is a small triangular space common to both sides known as the **submental triangle.**

Identify the **external maxillary (facial) artery** and the **anterior facial vein** at the point where they cross the lower border of the mandible. This is about ¾ in. anterior to the angle, the artery usually lying somewhat anterior to the vein. Observe that the vein crosses the digastric triangle superficially and joins a branch of the **posterior facial (retromandibular) vein** which emerges from the parotid gland to form the **common facial vein.** This crosses the digastric externally and enters the carotid triangle, to terminate, usually, in the internal jugular vein. Occasionally, it joins the external jugular or, more rarely, the anterior jugular. The course of the facial artery in the digastric triangle is at present hidden by the submaxillary (submandibular) gland, which should now be cleaned (Fig. 4).

The large superficial portion of the **submandibular gland** occupies most of the space of the digastric triangle. Displace the gland downward and medially, and observe that a thin-walled duct emerges from the deep surface and passes forward under cover of the posterior border of the mylohyoid muscle. Accompanying the duct is a narrow process of the glandular substance, which is known as the deep portion of the gland.

Clean the portion of the **facial artery** which lies in the digastric triangle. Arising in the carotid triangle as a branch of the **external carotid,** this vessel enters the digastric triangle by passing deep to the stylohyoid and digastric muscles. It passes upward and laterally in a groove on the deep surface of the submandibular gland and then bends downward on the inner surface of the mandible to the lower border of that bone, around which it turns to reach the face. In the digastric triangle, it gives rise to **glandular branches** and to a **submental branch,** which passes forward to be distributed to the digastric and mylohyoid muscles. In close relation to the submental artery is the terminal part of the **mylohyoid nerve,** whose origin as a branch of the mandibular nerve will be seen later. Descending along the inner surface of the mandible, it reaches the digastric triangle, where it supplies the mylohyoid muscle and the anterior belly of the digastric (Fig. 4).

Clean the **mylohyoid muscle.** This is a flat sheet of muscle which forms the floor of the digastric and submental triangles. Arising from the **mylohyoid line** on the inner surface of the **mandible,** its fibers pass downward and medially to be inserted into the body of the **hyoid bone** and a **median raphe** which extends from the hyoid bone to the lower end of the mandibular symphysis.

Attention should now be turned to the **carotid triangle.** Dissect in the fascia about ¼ in. above the greater cornu of the hyoid bone and expose the **hypoglossal nerve** where it rests against the hyoglossus muscle. Traced forward, it will be found to pass deep to the stylohyoid and then to disappear under cover of the mylohyoid. Traced backward, it bends upward to disappear under cover of the posterior belly of the digastric. Just below the digastric, it is crossed externally by the occipital artery. The **hyoglossus** is one of the extrinsic muscles of the tongue. It is, for the most part, covered at present by the digastric and the mylohyoid, but a small portion of it enters into the floor of the carotid triangle, its fibers running upward from the greater cornu of the hyoid bone. Close to the posterior border of this muscle, the hypoglossal nerve appears to give rise to a small branch which runs downward and forward to supply the thyrohyoid muscle (Fig. 5). This branch arises from the first cervical nerve and accompanies the hypoglossal nerve along its course.

The further dissection of the carotid triangle consists largely in the removal of a portion of the **carotid sheath.** This is the fascial sheath which encloses the carotid arteries, the internal jugular vein, and the vagus nerve. It is not a distinct membranous sheath but merely a condensation of fascia in which these structures are embedded.

The **internal jugular vein,** unless it is unusually large and filled with blood, will appear only in the upper angle of the carotid triangle, since the lower part of its course is completely overlapped by the sternomastoid. The lower part of the common carotid artery is also covered by the sternomastoid, but its terminal portion may now be exposed, just in front of the sternomastoid and behind the thyroid cartilage. The **common carotid** ends at about the level of the upper border of the thyroid cartilage by dividing into **internal** and **external carotids.** Clean the external carotid and its branches, in so far as they lie within the carotid triangle (Fig. 4). Note the **carotid sinus,** a dilatation usually at the termination of the common carotid or the beginning of the internal carotid, which is important in regulation of systemic blood pressure.

At its origin, the external carotid lies anterior to the internal. It ascends in the neck, inclining somewhat posteriorly, so that it comes to lie lateral to the internal carotid and passes from view under cover of the posterior belly of the digastric. The first branch of the **external carotid** is usually the **ascending pharyngeal.** This is a small vessel which arises from the inner surface of the external carotid and ascends deeply on the pharyngeal wall; it is best left for study until a later stage in the dissection.

The **superior thyroid artery** arises a short distance above the origin of the external carotid and runs forward, medially, and then downward, eventually to reach the thyroid gland, under cover of the omohyoid muscle. It gives rise near its origin to a small **hyoid branch** and, shortly after it bends downward, to a larger **superior laryngeal branch,** which runs forward to pierce the thyrohyoid membrane and enter the larynx.

The **lingual artery** arises at about the level

posterior belly of the digastric to reach the digastric triangle, where its further course has already been seen.

From its posterior aspect, the external carotid gives rise, close to the lower border of the digastric muscle, to the **occipital artery.**

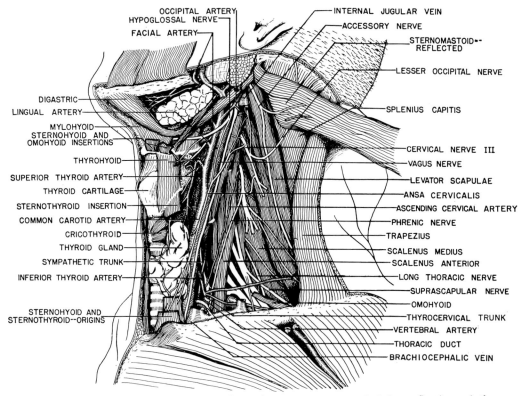

Fɪɢ. 5. Dissection of the neck to show the structures revealed by reflection of the sternomastoid muscle. The distal courses of the greater auricular, cutaneous nerve of the neck, and the supraclavicular nerves have been removed. The nerve to the subclavius muscle originates from the upper trunk of the brachial plexus, near the origin of the suprascapular nerve, and courses caudad medial to the cut end of the omohyoid muscle. The greater part of the internal jugular vein has been removed.

of the greater cornu of the hyoid bone and runs forward, usually with a slight upward bend, to disappear under cover of the hyoglossus muscle.

The **facial artery** arises slightly above the lingual or, not uncommonly, by a common stem with the latter vessel and, running forward and upward, passes under cover of the

This vessel runs backward and upward, crossing the internal jugular vein externally; its further course will be exposed later.

Attempt to display the **internal** and **external laryngeal nerves.** These are the terminal branches of the **superior laryngeal branch of the vagus,** but that fact cannot be demonstrated at present. Both run downward and forward deep to both internal and external carotid arteries. The internal nerve passes deep to the lingual artery near the origin of that vessel and pierces the thyrohyoid membrane in company with the superior laryngeal artery. The external laryngeal nerve is considerably smaller and will be found at a slightly lower level. Crossing deep to the superior thyroid artery, it passes under cover of the sternothyroid muscle to supply the cricothyroid, one of the intrinsic muscles of the larynx (Fig. 4).

Structures under Sternomastoid · · · · · · · · · · ·

Study the **sternomastoid,** noting origin and insertion; then, by flexing the head and neck forward and rotating the head from side to side, the sternomastoid can be freed and elevated to expose the underlying structures without cutting this muscle. If the dissection of the posterior triangle of the neck is done in conjunction with that of the axilla and it is desired to remove the clavicle, make a cut through the **periosteum** along the ventral surface of the clavicle, extending from the medial border of the deltoid through the lower fibers of the clavicular and the sternocostal attachments of the sternomastoid. By blunt dissection, reflect the periosteum from the surfaces of the clavicle between the **deltoid** and the **sternomastoid.** Insert the handle of a forceps between the periosteum and the caudal edge of the clavicle and, while depressing the subjacent structures, saw through the clavicle at the medial edge of the deltoid. Dissect free and elevate the lower fibers of the sternomastoid to expose the sternoclavicular articulation.

The **sternoclavicular articulation** is the diarthrodial joint at which the medial end of the clavicle meets the clavicular notch of the manubrium sterni and the upper border of the first costal cartilage. It is surrounded by a strong fibrous capsule, whose anterior surface should now be cleaned. The anterior portion of the fibrous capsule is known as the **anterior** sternoclavicular ligament. Cut through the entire circumference of the **capsule** close to the sternum to detach the clavicle. Observe that the fibers forming the posterior part of the capsule (**posterior sternoclavicular ligament**) are thicker and tougher than the anterior ones and that posteriorly the capsule is in close relation to the origins of the sternohyoid and sternothyroid muscles. This can be seen by elevating and reflecting craniad the sternomastoid and removing the medial segment of the clavicle. Note also that the interior of the joint is separated into two distinct cavities by an **articular disc** of fibrocartilage, which intervenes between the clavicle and the first rib and sternum.

The success of the later dissection of the neck depends to a large extent on the completeness of the freeing of the sternomastoid; free the muscle clear back to its attachment to the skull. As this muscle is elevated, observe that there may be, in relation to its deep surface in the region below and behind the angle of the mandible, a considerable aggregation of large **deep cervical lymph glands.** When these have been observed, they should be carefully but completely removed, together with the mass of fatty areolar tissue in which they are embedded. As this is done, secure the **accessory nerve.** This nerve emerges from under cover of the posterior belly of the digastric, behind the internal jugular vein, and runs downward and posteriorly across the deep surface of the **sternomastoid** to enter the posterior triangle. As it crosses the deep surface of the sternomastoid, it gives branches of supply to that muscle. Entering the deep surface of the sternomastoid in close relation to the accessory nerve is the **sternomastoid branch of** the **occipital artery.** This vessel occasionally arises as a direct branch of the external carotid, in which case it, as well as the occipital, will be found to cross the hypoglossal nerve externally.

Clean the internal jugular vein. The **internal jugular** emerges from under cover of the digastric and descends through the neck deep to the sternomastoid; it terminates behind the sternoclavicular articulation by joining the subclavian vein to form the brachiocephalic vein. It is crossed externally by the intermediate tendon of the omohyoid muscle and often by the descending cervical root of the ansa cervicalis. It is enclosed in the carotid sheath, where it lies lateral to the internal carotid artery above and the common carotid below. The tributaries of the internal jugular vein, with the exception of the common facial vein, correspond roughly to the lower branches of the external carotid artery.

Clean the **ansa cervicalis.** This is a nerve loop which is formed by the descending branch **(superior ramus)** of the first cervical nerve (called the **descendens hypoglossi** since it accompanies the hypoglossal nerve in part of its course) and a branch **(inferior ramus)** derived from the second and third cervical nerves **(descendens cervicalis).** The superior ramus emerges from under cover of the digastric and descends in close relation to the external aspect of the carotid sheath. The inferior ramus arises from the second and third cervical nerves and runs downward and forward, passing either superficial or deep to the internal jugular vein; it joins at an extremely variable level the superior ramus to form the loop

of the ansa cervicalis. From the lower end of this loop, branches descend to supply the **sternohyoid,** the **sternothyroid,** and **both bellies of** the omohyoid (Fig. 5).

Attention should next be directed to the **cervical plexus.** This is a looped nerve plexus derived from the anterior primary divisions of the first four cervical nerves; it lies under cover of the upper part of the sternomastoid muscle. The first nerve is small, and it will be exposed in a later dissection. It emerges above the transverse process of the atlas and turns downward in front of that process to join the second nerve. The second, third, and fourth nerves are each successively larger and enter the present area of dissection by passing laterally and downward from between the anterior and posterior tubercles of the transverse processes of the corresponding cervical vertebrae. The plexus proper takes the form of **three loops.** The **first** is that already noted between the first and second nerves and lies in front of the transverse process of the atlas. The **second loop** is formed by the second and third nerves, and the **third** by the third and fourth nerves. The cutaneous branches of the cervical plexus, which have already been seen in the dissection of the posterior triangle, should now be traced back to their origins. The **lesser occipital, great auricular,** and **cervical cutaneous nerves** all arise from the loop between the second and third nerves. **Anterior, middle,** and **posterior supraclavicular nerves** arise from the third loop, usually by a common stem. From this loop are also derived **muscular twigs,** which cross the posterior triangle to reach the deep surface of the **trapezius.**

Muscular branches arise also from the roots of the cervical plexus. The largest of these is the **phrenic nerve.** This nerve is derived principally from the fourth cervical and passes downward and medially on the anterior surface of the **scalenus anterior** to enter the thoracic cavity behind the brachiocephalic vein. It usually receives a twig from the fifth cervical nerve, and often one from the third. From the second and third nerves arise the two roots of the inferior ramus, whose part in the formation of the ansa cervicalis has been stated. The first cervical gives rise to a branch which passes forward deep to the internal jugular vein to join the hypoglossal nerve under cover of the posterior belly of the digastric. The remaining branches of the cervical plexus are small muscular twigs which pass from the second, third, and fourth nerves directly into the longus colli, longus capitis, and scalenus medius for the supply of those muscles.

Free and elevate the intermediate tendon of the omohyoid and reflect the anterior belly upward. Divide the sternohyoid and sternothyroid muscles just above the manubrium sterni and reflect them upward. Then clean and study the common carotid artery and the vagus nerve, both of which are enclosed in the carotid sheath (Fig. 5).

On the right side, the **common carotid** arises behind the sternoclavicular articulation as a branch of the brachiocephalic artery. On the left side, it arises in the thorax as a branch of the aorta and enters the neck behind the sternoclavicular articulation. Its course in the neck is similar on the two sides, extending from the sternoclavicular articulation upward and somewhat posteriorly to the level of the upper border of the thyroid cartilage, where it terminates by dividing into **internal** and **external carotids.** It has no other branches. Except at its termination, it is covered externally by the sternomastoid. It is further covered anteriorly, in the lower part of its course, by the omohyoid, sternothyroid, and sternohyoid muscles. Laterally, it is in relation to the internal jugular vein. Medially, it is in relation to the trachea and, in the middle portion of its course, to the thyroid gland. Posteriorly, it rests against the prevertebral muscles (longus colli and longus capitis).

The **vagus nerve** lies in the most posterior part of the carotid sheath. It is medial to the internal jugular vein and lateral to the internal carotid artery above and the common carotid below. It passes into the thorax behind the sternoclavicular articulation, lying, on the left side, between the common carotid artery and the brachiocephalic vein and, on the right side, between the brachiocephalic artery and the brachiocephalic vein.

Clean the **subclavius muscle,** which extends from the first rib to the periosteum of the clavicle. Attempt to locate the **nerve to** the **subclavius.** Note the **costoclavicular ligament,** a strong band of fibers extending laterally from the first rib to the periosteum over the costal tubercle on the inferior surface of the clavicle. The brachial plexus should now be reviewed in its entirety and its relations to the clavicle reestablished by replacing the clavicle during this review (Fig. 2).

When review of the brachial plexus is completed, the superior extremity, together with its girdle, can be removed, if the extremity is to be taken from the body and studied elsewhere. *However, if possible leave the extremity attached to the body so the relationships can be maintained for future study and review.* If the removal is essential, it can be accomplished by dividing the **serratus anterior** by a vertical incision at about the midaxillary line. Then sever the three **trunks of** the **brachial plexus,** the first part of the **axillary artery,** and the **axillary vein.** The upper trunk of the brachial plexus should be cut proximad to the origin of the **suprascapular nerve.**

Root of Neck ·

The **subclavian artery** lies deep in the root of the neck. On the right side, this vessel arises behind the sternoclavicular articulation as one of the end branches of the brachiocephalic artery; on the left side, it arises in the thorax as a branch of the aorta and enters the neck behind the sternoclavicular articulation, where it lies behind and slightly lateral to the common carotid. The subclavian artery in the neck is divided for descriptive purposes into three parts. Since this subdivision is based on the relation of the artery to the scalenus anterior, it is best first to clean and study that muscle.

The **scalenus anterior** arises by a series of slips from the anterior tubercles of the **transverse processes** of the third, fourth, fifth, and sixth cervical vertebrae. Descending under cover of the sternomastoid, its fibers narrow to a tendinous insertion on the **scalene tubercle** on the upper surface of the first rib. Its anterior surface is crossed from above downward and medially by the **phrenic nerve.** Parallel to the phrenic but somewhat more medial, the ascending cervical artery will be found on the anterior surface of the muscle. At its insertion, the scalenus anterior is crossed anteriorly by the **subclavian vein,** and at a slightly higher level by the **transverse cervical** and **transverse scapular arteries** (Fig. 6).

The **first part of** the **subclavian artery** extends from a point behind the sternoclavicular articulation upward and laterally to the medial border of the scalenus anterior; the **second part** runs laterally behind the scalenus anterior; the **third part** runs laterally and slightly downward from the lateral border of the scalenus anterior to the outer border of the first rib, where it becomes the axillary artery.

Clean and study the **first part of** the **subclavian artery.** Observe that this part of the artery is covered anteriorly by the clavicle and the sternomastoid and is crossed by the **phrenic**

and **vagus nerves,** the **vertebral vein** and part of the sympathetic chain, the **ansa subclavia.** On the left side, it is also crossed anteriorly by the terminal part of the thoracic duct. The **thoracic duct** emerges from behind the left common carotid artery at about the level of the lower border of the thyroid gland and runs laterally and downward, passing behind the vagus nerve and in front of the subclavian artery, to join the terminal part of the internal jugular, or the subclavian vein, or the beginning of the brachiocephalic vein (Fig. 6).

The first branch of the subclavian is the **vertebral artery.** This vessel ascends almost vertically to enter the costotransverse foramen of the sixth cervical vertebra behind the most lateral part of the longus colli muscle. The **vertebral vein** descends in front of the vertebral and subclavian arteries to join the brachiocephalic vein; it is frequently very large and may obscure the dissection of the arteries, in which case it should be removed.

Slightly more laterally, the thyrocervical trunk and the internal thoracic artery arise from the first part of the subclavian. The **thyrocervical trunk** runs upward for a short distance and usually divides into the **transverse cervical,** the **transverse scapular,** and the **inferior thyroid arteries.** The former two vessels pass laterally across the scalenus anterior. The inferior thyroid may be regarded as the main continuation of the thyrocervical trunk. It continues to ascend and then bends medially and downward, passing in front of the vertebral artery and behind the common carotid and the vagus to reach the thyroid gland. Near its origin the inferior thyroid gives rise to the **ascending cervical artery,** a small but constant branch which ascends on the scalenus anterior. The **internal thoracic** artery runs downward and forward from the subclavian to reach the anterior thoracic wall behind the first costal cartilage. Near its origin it comes into relation with the phrenic nerve, which may cross it either anteriorly or posteriorly.

Insert a probe beneath and elevate the lower part of the scalenus anterior muscle to observe the **second part of** the **subclavian artery.** Observe that both the **first** and **second parts of** the **subclavian** rest inferiorly and posteriorly against the **pleura,** by which they are separated from the lung. The **apices** of the pleura and lung rise for a considerable distance above the first rib on each side into the root of the neck. The only branch of the **second part of** the **sub-**

The sternohyoid and sternothyroid muscles should be retracted laterally to study the thyroid gland, trachea, and esophagus. The **thyroid** is a bilobed gland which lies in relation to the front and sides of the upper part of the trachea. It consists of two **lateral lobes** and a much smaller median connecting portion, the **isthmus,** which crosses the front of the trachea. The greatest extent of the lateral lobes is superiorly, where they may reach as high as the middle of the thyroid cartilage. Anterolaterally, the gland is covered by the infrahyoid muscles; posterolaterally, it is in relation to the common carotid

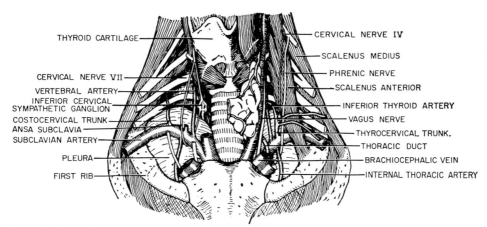

THYROID CARTILAGE—

CERVICAL NERVE VII—
VERTEBRAL ARTERY—
INFERIOR CERVICAL
SYMPATHETIC GANGLION—
COSTOCERVICAL TRUNK—
ANSA SUBCLAVIA—
SUBCLAVIAN ARTERY—

PLEURA—

FIRST RIB—

—CERVICAL NERVE IV
—SCALENUS MEDIUS
—PHRENIC NERVE
—SCALENUS ANTERIOR
—INFERIOR THYROID ARTERY
—VAGUS NERVE
—THYROCERVICAL TRUNK.
—THORACIC DUCT
—BRACHIOCEPHALIC VEIN
—INTERNAL THORACIC ARTERY

FIG. 6. Deep dissection of the root of the neck. The scalenus anterior and the thyroid gland have been removed on the right side.

clavian is the **costocervical trunk.** This vessel runs upward and posteriorly across the pleura and terminates by dividing into the **deep cervical** and **superior intercostal arteries.** The former ascends behind the scalenus medius to reach the deep muscles at the back of the neck. The superior intercostal descends on the posterior thoracic wall.

The **third part of** the **subclavian artery** rests upon the upper surface of the **first rib** and is in relation posteriorly to the scalenus medius and the lower trunk of the brachial plexus. It usually has no branches but occasionally gives rise to the transverse cervical or the suprascapular artery, or both.

artery. In the median line, the isthmus is covered externally only by skin and fascia.

The extensive blood supply of the thyroid gland is provided by the **superior** and **inferior thyroid arteries,** which anastomose freely with each other and with similar vessels of the opposite side. The blood is drained from the gland by the **superior** and **inferior thyroid veins.** The inferior thyroid vein does not accompany the artery but descends in front of the trachea to enter the thorax. It may be single or paired. There is frequently present a **middle thyroid vein,** which passes laterally into the internal jugular vein.

Cut across the isthmus of the **thyroid gland**

and reflect the two halves of the gland laterally. Study its posterior surface and attempt to identify the **parathyroid glands.** There are two pairs of these, a **superior** and an **inferior.** They are small, flattened oval bodies, closely applied to the posterior surfaces of the lateral lobes of the thyroid, and sometimes embedded within the thyroid substance. They may frequently be distinguished from the thyroid by their lighter color.

The **trachea** is a median tubular organ which begins at the lower border of the cricoid cartilage. From the **cricoid cartilage,** the trachea descends through the lower part of the neck into the thorax. Its lumen is kept permanently open by a series of cartilaginous rings in its wall. Observe that these rings are incomplete posteriorly, where the trachea rests against the anterior surface of the esophagus.

Only a very incomplete view of the esophagus may be obtained while the trachea is still in place. The **esophagus** is a hollow organ which begins at the level of the lower border of the cricoid cartilage as a direct continuation of the **pharynx** and descends into the thorax. It lies immediately behind the trachea and in front of the bodies of the vertebrae and the prevertebral muscles. It is flattened from before backward, its lumen being open only when food is passing through it.

Dissect in the groove between the esophagus and the trachea and expose the **recurrent** (inferior laryngeal) **nerve,** which ascends in this groove to reach the larynx. The origin of the left recurrent as a branch of the left vagus is within the thoracic cavity and cannot be seen at present. The right recurrent arises from the right vagus as the latter nerve crosses the subclavian artery. From its point of origin, the right recurrent turns medially and upward, passing behind the beginnings of the right subclavian and common carotid arteries, to reach the interval between the esophagus and trachea.

Back •

For the dissection of the back, the body lies prone with a block elevating the thorax and the head hanging freely, so that the back of the neck is stretched. Certain surface points should be identified before the skin is reflected. In the midline at the base of the skull is the **external occipital protuberance.** Laterally, behind the lower part of the auricle, is the **mastoid process.** Arching between the external occipital protuberance and the mastoid on either side, the **superior nuchal line** may be palpated. In the median line of the back, the **spinous processes** of most of the vertebrae are apparent. The highest vertebral spine which is ordinarily palpable is that of the sixth cervical vertebra. The higher cervical spines are separated from the skin by the **ligamentum nuchae,** a strong fibrous band which stretches in the median plane from the external occipital protuberance to the seventh cervical spine and is attached deeply to the spinous processes of all the cervical vertebrae. Below the last lumbar spine, the posterior surface of the **sacrum** is subcutaneous, and below it, between the buttocks, is the **coccyx.** Identify also the **crest of the ilium,** arching laterally from the posterior superior iliac spine. The posterior part of the iliac crest is often covered by a fairly thick layer of subcutaneous fat.

Locate the **vertebral border of** the **scapula.** Running laterally and upward from this border the **spine of** the **scapula** is subcutaneous throughout its length. It ends in the broad **acromion process,** which forms the bony prominence of the shoulder.

When these points have been observed, make the following incisions through the skin: (1) a median longitudinal incision starting at the external occipital protuberance and ending at the tip of the coccyx; (2) from the upper end of the first incision, one laterally and downward across the back of the skull behind the ears to the mastoid process; (3) from the first incision, one at the level of the first lumbar spine upward and laterally to the posterior axillary fold and then along this fold to the back of the arm; (4) from the first incision, one at the level of the seventh cervical spine straight laterally to the tip of the acromion; (5) from the lower end of the first incision, one upward and laterally to the posterior iliac spine and then along the iliac crest to the posterior axillary line. By these incisions, three large flaps of skin will be marked out on each side. These flaps should now all be reflected laterally.

The reflection of skin will expose the **superficial fascia** of the back. It has no specific characteristics but resembles the superficial fascia in other parts of the body. Before removing the superficial fascia, dissect some of the cutaneous nerves to demonstrate their segmental arrangement. Then reflect the superficial fascia, together with the deep fascia, in cleaning the superficial muscles of the back.

The **cutaneous nerves** of the back are derived from the **posterior primary divisions** of the cervical, thoracic, and lumbar spinal nerves. With the exception of the **great occipital nerve,**

they are small, but some of them will be seen piercing the superficial muscles of the back in linear series not far lateral to the median line, as these muscles are cleaned.

Superficial Structures of Back

The most superficial muscles of the back are the trapezius and the latissimus dorsi. Clean the trapezius by removing in a single layer the superficial and deep fascia which cover its external surface. As the uppermost part of the muscle is being cleaned, secure the **great occipital nerve.** This large cutaneous nerve is the terminal part of the posterior primary division of the second cervical nerve. It pierces the trapezius a little below and lateral to the external occipital protuberance and runs upward in the fascia to be distributed to the back of the scalp. It is accompanied in its distribution by the terminal branches of the **occipital artery** (Fig. 7).

The **trapezius** is a flat triangular muscle which arises by a long linear origin from the medial third of the **superior nuchal line,** the entire length of the **ligamentum nuchae,** and the **spinous processes** of all 12 thoracic vertebrae. Its fibers converge laterally to a V-shaped insertion on the posterior border of the lateral third of the **clavicle,** the medial border of the **acromion,** and the upper border of the **scapular spine.**

Clean the **latissimus dorsi** and the **posterior lamella of** the **lumbodorsal fascia.** The deep fascia known as the lumbodorsal fascia differs from the deep fascia ordinarily found surrounding muscles in that the fascia is here resolved into dense aponeurotic sheets. The lumbodorsal fascia, in the lumbar region of the back, is disposed in two layers or lamellae, between which the deep muscles of the back are enclosed. The more superficial of these layers (**posterior lamella**) must be cleaned at the same time as the latissimus dorsi, since the muscle takes origin in part from this layer of fascia. In removing the superficial fascia from the region just lateral to the lumbar vertebral spines, care must be taken to avoid cutting through and removing at the same time the posterior lamella of the lumbodorsal fascia. It may be recognized by the glistening aponeurotic appearance of its external surface. It is attached medially to the lumbar and sacral spines and stretches laterally as a broad aponeurotic sheet.

The **latissimus dorsi** is a broad flat muscle which covers the lower lateral part of the back. It is overlapped to a slight extent by the lowest part of the trapezius. It has a wide origin from the **spinous processes** of the lower five or six thoracic vertebrae, the **posterior lamella of** the **lumbodorsal fascia,** the **outer lip of** the posterior half of the **iliac crest,** and by small pointed slips from the outer surfaces of the **lower** three or four **ribs,** where it is in close relation to the lower slips of origin of the external oblique muscle of the abdomen. The fibers converge upward and laterally to a flat tendon which winds around the lower border of the teres major muscle to be inserted into the **intertubercular sulcus of** the **humerus.** The manner of its insertion cannot be investigated at present. The upper part of the lateral border of the latissimus dorsi forms the posterior fold of the axilla.

The relationship of the trapezius and latissimus dorsi muscles to other structures on the back creates two triangles of clinical importance. The upper, **triangle of auscultation,** is that space bounded by the trapezius muscle, the latissimus dorsi, and the vertebral border of the scapula. This space, on each side of the back, may become enlarged over the sixth and seventh ribs and their interspaces when the arms are folded over the chest and the trunk is bent forward. It is used for clearer diagnostic listening to the structures within the thoracic cavity. A lower triangular area on each side,

the **lumbar triangle,** is formed by the lower lateral border of the latissimus dorsi, the posterior edge of the external oblique muscle, and the ilium. The internal oblique muscle forms the floor of this triangle, which is a point of potential weakness in the abdominal wall.

The trapezius should now be reflected. It is essential for the proper display of the deeper layers of muscle that as each succeeding muscle is reached, its external surface be completely cleaned and that as each muscle is cut and reflected, it be completely reflected back to its bony attachments. Detach the uppermost fibers of the trapezius from the occipital bone and make a longitudinal incision through the trapezius parallel and about $\frac{1}{4}$ in. lateral to the median line of the body. Reflect the muscle laterally to its insertion. As this muscle is turned laterally, the nerves and vessels which supply the trapezius will be found ramifying on its deep surface.

The **trapezius** is supplied by the **accessory nerve,** supplemented by some twigs from the **third and fourth cervical nerves.** These reach the deep surface of the muscle by passing across the posterior triangle of the neck. They are accompanied by the **ascending (superficial) branch of** the **transverse cervical artery** (Fig. 7).

Clean and study the **rhomboid muscles.** These two muscles are sometimes more or less fused with one another. The **rhomboideus minor** is a narrow flat muscle taking origin from the lower parts of the **ligamentum nuchae** and the **spinous process of** the **seventh cervical vertebra.** Its fibers run downward and laterally to be inserted into the **vertebral border of** the **scapula** opposite the scapular spine. The **rhomboideus major** is a much wider flat muscle immediately below the minor. It takes origin from the upper four or five **thoracic spines** and is inserted into the **vertebral border of** the **scapula** below the scapular spine.

Clean the **levator scapulae.** This is a long flat muscle which arises by four pointed slips from the posterior tubercles of the **transverse processes of** the upper four **cervical vertebrae.** It is inserted into the **vertebral border of** the **scapula** above the scapular spine. The levator scapulae helps to form the floor of the poste-

through both rhomboid muscles by a vertical incision about ½ in. lateral to their origins and reflect them outward. As the muscles are being reflected, find and clean the **dorsal scapular nerve** and **deep branch of** the **transverse**

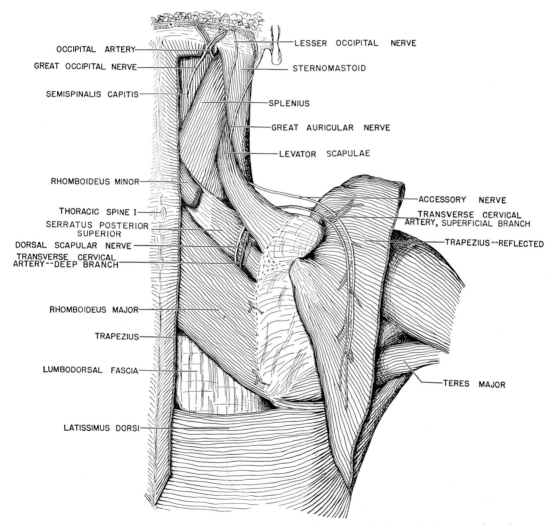

OCCIPITAL ARTERY
GREAT OCCIPITAL NERVE
SEMISPINALIS CAPITIS
RHOMBOIDEUS MINOR
THORACIC SPINE I
SERRATUS POSTERIOR SUPERIOR
DORSAL SCAPULAR NERVE
TRANSVERSE CERVICAL ARTERY--DEEP BRANCH
RHOMBOIDEUS MAJOR
TRAPEZIUS
LUMBODORSAL FASCIA
LATISSIMUS DORSI

LESSER OCCIPITAL NERVE
STERNOMASTOID
SPLENIUS
GREAT AURICULAR NERVE
LEVATOR SCAPULAE
ACCESSORY NERVE
TRANSVERSE CERVICAL ARTERY, SUPERFICIAL BRANCH
TRAPEZIUS--REFLECTED
TERES MAJOR

FIG. 7. Dissection of the upper part of the back after reflection of the trapezius. A segment of the rhomboideus minor has been removed.

rior triangle of the neck. Its origin is covered by the upper part of the sternomastoid, and its insertion by the trapezius.

Detach the scapular insertion of the levator scapulae and reflect this muscle upward. Cut

cervical artery. This nerve and artery leave the posterior triangle at the anterior border of the levator scapulae and descend together in a line slightly medial to the vertebral border of the scapula and deep to the levator scapulae and the two rhomboids. The **dorsal scapular nerve** is the nerve of supply for the rhomboids.

Cut the latissimus dorsi about 1 in. from its origin on the lumbodorsal fascia and reflect it laterally. This muscle is much thicker toward its insertion than it is at its origin.

Clean the posterior serrate muscles. These are two thin flat muscles which are often more tendinous than muscular. The **serratus posterior superior** is subjacent to the rhomboids, and its fibers run in the same direction as do those of the rhomboids. It arises from the lower part of the ligamentum nuchae, the spines of the seventh cervical, and the upper two or three thoracic vertebrae and is inserted by four slips into the external surfaces of the second, third, fourth, and fifth ribs. The **serratus posterior inferior** is covered externally by the latissimus dorsi. It arises from the posterior lamella of the lumbodorsal fascia in the region of the lower thoracic and upper lumbar vertebrae. Its fibers run upward and laterally to be inserted into the external surfaces of the lower four ribs. When the posterior serrate muscles have been studied, they may be removed. As this is done, attempt to identify the small branches of the **intercostal nerves** which emerge from the intercostal spaces to supply them.

As has been seen, the **trapezius** derives its main nerve supply from a cranial nerve, the **accessory.** The other muscles of the back which have been studied so far derive their nerve supply from the **anterior primary divisions** of spinal nerves. The **deeper muscles** of the back, yet to be displayed, are all supplied by the **posterior primary divisions** of spinal nerves, and it should be remembered that they are the only muscles in the body which are so supplied.

Clean the **splenius** muscle. This is a flat muscle which takes origin from the lower half of the **ligamentum nuchae** and the **spines of** the seventh **cervical and** first five or six **thoracic**

vertebrae. Its fibers run upward and laterally and, toward its insertion, the muscle becomes separated into two parts. The large upper portion, the **splenius capitis,** has a linear insertion on the **mastoid process** and the lateral part of the **superior nuchal line.** The lower portion, the **splenius cervicis,** is inserted by two or three tendinous slips into the **posterior tubercles of** the **transverse processes** of the upper two or three cervical vertebrae, where it is in close relation to the slips of origin of the levator scapulae. The insertion of the splenius is for the most part covered by the sternomastoid. Detach the splenius from its origin and reflect both parts to their insertions.

Deep Muscles of Back

The **vertebral groove** is occupied by a thick, elongated mass of muscle which is known collectively as the **sacrospinalis.** This muscle mass is thickest in the lower thoracic and lumbar regions. Here it is enclosed between the two lamellae of the **lumbodorsal fascia.** The **posterior lamella** of the lumbodorsal fascia has already been exposed. It is attached medially to the lumbar and sacral spines and stretches laterally across the external surface of the sacrospinalis to become continuous, finally, with the fascial sheaths of the internal oblique and transversus muscles of the anterior abdominal wall. Superiorly, it gradually thins out and in the upper thoracic region is hard to recognize as a distinct membranous layer. The **anterior lamella** is attached medially to the tips of the transverse processes of the lumbar vertebrae and stretches laterally across the anterior or deep surface of the sacrospinalis. The extent of the **lumbodorsal fascia** may be demonstrated by inserting a hypodermic needle through the posterior lamella of this fascia in the lumbar region and forcibly blowing in air. As this fascial compartment is extended, note its lateral and cephalic extent. For its display, the following dissection should be undertaken.

Make a longitudinal incision through the posterior lamella, parallel and about ½ in. lateral to the median line, from the level of the first lumbar spine to that of the fourth. From each end of this incision carry a horizontal incision laterally for about 1½ in. The rectangular flap of fascia thus marked out should be turned laterally to expose the posterior surface of the lumbar part of the sacrospinalis. If the **sacrospinalis** is now pushed medially, the **anterior lamella of** the **lumbodorsal fascia** will be exposed. Push the fingers medially, in front of the sacrospinalis, across the exposed surface of the anterior lamella and observe that this layer of the fascia is attached medially to the **transverse processes** of the lumbar vertebrae, which also lie anterior to the sacrospinalis. Observe also that the anterior and the posterior lamellae of the fascia fuse with one another along the lateral border of the sacrospinalis. It is this lateral fused portion of the lumbodorsal fascia which comes into relation with the muscles of the anterior abdominal wall. Finally, make a short longitudinal incision through the exposed portion of the anterior lamella. If the lips of this incision are spread apart, the posterior surface of the **quadratus lumborum muscle** will be exposed. This is a muscle in the posterior wall of the abdominal cavity.

Clean and study the **sacrospinalis.** Inferiorly, the entire mass has a common large fleshy origin from the spines of all the lumbar vertebrae, the dorsum of the sacrum, the posterior sacroiliac ligament, the most posterior part of the iliac crest, and the deep surface of the lowest part of the posterior lamella of the lumbodorsal fascia. As the fibers pass upward from their origin, the muscle becomes separated into three parallel longitudinal columns. The most lateral column is known as the **iliocostalis,** the middle one as the **longissimus,** and the smallest and most medial is the **spinalis.** A detailed dissection of each slip and subdivision of the

sacrospinalis is not essential, but sufficient cleaning and study should be done to demonstrate the following facts.

The line of division between the iliocostalis and the longissimus is indicated by the line along which the **posterior cutaneous nerves** emerge. The **iliocostalis** is subdivided from below upward into three parts: the **iliocostalis lumborum,** the **iliocostalis (thoracis) dorsi,** and the **iliocostalis cervicis.** The **iliocostalis lumborum** arises from the common origin and is inserted by a series of slips into the lower six or seven ribs at their angles. The **iliocostalis thoracis** receives additional slips of origin from the lower six ribs just medial to their angles and is inserted into the angles of the upper six ribs. The **iliocostalis cervicis** receives slips of origin from the upper ribs and is inserted into the transverse processes of the lower three or four cervical vertebrae. The slips of insertion of the iliocostalis can be seen while the muscle is in position, but the slips of origin are covered by the main mass of the muscle. They may be exposed by rolling the entire muscle laterally. It should be noted that there is no actual structural separation between the three parts of the iliocostalis; the subdivision is an arbitrary matter of anatomical nomenclature.

The **longissimus** is similarly subdivided into three parts for purposes of anatomical description. These are the longissimus thoracis, the longissimus cervicis, and the longissimus capitis. The **longissimus thoracis** arises at the common origin of the sacrospinalis and is inserted by means of two long series of muscular slips. The more lateral series is inserted into the transverse processes of the lumbar vertebrae and into the lower ten ribs lateral to their tubercles; the more medial series is inserted into the accessory tubercles of the lumbar vertebrae and the tips of the transverse processes of the thoracic vertebrae. The **longissimus cervicis** receives slips of origin from the transverse processes of the upper thoracic vertebrae and is inserted into the posterior tubercles of the transverse processes of the second to the sixth cervical vertebrae. The **longissimus capitis** arises from the transverse processes of the upper three or four thoracic vertebrae and the articular processes of the lower cervical vertebrae. As its fibers pass upward, they form a narrow bandlike muscle which is inserted into the posterior part of the mastoid process under cover of the splenius capitis and sterno-mastoid muscles.

The various subdivisions of this group may be exposed by inserting a finger under the whole muscle mass at the level of the second or third lumbar vertebra. Then transect the whole muscle mass at this level and pull it laterally. Use the handle of a forceps or a scalpel to separate the various individual insertions of the iliocostal and longissimus groups.

The **spinalis** is much the smallest of the three parts of the sacrospinalis. Its fibers run upward from the upper lumbar and lower thoracic spinous processes to be inserted into the spinous processes of a variable number of the upper thoracic vertebrae.

Free and elevate the longissimus capitis laterally to identify the **occipital artery.** This vessel ordinarily crosses the deep surface of the longissimus capitis just below its insertion. Occasionally it crosses the longissimus superficially. The **occipital artery** arises from the external carotid in the anterior triangle of the neck. Emerging from the deep surface of the mastoid process, it will now be seen running medially and upward in the interval between the splenius and semispinalis muscles. Near the medial border of the upper part of the splenius, it becomes superficial by piercing the trapezius or by winding around the lateral border of that muscle. It is distributed to the back of the scalp, in company with the **greater occipital nerve.**

Clean the **semispinalis capitis,** which has been exposed by the reflection of the trapezius and splenius. This is a large muscle which takes origin by a series of tendinous slips from the articular processes of the fourth, fifth, and sixth cervical vertebrae and the transverse processes of the first five or six thoracic verte-brae. It has a thick, fleshy insertion into the occipital bone between the superior and inferior nuchal lines just lateral to the external occipital crest. Observe that the semispinalis is pierced by the **greater occipital nerve** and that in the cervical region the semispinales of the two sides are separated from each other only by the **ligamentum nuchae.**

The deepest muscles of the back are several groups of numerous small muscular slips (transversospinales) which connect the various individual vertebrae with each other. Those are the **semispinalis cervicis, semispinalis thoracis, multifidus, rotatores, levatores costarum, interspinales,** and **intertransversarii.** The beginner may be forgiven for neglecting to dissect all of these muscles. A few of these muscles should be cleaned and identified at the different vertebral levels.

Suboccipital Triangle

Use the handle of a forceps and by blunt dissection retract the **semispinalis capitis** muscle laterally from the **ligamentum nuchae.** Identify the course of the **greater occipital** and the posterior division of the **third cervical nerves** medial to, or occasionally passing through, the substance of this muscle. Transect this muscle at a right angle to the course of its fibers about the level of the spine of the second or third cervical vertebra. Reflect the cut ends of the muscle upward and downward. This will expose the **rectus capitis major** and **minor** and the **superior** and **inferior oblique** muscles. The rectus major, superior, and inferior oblique muscles form the sides of a small triangle (**the suboccipital triangle**) on each side. Insert a probe or the sharp end of a forceps through the fascia and ligaments in the floor of the upper part of this triangle, and a potential space will be felt between the base of the **occipital bone** and the **arch** of the **atlas.** Clean away the fascia and ligaments from this area and identify the course of the **vertebral artery** over the **arch of** the **atlas.** The posterior division of the first cervical nerve will be seen sending branches to the four small muscles of the suboccipital area. These muscles extend from the axis to the atlas and from the atlas to the base of the occipital bone.

Vertebral Canal and Spinal Cord

Preparatory to opening the vertebral canal, the **laminae** and **spinous processes** of the vertebrae must be cleaned as completely as possible. This is done by retracting the larger, longer muscles laterally and removing the smaller ones which fill the vertebral groove on each side. In doing this, retain a few of the posterior primary divisions of the thoracic nerves, so that they may later be traced to the main trunk of the nerves from which they arise. The **vertebral canal** is then to be opened by removal of the entire series of the laminae and spinous processes from the level of the second cervical vertebra down to the middle of the sacrum. The successive laminae and spines will be held together by the **ligamenta flava** and the **interspinous ligaments** and may be removed in one piece. Cut through the **laminae** on each side with a chisel. The chisel cut should be made at a right angle to the edge of the lamina on each side, just medial to the articular process. Change to the cephalic or caudal border of the laminae to make the cuts along the convexity or concavity of the vertebral contours. In dealing with the sacrum, remember that the posterior wall of the sacral canal is very thin and that it is desired only to remove this wall, *not* to cut through the body of the sacrum.

When the vertebral canal is opened, a narrow space loosely filled with fat will be exposed, which lies between the periosteum of the vertebrae and the dura mater of the spinal cord. In the fat of this space are the spinal arteries and the **internal vertebral venous plexus.** The **spinal arteries** are a paired series of vessels which enter the canal at the intervertebral foramina. The venous plexus is drained by spinal veins, which leave the canal through the intervertebral foramina. The vessels supplying the spinal cord and the meninges are not all of the same size. At certain vertebral levels, the arteries and veins are larger than at other levels. These are the more important vessels supplying the spinal cord.

Clean the external surface of the dura mater spinalis by removing the fat and the venous plexus. The **dura mater** is the most external and the strongest of the three coverings (meninges) of the spinal cord. At the foramen magnum, it is firmly bound to the occipital bone and becomes continuous with the inner layer of the cranial dura. In the vertebral canal, as now exposed, it lies loosely and takes the form of a fibrous tube. At about the level of the second piece of the sacrum, it contracts to a filament, the **coccygeal ligament,** which extends downward through the sacral canal to be attached to the dorsum of the coccyx. Observe the series of lateral prolongations of the dura, which pass into the intervertebral foramina; within these are enclosed the roots of the spinal nerves.

Open the dura by a longitudinal incision along its entire length; reflect the cut edges laterally and pin them to the sides of the vertebral canal to expose the **arachnoid.** This is the second of the spinal coverings. It is a thin, delicate membrane of gauzy texture. At the foramen magnum, it is continuous with the cranial arachnoid; inferiorly, it extends as far as does the dura and ends by joining the **filum terminale,** the thread which forms the core of the coccygeal ligament. The arachnoid also shows a series of lateral prolongations, which surround the roots of the spinal nerves and blend with the dura in the intervertebral foramina. Between the dura and the arachnoid is a narrow interval, the **subdural space,** which contains in life a fluid similar to lymph. The subdural space is traversed by filamentous strands by which the arachnoid is loosely attached to the inner surface of the dura.

Slit the arachnoid longitudinally to expose the **pia mater,** the **spinal cord,** and the roots of the **spinal nerves.** The pia is the innermost of the three meninges. It is a delicate membrane which closely invests the outer surface of the spinal cord and the roots of the nerves, from which it cannot readily be separated. It is best regarded as an integral part of the spinal cord. The **subarachnoid space** is more capacious than is the subdural space, particularly in the lumbar region, where it encloses the great group of lumbar and sacral nerve roots known as the **cauda equina.** The subarachnoid space contains the **cerebrospinal fluid.**

Study the external form of the spinal cord. The **spinal cord** (medulla spinalis) begins at the **foramen magnum,** above which it is directly continuous with the medulla oblongata of the brain, and ends at about the level of the lower border of the **first lumbar vertebra.** The tapering inferior end of the cord, from which the sacral nerve roots arise, is known as the **conus medullaris.** From the tip of the conus a thread-like structure, the **filum terminale,** is continued downward through the subarachnoid space; below the termination of the dura, the filum terminale is enclosed within the coccygeal ligament. Observe that the diameter of the spinal cord is not the same throughout but is greatest in the lower cervical region, where it exhibits the **cervical enlargement,** and in the lower thoracic region, where it exhibits the **lumbar enlargement.** This is due to the large size of the lower cervical and the lumbar nerves, which arise from these two regions.

From the spinal cord arise, each by two roots, eight pairs of cervical nerves, twelve pairs of thoracic nerves, five pairs of lumbar nerves, five pairs of sacral nerves, and one pair of coccygeal nerves. Transect the spinal cord and its meningeal coverings at the level of the second and sixth thoracic vertebrae. Cut the spinal nerves on each side, about 1 in. lateral to this segment, and remove the segment of spinal cord, its meningeal coverings, and the attached nerve roots from the spinal canal. Open the meningeal coverings by a longitudinal incision along the length of the ventral surface of this segment. The **posterior roots** are made up of **afferent** (sensory) **nerve fibers** and arise from the posterolateral sulcus on the posterior aspect of the cord. The **anterior roots** are made up of **efferent** (motor) **nerve fibers** and arise from the anterolateral sulcus on the anterior aspect of the cord. Each root does not arise as a single structure but as a linear series of filaments, which unite to form a single root. The two roots of each nerve remain distinct within the vertebral canal and unite only upon reaching the intervertebral foramina. On each posterior root, just proximal to the point of union, is a swelling, the **spinal ganglion.** These ganglia, with the exception of those of the sacral nerves, are also situated within the intervertebral foramina.

The length of the spinal nerve roots increases steadily from above downward, since the length of the cord is so much less than is that of the vertebral canal. Observe that the cervical roots pass almost directly laterally to reach the intervertebral foramina, while in the thoracic region the roots take a course of constantly increasing obliquity, downward and laterally. The lumbar and sacral roots, which arise in close succession from the lower part of the cord, pass almost vertically downward through the subarachnoid space in a brushlike aggregation of filaments which is known as the **cauda equina.**

With the bone forceps, chip away the articular processes forming the posterior boundary of one or two of the intervertebral foramina in the lower thoracic region to expose the spinal ganglion and the trunk of the spinal nerve. The nerve trunk and the ganglion are enclosed in a prolongation of the dura mater, which must be carefully cleared away. Observe that the **trunk of** the **spinal nerve** is very short, as each divides almost at once into **an anterior and a posterior primary division.** In nearly all cases, the anterior primary division is much the larger. The posterior primary division passes directly backward through the deep muscles of the back. The anterior primary division passes laterally. The anterior primary divisions of the thoracic nerves are the **intercostal nerves;** the anterior primary divisions of the cervical, lumbar, and sacral nerves take part in the formation of the cervical, brachial, lumbar, and sacral plexuses.

In the lower thoracic region, dissect the connections between the anterior divisions of the spinal nerves and the sympathetic ganglia in the thorax. These connections are the **white** and **gray rami communicantes,** and their structure and relations can be seen much better when the thorax is dissected (p. 114).

In the upper part of the spinal cord, above the level of the fifth cervical nerve roots, note the fibers forming the **spinal part of** the **accessory nerve.** These fibers arise from the lateral part of the spinal cord and form a single trunk which ascends between the denticulate ligament and the posterior roots of the spinal nerves to enter the skull through the foramen magnum.

Head and Neck ·

Face

The surface features of the face are those with which the dissector is, for the most part, already thoroughly familiar. The **mental protuberance,** the lower border, and the **angle of** the **mandible** are readily palpable through the skin. The prominence of the cheek is formed by the **zygomatic bone,** which extends posteriorly to join the zygomatic process of the temporal bone in the formation of the **zygomatic arch,** also subcutaneous. The lips are covered with a **mucous membrane,** which is continuous externally with the skin of the face and internally with the mucous membrane lining the mouth. At the nostrils, the skin of the face is continuous with the mucous lining of the nasal cavities. The free margins of the upper and lower eyelids together form a slitlike orifice known as the **rima palpebrarum.** At the rima, the skin of the face is continuous with the conjunctiva. The **conjunctiva** is a delicate membrane which forms the inner linings of both eyelids and is further reflected over the anterior part of the eyeball, the conjunctiva as a whole enclosing a space open to the exterior at the rima palpebrarum and known as the conjunctival sac. The **conjunctival sac** lies between the inner surfaces of the eyelids and the anterior surface of the eyeball. In the free margin of each eyelid, close to its medial end, is a small opening at the summit of a slight elevation. The elevation is the papilla lacrimalis, and the opening the **puncta lacrimalis.** It marks the beginning of the **lacrimal duct,** which conveys the tears from the conjunctival sac.

Make the following incisions through the

skin: (1) a median longitudinal from the occipital protuberance and running downward across the forehead, along the bridge of the nose, and ending at the mental protuberance; (2) a transverse incision starting from the first incision at the level of the rima palpebrarum and running laterally and backward to a point just in front of the external auditory meatus (this incision must bifurcate in the region of the upper and lower eyelids, so that it will pass through the skin of each lid just above and below the rima); (3) a transverse incision running from the angle of the mouth laterally and backward to the posterior border of the ramus of the mandible (from the angle of the mouth, this incision should be extended medially along the red margins of the upper and lower lips); (4) a transverse incision along the lower border of the mandible from the symphysis to a point slightly behind the angle. By this means, three flaps of skin will be mapped out, which should all be reflected laterally and backward from the median line. Some difficulty will be met in reflecting the skin of the face, since the superficial muscles of the face are inserted for the most part into the skin; the strands of these muscles should be cut away from the deep surface of the skin and the skin reflected cleanly. In the temporal region, the **superficial temporal vessels** lie immediately subjacent to the skin and will be reflected with it if care is not taken.

The superficial muscles of the face are known as the **muscles of facial expression.** These muscles, for the most part, take origin on one of the bones of the face and are inserted into the skin and superficial fascia. Since they are difficult to demonstrate satisfactorily in the cadaver, only a few of them will be dissected. The proper plane for reflecting the skin, particularly in those specimens where a large amount of subcutaneous fat is present, can be achieved by removing the skin and subcutaneous tissue from the outer surface of the upper part of the platysma muscle, which has been exposed, and continuing this plane of dissection upward on the face.

The **orbicularis oculi** is a circular muscle which surrounds the rima palpebrarum. Its fibers lie just beneath the skin in the upper and lower eyelids, but it is more extensive than the lids and also covers the bony rim of the orbit, from which some of its fibers take origin.

The **frontalis** is a thin flat muscle which lies just under the skin of the forehead. Its fibers arise from the galea aponeurotica, the aponeurosis covering the vertex of the skull, and are inserted into the skin of the eyebrows and the root of the nose, blending to some extent with the upper part of the orbicularis oculi.

The **nasalis** is a small muscle which arises at the side of the bridge of the nose and runs downward and laterally to be inserted in the skin at the junction of the wing of the nose and the cheek.

The **orbicularis oris** surrounds the opening of the mouth and is the main intrinsic muscle of the lips. Its fibers are derived largely from the other superficial muscles yet to be observed and are inserted both into the skin covering the lips externally and into the mucous membrane lining the lips internally.

The **quadratus labii superioris** arises by three heads, a zygomatic head (zygomaticus minor) from the lowest part of the external surface of the zygomatic bone, an infraorbital head (levator labii superioris) from the infraorbital margin of the maxilla, and an angular head (levator labii superioris alaeque nasi) from the root of the nose. The fibers of the three heads converge toward the upper lip, into the skin of which they are inserted, many of them joining the orbicularis oris.

The **zygomaticus major** is a flat, bandlike muscle arising from the external surface of the zygomatic bone lateral to the origin of the zygomatic head of the quadratus labii superioris and passing to the angle of the mouth.

The **risorius** is a purely superficial muscle

arising from the superficial fascia over the parotid gland. It passes forward across the cheek to the angle of the mouth, where it blends with the orbicularis oris.

The **triangularis** arises from the lower part of the external surface of the anterior half of the mandible and converges upward toward the angle of the mouth, where it is in part inserted directly into the skin and in part joins the orbicularis oris.

The muscles just described, as well as the deeper muscles of the same group, are all supplied by branches of the **facial nerve.** Since these branches enter the deep surfaces of the muscles, they will not have been injured if the dissection has been carefully done. Attempt now to demonstrate the branches of distribution of the facial nerve.

As the trunk of the **facial nerve** emerges from the **stylomastoid foramen,** it passes di-

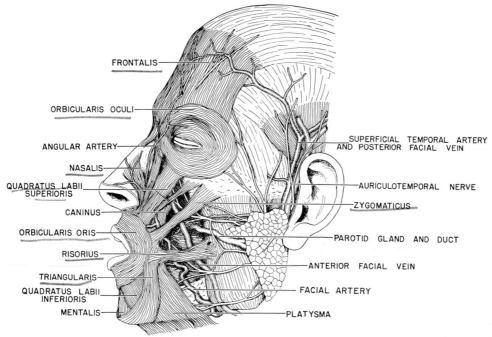

FIG. 8. Superficial dissection of the face. The branches of the facial nerve, which are seen emerging from the borders of the parotid gland, are not labeled.

The **quadratus labii inferioris** arises from the external suface of the mandible below the canine and premolar teeth and runs upward and medially into the orbicularis oris.

The **platysma** lies for the most part in the neck. Its more posterior fibers, however, run upward across the mandible, behind the triangularis, and blend with the triangularis, the risorius, and the orbicularis oris. The anatomy of the other facial muscles should be reviewed in one of the descriptive texts.

rectly into the **parotid gland.** Within the substance of the gland, it breaks up into numerous branches which emerge separately onto the face from under cover of the superior and anterior borders of the parotid. For this reason, it is best first to clean carefully the external surface of the parotid and to identify the branches of the facial nerve as the borders of the gland are cleaned (Fig. 8).

The **parotid gland** occupies the interval between the posterior border of the ramus of the mandible and the anterior border of the sterno-mastoid muscle and mastoid process. A flattened portion is also prolonged forward over the external surface of the ramus of the mandible and posterior part of the masseter muscle. The **duct of** the **parotid** is usually of considerable size. It emerges from the anterior border of the gland and crosses the cheek anteriorly about ½ in. below the zygomatic arch. It pierces the middle of the cheek to open into the **cavity of** the **mouth** at the parotid papilla, on the level of the second upper molar tooth. The parotid gland is enclosed in a sheath of fairly dense fascia which is continuous anteriorly with the deep fascia covering the external surface of the masseter muscle.

Emerging from under cover of the superior border of the gland will be found the **temporal** and **zygomatic branches of** the **facial nerve.** The temporal branch runs upward over the temporal fascia to be distributed to the auricularis superior and anterior (two small, unimportant muscles of the external ear) and to the frontalis. The zygomatic branch runs upward and forward across the zygomatic bone to reach the orbicularis oculi.

Emerging from under cover of the anterior border of the parotid are the **buccal** and **mandibular** branches of the facial nerve. The buccal branches, of which there are usually two or three, pass forward across the cheek to supply the zygomaticus, quadratus labii superioris, nasalis, orbicularis oris, risorius, caninus, and buccinator. The mandibular branch passes forward just above the lower border of the mandible to reach the triangularis and quadratus labii inferioris. The various branches of the facial, particularly the buccal and mandibular branches, usually communicate with one another on the face by small connecting loops. The **cervical branch** of the facial descends into the neck below the angle of the mandible to supply the **platysma.**

The substance of the parotid gland should now be carefully cut away, a bit at a time, to expose the structures which are embedded in it. These are the trunk of the **facial nerve** and the beginning of its branches, the terminal part of the **external carotid artery,** and the **posterior (retromandibular) facial vein.**

The **facial nerve** should be exposed first, since it winds superficially around the external carotid and the retromandibular vein. Shortly after emerging from the stylomastoid foramen, the facial gives rise to a small **posterior auricular branch** which passes upward and backward on the external surface of the mastoid process to supply the posterior auricular and occipitalis muscles. Just below this, the trunk gives off a branch which descends deeply to supply the stylohyoid and the posterior belly of the digastric. The trunk of the facial, still within the substance of the parotid, then usually divides into two trunks, an upper and a lower. From the **upper trunk** arise **temporal, zygomatic,** and **buccal** branches; from the **lower trunk, buccal, mandibular,** and **cervical** branches (Fig. 9).

The **retromandibular vein** is formed in the region of the root of the zygomatic arch by the union of **superficial temporal** and **middle temporal veins.** It descends through the substance of the parotid, usually crosses the digastric superficially, and terminates at about the level of the angle of the mandible by dividing into two branches, one of which usually passes forward to join the anterior facial in the common facial, while the other crosses the sternomastoid to join the external jugular vein. It lies superficial to the external carotid artery and may be removed, if desired, in cleaning the artery.

Ascending from the carotid triangle of the neck deep to the stylohoid and the posterior belly of the digastric, the **external carotid** artery becomes embedded in the deepest part of the parotid gland, where it is crossed externally by the facial nerve. It ascends behind the posterior border of the ramus of the mandible and terminates behind the neck of the mandible by dividing into the **maxillary** and **superficial temporal arteries.** Deeply it is in relation to the styloid process, which separates it from the internal carotid artery. Just above the posterior belly of the digastric, it gives rise to

the level of the upper tip of the auricle, divides into frontal and parietal branches which ramify in the scalp over the frontal and parietal bones. Near its origin, it gives rise to the **transverse facial artery,** which passes forward across the face just above the parotid duct. At a slightly higher level, the superficial temporal gives rise

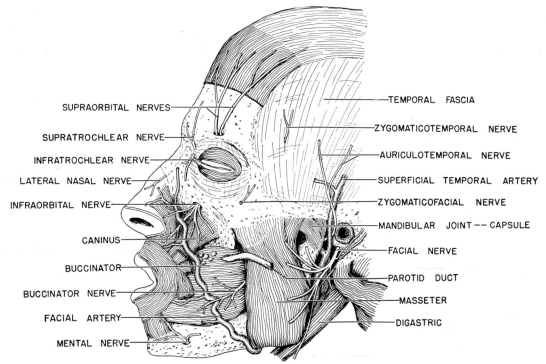

SUPRAORBITAL NERVES

SUPRATROCHLEAR NERVE

INFRATROCHLEAR NERVE

LATERAL NASAL NERVE

INFRAORBITAL NERVE

CANINUS

BUCCINATOR

BUCCINATOR NERVE

FACIAL ARTERY

MENTAL NERVE

TEMPORAL FASCIA

ZYGOMATICOTEMPORAL NERVE

AURICULOTEMPORAL NERVE

SUPERFICIAL TEMPORAL ARTERY

ZYGOMATICOFACIAL NERVE

MANDIBULAR JOINT -- CAPSULE

FACIAL NERVE

PAROTID DUCT

MASSETER

DIGASTRIC

FIG. 9. Deep dissection of the face. The parotid gland has been entirely removed.

a small **posterior auricular branch,** which accompanies the posterior auricular branch of the facial nerve across the external surface of the mastoid process.

Only the beginning of the maxillary artery can be exposed at the present time. It passes forward and medially, deep to the neck of the mandible, to enter the infratemporal fossa.

Clean the superficial temporal artery, securing at the same time the auriculotemporal nerve. The **superficial temporal artery** ascends immediately in front of the ear and, at about

to the **middle temporal artery,** which runs forward to pierce the temporal fascia and enter the temporal muscle.

The **auriculotemporal nerve** is a cutaneous nerve derived from the **mandibular division of the trigeminal.** It emerges on the face from behind the condyle of the mandible and turns upward, in close relation to the superficial temporal artery, to be distributed to the skin of the upper part of the auricle and the greater part of the temporal region (Figs. 8 and 9).

The **facial artery** reaches the face by winding over the lower border of the mandible about ¾ in. in front of the angle. From this point, it passes upward and forward across the face, pursuing a somewhat tortuous course, to the medial angle of the eye, where its terminal portion is known as the **angular artery.** In its course across the face, it usually passes deep to the risorious, zygomaticus, and quadratus labii superioris, which should be elevated or their fibers divided to expose the artery. From the anterior aspect of the facial artery originate the **superior** and **inferior labial arteries,** which run forward and medially in the substance of the upper and lower lips to anastomose with similar branches of the opposite side, and to a **lateral nasal branch** to the side of the nose. From its posterior aspect arise irregular branches to the skin and muscles of the cheek.

Clean the **masseter** muscle. This is a thick quadrilateral muscle belonging to the group known as the muscles of mastication, which covers the ramus of the mandible externally. It arises from the lower border and internal surface of the **zygomatic arch** and is inserted on the external surface of the **ramus** and of the **body of** the **mandible** near the angle. Its nerve supply, which crosses the mandibular notch to enter the deep surface of the muscle, is derived from the mandibular division of the trigeminal nerve. This nerve will be dissected later.

The cutaneous nerves of the face are all derived from the **trigeminal** or fifth cranial **nerve.** The three divisions of this nerve are the **ophthalmic, maxillary,** and **mandibular nerves,** and cutaneous branches of each of these appear on the face. Their terminal ramifications are superficial, since they reach the skin, but the main trunks, which should now be exposed, enter the face deeply, most of them emerging from foramina in the facial bones. In exposing the nerves, the various superficial muscles of facial expression which cover them should be separated or retracted (Fig. 9).

The cutaneous branches of the **ophthalmic nerve** are the **supraorbital, supratrochlear, infratrochlear,** and **external nasal nerves.** The largest of these is the supraorbital. It leaves the orbit at the supraorbital notch or foramen and passes upward on the frontal bone under cover of the frontalis muscle. Its branches of distribution pierce the frontalis to supply the skin of the forehead. The supratrochlear nerve is small; it emerges from the upper medial angle of the orbit, under cover of the frontalis and the orbicularis oculi, to supply the skin in the region of the glabella. The **infratrochlear nerve,** also small, appears on the face just above the medial angle of the eye and supplies the skin of the eyelids and the upper part of the side of the nose. The **external nasal nerve** emerges between the nasal bone and the nasal cartilage and supplies the skin of the bridge of the nose.

The cutaneous branches of the **maxillary nerve** are the **infraorbital, zygomaticofacial,** and **zygomaticotemporal nerves.** The infraorbital is the terminal part of the maxillary nerve proper. It emerges from the infraorbital foramen and breaks up, under cover of the infraorbital head of the quadratus labii superioris, into a number of branches which supply the skin of the upper lip, the wing of the nose, and the upper part of the cheek. The zygomaticofacial nerve emerges through a small foramen in the zygomatic bone to supply the skin over the malar prominence. The zygomaticotemporal is a minute nerve which pierces the temporal fascia to supply a small area of skin in the anterior part of the temporal region.

The cutaneous branches of the **mandibular nerve** are the **auriculotemporal,** the **buccinator (buccal),** and the **mental nerves.** The auriculotemporal nerve has already been exposed. The buccal nerve emerges from under cover of the anterior border of the masseter and runs downward and forward to supply the skin of the lower part of the cheek. The mental nerve emerges from the mental foramen of the mandible, under cover of the triangularis, to supply the skin of the chin and lower lip.

The locations of two of the larger nerve trunks may be facilitated by finding the foramina through which they emerge. Insert the more pointed end of a probe through the facial muscles about ¼ in. caudad to the midpoint of the lower orbital ridge. Move the probe around until it enters the **infraorbital foramen.** The **mental foramen** can be similarly found by passing the probe through the muscles over the mandible at the level of the root of the second premolar tooth. When the foramina have been located, separate the fibers of the overlying muscles and secure the nerves emerging through these foramina.

The only deeper muscles of facial expression to which attention need be paid are the **caninus** and the **buccinator.** The caninus lies under cover of the quadratus labii superioris. It arises from the canine fossa of the maxilla and descends to the angle of the mouth, where some of its fibers are inserted directly into the skin and others join the orbicularis oris. The buccinator lies in the substance of the cheek. It arises from the molar portion of the alveolar process of the maxilla, the external surface of the mandible just below the molar teeth, and the **pterygomandibular raphe.** The latter is a fibrous band which extends from the pterygoid hamulus to the upper border of the mandible at the junction of the body and the ramus. From this origin, the fibers pass forward to be inserted into the mucous membrane of the mouth near the angle of the mouth and to join the orbicularis oris. Posteriorly, just in front of the masseter, the buccinator is covered externally by a thick mass of fatty tissue, the **suctorial pad,** which should be removed in cleaning the muscle. The buccinator is pierced by the **parotid duct** and by small branches of the buccinator nerve which supply the mucous membrane lining the cheek. Both the **caninus** and the **buccinator** are supplied by **buccal branches of** the **facial nerve.**

Temporal and Infratemporal Regions

The **temporal fascia** is a strong membranous fascia which covers externally the temporal muscle. Superficial to this fascia are two thin muscles of the facial group, the superior and anterior auricular. They should be removed in cleaning the temporal fascia. The temporal fascia is attached above to the superior temporal line and below to the upper border of the zygomatic arch and the posterior border of the zygomatic bone. It is thickest inferiorly, where it splits into two layers between which is enclosed a small amount of fatty tissue. Review the relations of the fascia over the temporal and infratemporal regions to that in the cervical region.

Remove the temporal fascia and clean the external surface of the **temporal muscle,** one of the muscles of mastication. It arises from the whole of the temporal fossa, with the exception of that part formed by the **zygomatic bone,** and is inserted into the borders and the entire internal surface of the coronoid process of the **mandible.** To expose the insertion of the temporal, the masseter muscle should be reflected. Insert the handle of a forceps between the zygomatic arch and the outer surface of the temporal muscle. While depressing the subjacent structures, saw through the **zygomatic arch** at the anterior and posterior ends of the origin of the masseter and reflect the arch with the attached masseter downward to the insertion of that muscle, by elevating the branches of the facial nerve and passing the masseter muscle and zygomatic arch beneath these nerves. The anterior saw cut must pass posteriorly from below upward to avoid injury to the lateral wall of the orbit. As the **masseter** is reflected, a small bit of the muscle substance should be left attached to the nerve which enters its deep surface, so that the nerve may be later recognized and traced to its origin. Note the direction of the superficial (downward and backward) and the deep (downward and forward) fibers of the masseter muscle.

When the temporal muscle has been thoroughly cleaned, saw through the **coronoid process** of the mandible at its junction with the ramus and reflect the coronoid process with the temporal muscle laterally and upward toward the origin of the muscle. The reflection of the temporal is often complicated by the fact that its deep surface is connected by small muscle fasciculi with the deeper muscles of the region (buccinator and external pterygoid). Such fasciculi, if they exist, should be cut. The temporal is supplied by two (or three) **deep temporal nerves,** which will be found running upward on the temporal surface of the great wing of the sphenoid to enter its deep surface. They should be preserved.

Remove the facial muscles from the area of the mental foramen and locate the branches of the **mental nerve** and **artery.** Elevate the facial artery and facial vein from the mandible. Starting at the mental foramen, use a mallet and chisel, aided if necessary by bone forceps, and carefully chip away the outer table of the mandible to open the **mandibular canal** and expose the course of the **inferior alveolar nerve.** This nerve runs forward through the mandible and gives off **dental branches** to the roots of all the lower teeth and **gingival branches** to the mucous membrane of the gum, all of which pass through minute canals in the bone. The inferior alveolar artery accompanies the nerve and gives rise to small branches which correspond to those of the nerve.

In order to open fully the infratemporal fossa for dissection, it is necessary to remove the upper part of the ramus of the mandible. To do this, make two transverse cuts with a saw or bone forceps. The superior cut should pass through the neck of the mandible at its junction with the ramus. The inferior cut must cross the ramus transversely high enough to avoid cutting the **inferior alveolar nerve,** which enters the **mandibular foramen** on the inner surface of the ramus.

The **pterygoid plexus of veins,** which drains into the posterior facial vein, surrounds the maxillary artery together with its branches. The veins should be cut away as the other structures are cleaned.

Clean first the **external (lateral) pterygoid muscle,** taking care to preserve any nerves and arteries which may cross its external surface. The lateral pterygoid arises by two heads, which are separated from each other by a slight groove. The lower head, which is the larger, arises from the external surface of the **lateral pterygoid plate and** from the **tuberosity of** the **maxilla.** The upper head arises from the infratemporal surface of the **great wing of** the **sphenoid.** The fibers of both heads pass backward and laterally and converge to a tendinous insertion into a depression on the front of the **neck of** the **mandible** and a few fibers go to the articular capsule and disc.

The **buccal nerve,** will usually be found to emerge from between the two heads of the lateral pterygoid. The **deep temporal nerves** usually emerge from under cover of the upper border of the muscle, though the more anterior one may appear between the two heads. Descending from under cover of the inferior border of the lateral pterygoid, two relatively large nerves will be seen. The more anterior is the **lingual nerve;** it passes downward and forward to reach the inner surface of the mandible in the region of the last molar tooth. Just behind the lingual is the **inferior alveolar nerve,** which enters the mandibular foramen on the inner surface of the ramus; slightly above the mandibular foramen the inferior alveolar gives rise to a small branch, the **mylohyoid nerve,** which descends in the mylohyoid groove on the inner surface of the mandible to reach the digastric triangle.

The **internal (medial) pterygoid muscle** should now be cleaned. It arises by two heads. The external head, which is very much the smaller, arises from the **maxillary tuberosity** and the pyramidal process of the palatine bone. The large internal head arises from the **pterygoid fossa;** this origin is at present hidden by the lower head of the lateral pterygoid. The

lateral pterygoid muscle and lies medial to the neck of the mandible. The **second part** crosses the lower head of the lateral pterygoid, passing from the lower border of the muscle to the pterygomaxillary fissure in the region of the interval between the two heads of the muscle. The **third part** lies in the pterygopalatine fossa and cannot now be exposed. The relation of the second part of the artery to the lateral pterygoid is variable. In about 50 per cent of the cases, the artery crosses the external sur-

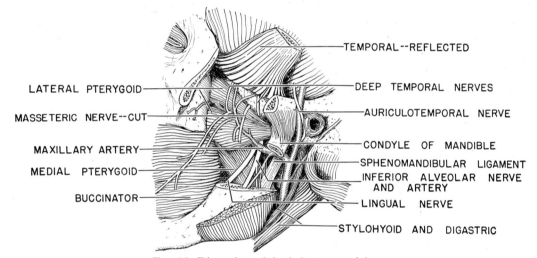

LATERAL PTERYGOID

MASSETERIC NERVE--CUT

MAXILLARY ARTERY

MEDIAL PTERYGOID

BUCCINATOR

TEMPORAL--REFLECTED

DEEP TEMPORAL NERVES

AURICULOTEMPORAL NERVE

CONDYLE OF MANDIBLE

SPHENOMANDIBULAR LIGAMENT

INFERIOR ALVEOLAR NERVE AND ARTERY

LINGUAL NERVE

STYLOHYOID AND DIGASTRIC

FIG. 10. Dissection of the infratemporal fossa.

main mass of the medial pterygoid lies below the lateral pterygoid; its fibers run downward, backward, and laterally to be inserted into the lower half of the internal surface of the **ramus of the mandible.**

The **maxillary artery** arises behind the neck of the mandible as one of the terminal branches of the external carotid and runs forward, upward, and medially through the **infratemporal fossa** to the pterygomaxillary fissure, through which it passes into the pterygopalatine fossa. It is divided for descriptive purposes into **three parts,** the first and second of which lie in the infratemporal fossa. The **first part** extends from the external carotid to the lower border of the

face of the muscle; in the other 50 per cent, it crosses the deep surface, in which eventuality it cannot be exposed until the lateral pterygoid is reflected. The structures that are supplied with blood by the maxillary artery are the same in either case, but the manner of origin of the branches is somewhat different in the two conditions.

In addition to two small branches, the **anterior tympanic** and the **deep auricular,** the first part of the **maxillary** gives rise to a large branch, the **inferior alveolar artery,** which enters the mandibular foramen in company with the inferior alveolar nerve. In cases where the second part crosses the lateral pterygoid externally, the further branches are as follows. The first part gives rise to the **middle meningeal artery,** which ascends deep to the lateral pterygoid to enter the **foramen spinosum.** The second part gives rise to a series of **muscular branches,** which supply the temporal, medial, and lateral pterygoid and masseter muscles and to the **buccal artery,** which accompanies the buccal nerve on to the cheek. In cases where the second part of the maxillary crosses the deep surface of the lateral pterygoid, the mid-

the **temporomandibular (lateral) ligament.** This ligament is attached above to the root of the zygoma and narrows inferiorly to its attachment on the lateral aspect of the condyle and neck of the mandible. Define the **sphenomandibular ligament.** This is an accessory ligament of the joint, which is not joined to the capsule but lies medial to it; it is a thin fibrous band which runs from the spine of the sphenoid to the lingula of the mandible. Cut through the circumference of the capsule and disarticulate

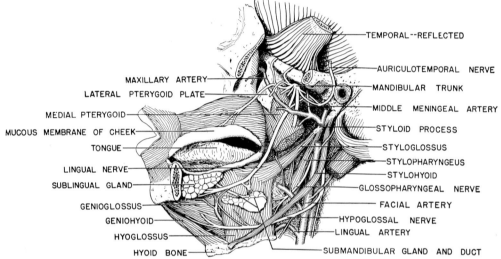

MAXILLARY ARTERY
LATERAL PTERYGOID PLATE
MEDIAL PTERYGOID
MUCOUS MEMBRANE OF CHEEK
TONGUE
LINGUAL NERVE
SUBLINGUAL GLAND
GENIOGLOSSUS
GENIOHYOID
HYOGLOSSUS
HYOID BONE

TEMPORAL--REFLECTED
AURICULOTEMPORAL NERVE
MANDIBULAR TRUNK
MIDDLE MENINGEAL ARTERY
STYLOID PROCESS
STYLOGLOSSUS
STYLOPHARYNGEUS
STYLOHYOID
GLOSSOPHARYNGEAL NERVE
FACIAL ARTERY
HYPOGLOSSAL NERVE
LINGUAL ARTERY
SUBMANDIBULAR GLAND AND DUCT

FIG. 11. Deep dissection of the submandibular and infratemporal regions. The lateral pterygoid muscle and the left side of the mandible have been removed.

dle meningeal artery arises from the second part and will be entirely covered by the lateral pterygoid, as long as that muscle remains in place. The branches described above as arising from the second part usually here arise from a large common stem on the first part of the maxillary and ascend on the external surface of the lateral pterygoid (Fig. 10).

Study the **mandibular articulation.** This is a **diarthrodial joint** at which the **condyle of the mandible** articulates with the **mandibular fossa of** the **temporal bone.** It is enveloped in a loose articular capsule, which is strengthened on its lateral aspect by the fibers constituting

the condyle. Observe the **cartilaginous articular disc,** which is interposed between the condyle and the temporal bone and divides the articular cavity into distinct superior and inferior parts.

With the disarticulation of the condyle, the **lateral pterygoid** may be reflected medially and forward. If the second part of the maxillary artery lies deep to the lateral pterygoid, it may now be seen, and the **middle meningeal artery** may be traced to the foramen spinosum. At the same time, the mandibular nerve and its branches will be exposed and should be cleaned (Fig. 11).

The **mandibular nerve** emerges from the cranial cavity through the **foramen ovale** and divides almost immediately into a small anterior and a large posterior division. The anterior division runs forward under cover of the lateral pterygoid for a short distance and then reaches the external surface of that muscle, either by passing between its two heads or, much less frequently, by winding over its upper border. From this point on, it is known as the **buccal nerve,** whose further course has already been seen. While still under cover of the lateral pterygoid, the anterior division gives rise to several muscular branches. These are the **deep temporal nerves,** which supply the temporal muscle, and the **nerves** of supply **to** the **masseter** and the **lateral pterygoid.**

The posterior division of the mandibular nerve descends for a short distance and divides into the **lingual,** the **inferior alveolar,** and the **auriculotemporal nerves.** The lingual and inferior alveolar nerves descend under cover of the lateral pterygoid to reach the external surface of the medial pterygoid, where they have already been seen. Observe that the lingual is joined, shortly below its origin, by another small nerve, which may be seen running downward and forward medial to the inferior alveolar nerve. This is the **chorda tympani.** It passes through the temporal bone, which it leaves at the petrotympanic fissure, to enter the infratemporal fossa and join the lingual nerve.

The **auriculotemporal nerve** usually arises by two roots which embrace the **middle meningeal artery** and join behind it. The nerve then passes posteriorly to wind laterally behind the mandibular joint and turn upward over the root of the zygoma, from which point its further course has been traced.

Attempt to demonstrate the **nerve** supply **to** the **medial pterygoid** muscle. This small nerve usually arises directly from the trunk of the mandibular just below the foramen ovale and enters the upper part of the medial pterygoid.

The **otic ganglion** should be noted on the medial side of the mandibular nerve, just below the foramen ovale. The nerves passing to and from this ganglion should be reviewed from one of the standard texts.

Cranial Cavity

As a preparation for the opening of the cranial cavity, the bony vault of the skull should be stripped bare. To do this, make a median sagittal incision through the scalp, including any skin which may remain on the back of the head, from the glabella to the external occipital protuberance and another at a right angle to this incision about the midpoint of the sagittal suture. The various layers of the scalp may then all be turned downward and laterally on each side, leaving the external surface of the bones of the cranial vault clean. Attempt to identify the various layers of the scalp. Any remnants of the temporal muscle should also be reflected downward from the upper part of the temporal fossa. Then tie a string around the cranium and mark on the bone with a pencil carried along the string the line on which the cranial cavity is to be opened. Anteriorly, this line should be about $\frac{3}{4}$ in. above the upper margin of the orbits and, posteriorly, about the same distance above the external occipital protuberance.

With a saw, cut through the **outer table** of the bones along this line. When the **diploe** is reached, do not use the saw, for the inner table should be broken through with a chisel. The **calvaria** may then be pulled off, and the external surface of the dura mater of the brain will be exposed.

Cranial Meninges and Dural Venous Sinuses

The **cranial dura** consists of two layers, the outer of which is actually the **periosteum** of the inner surface of the cranial bones. The inner, or **supporting, layer** of the cranial dura is analogous to the spinal dura, with which it is continuous at the foramen magnum. The two layers of the cranial dura are in most regions firmly attached to one another, but in certain places they separate to enclose blood spaces, the **sinuses of** the **dura mater.** The dural sinuses are in fact veins, but they differ from typical veins in that the actual wall of the vessel consists only of an endothelial layer, the chief support of the wall being provided by the dura mater in which the vessel is enclosed. The outer layer of the cranial dura is everywhere in close relation to the inner surface of the cranial bones. The inner layer, however, shows reduplications, or double folds, which project into the cranial cavity and partially subdivide it. These reduplications, which will be seen as the dissection proceeds, are the **falx cerebri,** the **tentorium cerebelli,** and the **falx cerebelli.**

Make a sagittal incision through the dura about ½ in. lateral to the midline on each side from the frontal to the occipital region; passing laterally from each end of these incisions, make transverse incisions and turn the flaps of dura thus marked out laterally to expose the **subdural space** and the **arachnoid.** The cranial arachnoid is a delicate membrane, through which the upper surface of the cerebral hemispheres will be readily seen. No special study of the cranial arachnoid need be made, but it may be removed with the brain.

Observe the numerous **cerebral veins,** which leave the upper surface of the cerebral hemispheres and pierce the arachnoid to enter the dura close to the median line. These veins carry blood to the superior sagittal sinus, which should now be opened. To do this, it is necessary only to make a median sagittal incision in the dura. The **superior sagittal sinus** is enclosed within the dura mater. It begins anteriorly at the crista galli of the ethmoid bone and extends posteriorly along the cranial vault in the median plane to the internal occipital protuberance, where it ends by joining the right (less frequently the left) **transverse sinus.** In its course it receives the superior cerebral veins.

Spread the cerebral hemispheres apart and observe the **falx cerebri.** This is a double fold of the inner layer of the dura mater, which stretches downward in the median plane between the two hemispheres. Superiorly, its two layers separate to enclose the superior sagittal sinus and to become continuous with the inner layer of the dura of the cranial vault on either side. Anteriorly, it is attached to the crista galli. Its inferior border is free, except in the posterior part of the cranial cavity. Enclosed within this lower free margin is the **inferior sagittal sinus.** Posteriorly, the falx cerebri is joined at its inferior margin to the tentorium cerebelli.

Cut the falx cerebri away from the crista galli and draw its free anterior portion upward and posteriorly out of the cleft between the two cerebral hemispheres. Tilt the head well backward and draw the **frontal lobes** of the cerebrum upward and backward from the floor of the anterior cranial fossa. As this is done, the minute filaments of the **olfactory nerves** may be seen piercing the cribriform plate of the ethmoid to reach the **olfactory bulb.** The **optic nerves** also will come into view, passing from the base of the diencephalon to the optic canals. They should be cut just posterior to the optic canals, or a transverse incision should be made through the middle of the **optic chiasma** and the anterior part of the chiasma with the attached optic nerves reflected anteriorly. Just below the optic canals the **internal carotid artery** will be seen, running posteriorly to reach the base of the brain. In the midline, between the two internal carotids, the **infundibulum** will appear. This narrow stalk, which connects the base of the brain with the **hypophysis,** must also be severed. If the temporal lobes of the cerebral hemispheres are now dislodged from the middle cranial fossa and both hemispheres tilted still farther upward and backward, the anterior part of the **tentorium cerebelli,** which roofs the posterior cranial fossa, will be seen; and, passing upward from the posterior fossa at the free margin of the tentorium, a portion of the brain stem, the **mesencephalon,** will appear. This should be cut through in a transverse plane, just above the tentorium cerebelli. The **cerebral hemispheres,** together with the **diencephalon** and the upper segment of the mesencephalon, will then be free and can be removed from the cranial cavity.

The **tentorium cerebelli** should now be examined. It is a transverse reduplication of the inner layer of the cranial dura, which is interposed between the posterior parts of the cerebral hemispheres and the cerebellum. Its outer border is attached to the anterior and posterior clinoid processes, the superior border of the petrous portion of the temporal bone, the posteroinferior angle of the parietal bone, and the transverse ridges of the occipital bone. Its inner or anterior border is free and forms the margin of an opening, the **tentorial notch,** through which the posterior cranial fossa communicates with the general cranial cavity. In the median line, the upper surface of the tentorium is joined to the inferior border of the posterior part of the falx cerebri.

Open the venous sinuses which are enclosed by the layers of the tentorium. In the median plane, along the line of junction of the tentorium and the falx, is the **straight sinus.** This sinus begins as a continuation of the inferior sagittal sinus at the tentorial notch, where it also receives the **great cerebral vein,** and passes straight backward to the internal occipital protuberance, where it ends, usually by joining the **left transverse sinus.** The transverse sinus of each side begins at the internal occipital protuberance and passes laterally, enclosed within the attached margin of the tentorium, along the occipital bone; at the lateral end of the superior border of the petrous part of the

temporal bone, it turns downward in the dura lining the wall of the posterior cranial fossa, where its further course may be seen after the tentorium has been removed. The **right transverse sinus** most commonly begins as a continuation of the superior sagittal sinus and the left as a continuation of the straight sinus. This relationship may, however, be reversed, or all four sinuses may communicate at the confluence of the sinuses.

The **superior petrosal sinus** is enclosed in the outer margin of the tentorium along the line of attachment of that margin to the superior border of the petrous part of the temporal bone. It begins just lateral to the posterior clinoid process, where it receives blood from the cavernous sinus, and ends by joining the transverse sinus at the point where the latter turns inferiorly.

Make a sagittal incision in the tentorium slightly to the left of the median line. Then raise the right half of the cut tentorium and observe the **falx cerebelli,** which passes downward in the median plane from the undersurface of the tentorium into the cleft between the cerebellar hemispheres. Then make incisions through the tentorium on each side, extending laterally and backward about ½ in. medial to the transverse sinus. Reflect the severed halves of the tentorium upward to expose the **cerebellum,** the **posterior segment of** the **mesencephalon,** the **pons,** and the **medulla oblongata.** These portions of the brain should now be lifted from the floor of the **posterior fossa.** As this is done, the remaining cranial nerves should be identified and divided close to their points of attachment to the brain.

Cranial Nerves

The **oculomotor nerves** are relatively large. They arise from the lower surface of the midbrain near the median line. The **trochlear nerves** are much smaller; they wind downward around the lateral border of the posterior part of the midbrain. Arising from the side of the pons will be seen the various filaments which make up the roots of the **trigeminal nerve.** At the posterior border of the pons, near the median line, is the origin of the **abducens nerve.** Slightly more laterally, the **facial** and **acoustic (statoacoustic) nerves** will be seen to leave the posterior border of the pons. In the median line, the **basilar artery** will be found running forward in close relation to the inferior surface of the pons; it also should be divided. Below and behind the pons the brain stem narrows to the **medulla oblongata.** Arising from the sides of the medulla are the roots of the **vagus, glossopharyngeal,** and **accessory nerves** and, from its inferior surface, the various filaments which join to form the **hypoglossal nerve.** When the roots of all these nerves have been severed close to their points of emergence from the brain, the medulla should be divided transversely just above the foramen magnum and the brain completely removed from the cranial cavity.

Compare the floor of the cranial cavity as it now appears with the internal base of a macerated skull. The differences which will at once appear depend on the fact that the inner layer of the cranial dura does not in all regions closely follow the contour of the bones but is separated to some extent from the outer layer by structures which are interposed between the two layers. This is particularly true in the **middle cranial fossa,** where it should be noted that nothing can be seen of the superior orbital fissure, the foramen rotundum, the foramen ovale, the carotid canal, or the foramen spinosum as long as the inner layer of the dura is intact, since all of these openings are bridged over internally by the **inner layer of the dura.** Certain of the cranial nerves pierce the inner layer of the dura at a considerable distance from the foramina by which they leave the skull and pass forward between the two layers to reach these foramina.

Observe the points at which the oculomotor, trochlear, trigeminal, and abducens nerves pierce the inner layer of dura. The **oculomotor** is most anterior, entering the dura at the side of the posterior clinoid process. The **trochlear nerve** enters the dura at the most anterior point of attachment of the tentorium cerebelli. The point of entrance of the **trigeminal nerve** is slightly posterior and inferior to that of the trochlear; it is covered superiorly by the narrow anterior part of the tentorium. The **abducens nerve** enters the dura well back on the floor of the posterior fossa. To follow the further course of these nerves, the inner layer of the dura must be carefully stripped away from the floor of the middle cranial fossa at the side of the hypophyseal fossa. As this is done, the cavernous sinus will be opened.

Brain

The following dissection should be done on an intact brain or on one in which only the mesencephalon was transected, so that the parts of the brain can be reapproximated for study. *This dissection does not include all of the structures which would be considered in a course of neuroanatomy.* It is designed to acquaint the student with some of the parts which can be seen grossly on the surface of, and in macroscopic sections cut from, the brain.

Without distributing the meningeal coverings which are still present on the brain, a study should be made of its main external parts to help in understanding the following dissections. Place the brain so that its inferior surface (base) can be studied (Fig. 12). Note that the cut end of the **spinal cord** is continuous with the **medulla oblongata.** The medulla is about 1 in. long and ends at the **pons,** which is also easily recognized as a prominent ridge of transverse fibers extending laterally into the hemispheres of the **cerebellum.** The **hindbrain** ends at the rostral border of the pons and the **midbrain** begins there.

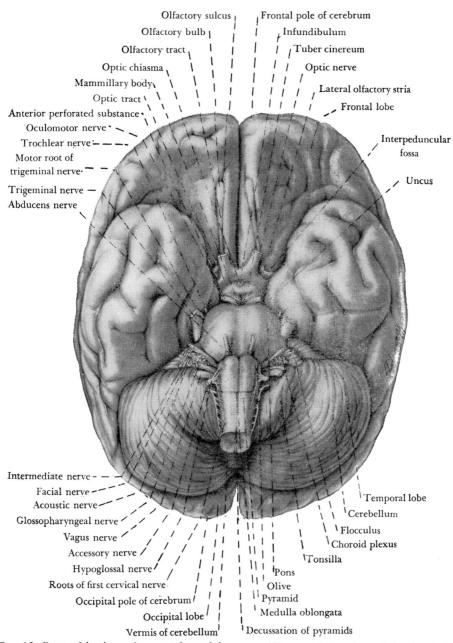

Olfactory sulcus
Olfactory bulb
Olfactory tract
Optic chiasma
Mammillary body
Optic tract
Anterior perforated substance
Oculomotor nerve
Trochlear nerve
Motor root of trigeminal nerve
Trigeminal nerve
Abducens nerve

Frontal pole of cerebrum
Infundibulum
Tuber cinereum
Optic nerve
Lateral olfactory stria
Frontal lobe
Interpeduncular fossa
Uncus

Intermediate nerve
Facial nerve
Acoustic nerve
Glossopharyngeal nerve
Vagus nerve
Accessory nerve
Hypoglossal nerve
Roots of first cervical nerve
Occipital pole of cerebrum
Occipital lobe
Vermis of cerebellum

Temporal lobe
Cerebellum
Flocculus
Choroid plexus
Tonsilla
Pons
Olive
Pyramid
Medulla oblongata
Decussation of pyramids

Fig. 12. Base of brain and roots of cranial nerves. (*By permission from Schaeffer* (*ed.*), *"Morris' Human Anatomy," 11/e, McGraw-Hill Book Company, Inc., Blakiston Division, New York, 1953.*)

The only parts of the midbrain visible are the cordlike right and left cerebral peduncles in front of the pons, diverging laterally as they ascend to the forebrain. The space between the peduncles is the interpeduncular fossa (Fig. 12).

The two **cerebral hemispheres** are the most conspicuous parts of the **forebrain** (prosencephalon). Each hemisphere is composed of four lobes: the **frontal, parietal, occipital,** and **temporal.**

Most, if not all, dura mater was probably removed from the surfaces of the brain at the time that it was taken out of the cranial cavity. Two of the other meninges—the **arachnoid** and the **pia mater**—should be present on the outer surface of the brain, and these should be studied. The outer parts of the brain can be seen through them, and it will be noted that the arachnoid is a thin, weblike covering which is continuous over the convolutions and processes of the brain. A space beneath and partially within the arachnoid, the **subarachnoid space,** contains cerebrospinal fluid during life. The arachnoid is most apparent where it extends over the convolutions and also where it forms pocketlike areas or cisterns. Identify the **cisterna magna** between the cerebellum and the medulla, and on the ventral surface of the brain, the **pontine, interpeduncular,** and **chiasmatic cisterns** near the pons, cerebellar peduncles, and optic chiasma, respectively. Additional small cisterns are formed in the subarachnoid spaces related to other parts of the brain. **Arachnoid granulations,** projections of the arachnoid outward, are present in certain areas, particularly on each side of the superior sagittal sinus. In the roof of the fourth ventricle, a median and two lateral apertures are found in the arachnoid for the outward passage of cerebrospinal fluid. These are the **foramina of Magendie** and **Luschka.** Now remove the arachnoid from the surfaces of the brain by gently tearing it away from the underlying structures, being particularly careful to avoid destroying the blood vessels and the cranial nerves while removing this layer.

The **pia mater** is closely applied to the outer surface of, and sends trabecular prolongations into, the parenchyma of the brain. Unlike the arachnoid, the pia even extends into the depths of the sulci, and it follows all the configurations of the brain.

With the aid of one of the descriptive textbooks, review the arterial circle at the base of the brain (the **circle of Willis**); the smaller branches from this circle supplying the basal parts of the brain; and study the course of the larger **anterior, middle,** and **posterior cerebral arteries.** Review the cerebral veins and their connections to the dural venous sinuses. Locate the cut end of the great cerebral vein (of Galen), extending upward near the splenium of the corpus callosum (Fig. 14).

Again study the base of the brain (Fig. 12) identifying additional structures not noted previously such as the pyramids, olive, uncus, mammillary body, infundibulum, tonsilla, flocculus, and lateral olfactory stria. Relocate the points of emergence of the cranial nerves as previously described on pages 43 and 44.

Then turn the brain over and carefully separate the two cerebral hemispheres, and while retracting them laterally, note the distribution of the cerebral arteries on the medial surface of the hemispheres and the whitish **corpus callosum** extending between the two hemispheres.

As a result of the growth of the cerebral hemispheres, the surface of the brain has become convoluted and folded in the form of elevations (**gyri**) and furrows (**sulci** and **fissures**). To aid in understanding this complex structure, examine the external surface of the cerebral hemispheres, and with the aid of one of the descriptive texts, identify the various gyri, sulci, lobes, and fissures. Although all of these have been named as landmarks, the following main ones should be identified. The **lateral (Sylvian) fissure,** the **central (Rolandic) sulcus,** the **parieto-occipital sulcus,** and the **calcarine fissure** (Figs. 13 and 14). The **precentral** and **postcentral gyri** on each side of the central sulcus, which are motor and sensory

and note the difference in thickness of the cortex in each of the various regions of the brain.

Next use a sharp knife and bisect the brain in the midsagittal plane, and then study the medial surface of the brain cut in the midsagittal section and identify the following structures

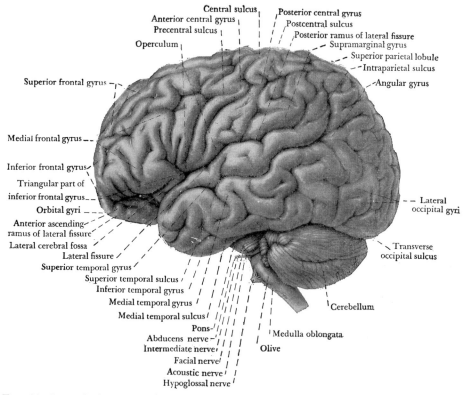

FIG. 13. Lateral view of brain. (*By permission from Schaeffer* (*ed.*), *"Morris' Human Anatomy,"* 11/e, *McGraw-Hill Book Company, Inc., Blakiston Division, New York,* 1953.)

respectively, should be identified. Next separate the margins of the lateral fissure and locate the **insula (island of Reil),** which is located between the frontal and temporal lobes (Fig. 18). Identify, from one of the descriptive texts, the motor, somesthetic, auditory, and visual centers of the cerebral hemispheres, and on one side remove a cube of tissue about 1 cm from each of these cortical centers. Then section each cube at right angles to the surface

(Fig. 14): the various gyri and sulci seen from this surface, the parts of the corpus callosum, the septum pellucidum, the fornix, cavity of the third ventricle with its choroid plexus, the massa intermedia, anterior commissure, the pineal and quadrigeminal bodies, the cerebellum, the cerebral aqueduct, and the fourth ventricle. Inferiorly identify the medulla, pons, cerebral peduncle, mammillary bodies, hypophysis, infundibulum, optic chiasma, lamina terminalis, and parolfactory area. In order to understand the inner structures of the brain, as well, and the size and shape of the ventricles, one half of the brain should be cut into a series of frontal sections and the other half sectioned in the horizontal plane. The latter sections should be made from that half of the brain from which the sections of cerebral cortex were taken. The

make successive cuts in the horizontal plane, each about ½ in. thick, until the structures shown in each half of Fig. 18 are found. Now, from both the coronal and horizontal sections attempt to follow the course of the **cerebral ventricles.** Note that the **choroid plexuses** may have been cut while sectioning the brain, but parts of them may still be present within the

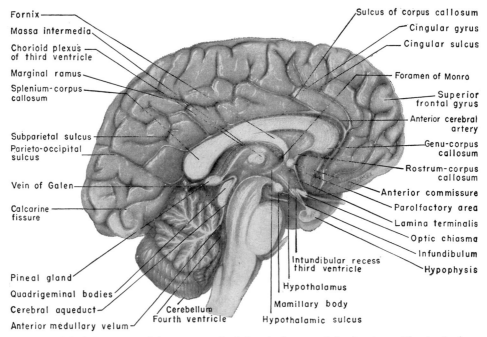

Fig. 14. Medial aspect of human cerebral hemisphere and brain stem. The brain has been sectioned through the longitudinal fissure. (*By permission from Peele, "The Neuroanatomical Basis for Clinical Neurology," McGraw-Hill Book Company, Inc., Blakiston Division, New York, 1954.*)

frontal sections should pass through the body of the corpus callosum, optic chiasma, and anterior commissure; the mammillary bodies, thalamus, and striate body; and the region of the splenium of the corpus callosum. Refer to Figs. 15 through 17 for the location of these landmarks. *In these figures, sections through both the right and left halves of the brain are shown, although in your dissection only one half will have been cut in the planes designated.* Next, take the other half of the brain and

ventricles. Start with the two **lateral ventricles,** noting their form and their extent into the lobes of the cerebral hemispheres (Figs. 14 to 18). Then locate the **foramen of Monro** (Fig. 14) by which they empty into the middle or **third ventricle,** the narrow compressed space between the two parts of the brain known as the thalamus (Figs. 14 and 16). Trace the third ventricle down through the **cerebral aqueduct** (Fig. 14) into the **fourth ventricle,** and note the openings in the roof of the fourth ventricle and the position of this ventricle in relationship to the cerebellum and medulla (Fig. 14). It may be necessary to remove the septum pellucidum from the undersurface of the corpus callosum of the hemisphere to observe the lateral ventricles to better advantage, and the outward bulge in their walls caused by the thalamus. The **septum pellucidum** consists of two thin sheets which extend from the concave

main middle part, the body or trunk. The anterior end, the **genu,** is folded downward and backward on itself. The posterior end, the **splenium,** is rounded and overlies the midbrain, extending backward as far as the highest point of the cerebellum. The splenium overlaps the tela choroida of the third ventricle and **pineal gland** (Fig. 14). The fibers of the corpus callosum mingle with the projection

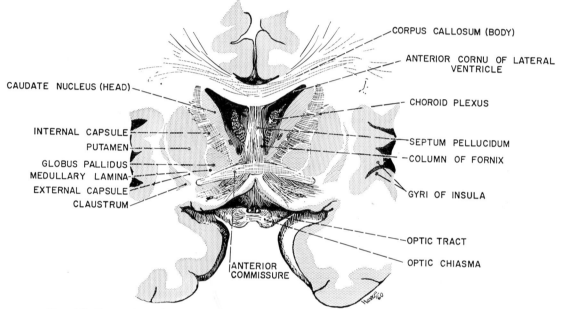

FIG. 15. Coronal section through the optic chiasma, anterior commissure, and body of the corpus callosum.

undersurface of the corpus callosum to the body of the fornix. The **fornix** is composed of two stout bands beneath the corpus callosum and over the thalamus which are made up of parts known as the crura, hippocampal commissures, body, and the columns (Figs. 14, 15, 16, and 18).

The largest central connection between the two cerebral hemispheres is the **corpus callosum** (Fig. 14). Its shape, size, and extent can be obtained from the frontal and horizontal sections (Figs. 15 to 18). The two ends of the corpus callosum are much thicker than the

fibers of the corona radiata. Those from the **genu** of the corpus callosum to the frontal lobe are the forceps anterior (minor), whereas those from the body form the **tapetum** and those from the splenium to the occipital lobe are the forceps posterior (major).

The two **thalami** consist of large, ovoid masses of gray matter along the side wall of, and extending caudad beyond, each third ventricle (Fig. 16). Note that the two anterior parts are close together, whereas the posterior extremities diverge with the pineal gland located between the two thalami (Fig. 18). The median, rounded posterior portion of the **thalamus** is known as the **pulvinar.** The gray substance of the thalamus is subdivided into anterior, medial, and lateral parts by a white layer, the **internal medullary lamina,** and just under the lateral surface is another white layer, the **external medullary lamina.** The nuclei are the medial, anterior medial, lateral, and posterior groups.

between the claustrum and the insula laterally and the caudate nucleus and the thalamus medially (Fig. 18). The lentiform nucleus is further subdivided into two parts by the **external medullary lamina:** the larger, more laterally placed **putamen** and the smaller, medially placed **globus pallidus.** The **internal medullary lamina** subdivides the globus pallidus into internal and external parts.

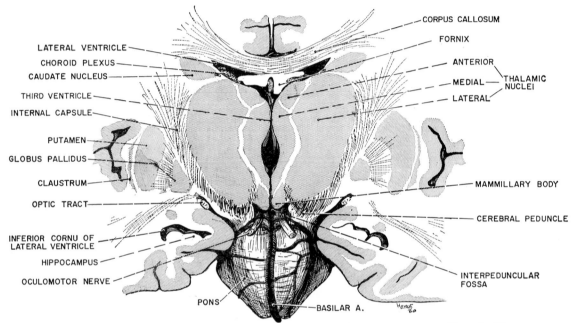

FIG. 16. Coronal section through the thalamus at the region of the mammillary bodies.

Deeply placed within the cerebral hemispheres are four masses of gray matter, the **basal ganglia.** These are known as the **caudate, lentiform,** and **amygdaloid nuclei** and the **claustrum** (Fig. 18). The caudate and lentiform nuclei together with fascicles of the internal capsule which separates them constitute the **corpus striatum.** The caudate nucleus, which is located adjacent to the lateral wall of the lateral ventricle, is arched and may be cut twice in a horizontal section (Fig. 18). This nucleus fuses anteriorly and inferiorly with the lentiform nucleus.

The **lentiform (lenticular)** nucleus is located

The claustrum is a thin plate of gray matter which is embedded in a thin layer of white matter. The **claustrum** separates the putamen from the insula laterally and is separated from the putamen by a layer of white fibers, the external capsule (Fig. 18).

The amygdaloid nucleus, at the pointed end of the caudate nucleus, is a small mass of gray matter.

The **internal capsule** separates the lentiform nucleus laterally from the caudate nucleus and from the thalamus medially (Fig. 18). It is roughly V-shaped. The angle at the bottom of the V is known as the genu; the frontal part

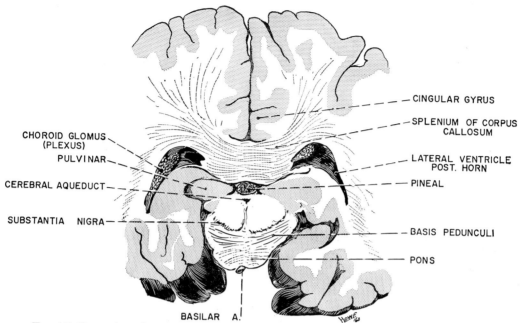

CINGULAR GYRUS

SPLENIUM OF CORPUS CALLOSUM

CHOROID GLOMUS (PLEXUS)

PULVINAR

LATERAL VENTRICLE POST. HORN

CEREBRAL AQUEDUCT

PINEAL

SUBSTANTIA NIGRA

BASIS PEDUNCULI

PONS

BASILAR A.

FIG. 17. Coronal section through the pons, pineal, and splenium of the corpus callosum.

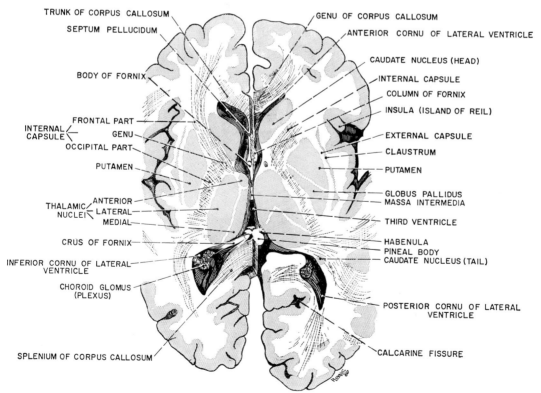

TRUNK OF CORPUS CALLOSUM

SEPTUM PELLUCIDUM

GENU OF CORPUS CALLOSUM

ANTERIOR CORNU OF LATERAL VENTRICLE

CAUDATE NUCLEUS (HEAD)

BODY OF FORNIX

INTERNAL CAPSULE

COLUMN OF FORNIX

INSULA (ISLAND OF REIL)

FRONTAL PART

INTERNAL CAPSULE

GENU

OCCIPITAL PART

EXTERNAL CAPSULE

CLAUSTRUM

PUTAMEN

PUTAMEN

THALAMIC NUCLEI

ANTERIOR

LATERAL

MEDIAL

GLOBUS PALLIDUS

MASSA INTERMEDIA

THIRD VENTRICLE

CRUS OF FORNIX

INFERIOR CORNU OF LATERAL VENTRICLE

HABENULA

PINEAL BODY

CAUDATE NUCLEUS (TAIL)

CHOROID GLOMUS (PLEXUS)

POSTERIOR CORNU OF LATERAL VENTRICLE

SPLENIUM OF CORPUS CALLOSUM

CALCARINE FISSURE

FIG. 18. Horizontal sections through the thalamus and corpus striatum. The section on the right was cut about ¼ in. deeper than the section on the left.

or anterior limb extends laterally and rostrally, whereas the occipital or posterior limb extends laterally and toward the occiput, between the lentiform nucleus and the thalamus.

Next remove the remains of the cerebral hemispheres from the brain stem and then note the structure of the **cerebellum** (Fig. 14). On its cut median surface, the gray matter stands out distinctly from the white matter. The central mass of white matter sends prolongations into the various lobes in the form of a branching tree. The name **arbor vitae** has been applied to the white matter. The other parts of the cerebellum to be noted are the paired **hemispheres** and the median unpaired portion, the **vermis.** The vermis extends around the cerebellum in an almost complete circle, forming the superior and inferior vermis. This division of the cerebellum into hemispheres and vermis is not morphologically correct, but it is of established usage. There are names applied to the various lobules and processes of the cerebellum.

For more detailed knowledge of the brain, the descriptive texts should be studied—not only to become familiar with those structures which are labeled but not described in this chapter but also to learn other important structures which are neither illustrated nor described here.

Cavernous Sinus

The **cavernous sinus** is a venous sinus which lies between the two layers of the dura at the side of the hypophyseal fossa. It receives blood from the **superior** and **inferior ophthalmic veins,** which enter it from the orbit by passing through the superior orbital fissure, and from the **sphenoparietal sinus,** which lies within the dura along the free margin of the lesser wing of the sphenoid bone. It drains posteriorly by means of the **superior** and **inferior petrosal sinuses.** The cavernous sinuses of the two sides are united by the anterior and posterior **inter-**

cavernous sinuses, which lie in the dura covering the hypophysis in front of and behind the infundibulum. In close relation to the lateral wall of the cavernous sinus are the trochlear and oculomotor nerves, the semilunar ganglion, and the ophthalmic and maxillary divisions of the trigeminal nerve. Projecting farther medially into the sinus are the abducens nerve and the internal carotid artery (Fig. 19).

Clean the **trigeminal nerve.** Shortly after it enters the dura, the root fibers of this nerve expand to form the **semilunar ganglion.** This large ganglion is covered by the inner layer of dura forming the lower lateral part of the wall of the cavernous sinus. From the ganglion, the **ophthalmic division** of the trigeminal passes forward in the lateral wall of the sinus to reach the superior orbital fissure. As is reaches the superior orbital fissure, the ophthalmic nerve divides into the lacrimal, frontal, and nasociliary nerves, but these probably cannot be identified until the orbit is opened. Below the ophthalmic, in the lower part of the lateral wall of the cavernous sinus, the **maxillary division** of the trigeminal runs forward to the **foramen rotundum.** The **mandibular division** passes directly downward from the posterior part of the ganglion to the **foramen ovale.**

The **oculomotor** and **trochlear nerves** pass forward in the upper part of the lateral wall of the cavernous sinus. The oculomotor is the highest of all the nerves, the trochlear lying between the oculomotor and the ophthalmic. Both of these nerves enter the orbit at the superior orbital fissure. The **abducens nerve** projects farther medially into the cavernous sinus; it runs forward medial to the ophthalmic nerve and lateral to the internal carotid artery to enter the orbit at the superior orbital fissure.

The **internal carotid artery** enters the cranial cavity at the internal opening of the carotid canal, which lies just above the foramen lacerum. Running forward between the two layers of the dura, the artery enters the wall of the cavernous sinus. Below the anterior clinoid process it turns upward, medially, and then backward to pierce the inner layer of the dura just below and behind the optic foramen. As it emerges from the dura, it gives rise to the **ophthalmic artery,** which passes forward into the orbit through the optic foramen, where it lies immediately below the optic nerve.

Observe that the **facial** and **statoacoustic** bral arteries join to form the **basilar artery** (Fig. 19). Separate the facial from the stato-acoustic nerve and attempt to identify the smaller, intervening **nervus intermedius.**

The transverse sinus has already been opened as far as the point in the peripheral attached margin of the tentorium cerebelli where it is joined by the superior petrosal sinus. Its terminal portion should now be

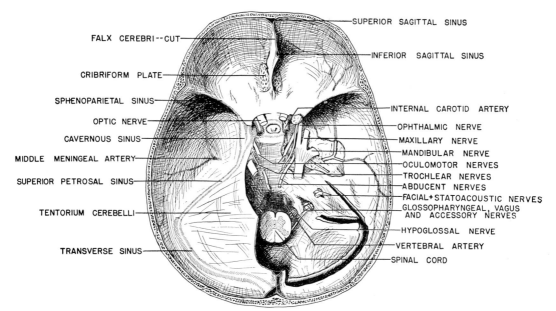

FIG. 19. The interior of the cranial cavity after removal of the brain. The tentorium cerebelli has been removed on the right side and the transverse, superior petrosal, and cavernous sinuses opened.

nerves leave the posterior cranial fossa by entering together the **internal auditory meatus** in the petrous part of the temporal bone. The **glossopharyngeal, vagus,** and **accessory nerves** enter the medial end of the **jugular foramen.** Medial to the jugular foramen, close to the anterolateral margin of the foramen magnum, is the **hypoglossal foramen,** by which the **hypoglossal nerve** leaves the cranial cavity. Observe that the **vertebral artery** enters the cranium on each side at the lateral margin of the **foramen magnum.** Passing forward and medially over the floor of the posterior fossa, the two verte-

opened. Observe that it pursues a curved course downward and medially, within the dura mater lining the posterior fossa, to the lateral part of the jugular foramen. The **transverse sinus** terminates in the **jugular foramen,** below which it is continuous with the internal jugular vein. The **inferior petrosal sinus** lies in the groove between the basal portion of the occipital bone and the petrous portion of the temporal. It runs from the lower posterior part of the cavernous sinus to the jugular foramen, where it joins the internal jugular vein.

Observe the distribution of the **middle**

meningeal artery. This vessel, a branch of the **maxillary artery,** enters the cranial cavity at the foramen spinosum and divides almost at once into anterior and posterior branches, which are distributed to the dura mater of the floors of the anterior and middle cranial fossae and of the cranial vault. These vessels are embedded in the outer layer of the dura but can usually be clearly seen through the dura without dissection. The dura of the posterior cranial fossa is supplied by one or two small **meningeal branches** of the **occipital artery,** which reach the dura by passing through the jugular foramen.

Orbit

The dissection of the orbit is approached by removing the **orbital plate** of the frontal bone. This is done by using a chisel to break through the orbital plate about 1 in. lateral to the crista galli. Then chip away the remaining part of the orbital plate—noting the position of the **frontal sinus** within this bone. Using the handle of a forceps, depress the periosteum and orbital contents downward in the front part of the orbital cavity. Then make two saw cuts down through the squamous portion of the frontal bone to the floor of the **anterior cranial fossa.** The first cut should be made opposite the end of the cribriform plate of the ethmoid, the second downward and medialward opposite the end of the lesser wing of the sphenoid. This cut section of the frontal bone should then be reflected forward. The lateral part of the cribriform plate of the ethmoid should be gently removed with the aid of a chisel or bone forceps to observe the **ethmoid air cells** and the course of the **anterior** and **posterior ethmoid vessels** and **nerves.** The lesser wing of the sphenoid may be chipped carefully away with bone forceps, so as to open completely the superior orbital fissure from above; it is advisable, however, to leave the bony rim of the optic foramen intact.

Carefully free and retract medialward the mucous membrane lining of the frontal and ethmoidal sinuses so that they can be studied later while dissecting the nasal cavity. Then remove the bone from the caudal wall of these sinuses to expose the orbit.

If the orbit has been carefully opened, the **periosteum** of its roof, which is very loosely attached to the bone, will remain intact. This periosteum should now be slit longitudinally and reflected to each side to expose the cavity of the orbit from above. The structures contained in the orbit are embedded in loose fatty tissue, which must be removed bit by bit as the dissection proceeds.

The structures which lie highest in the orbit and which should first be cleaned are three nerves, the **trochlear,** the **frontal,** and the **lacrimal,** all of which enter through the upper part of the superior orbital fissure. The trochlear nerve is the most medial; it passes forward and medially to end in the superior oblique muscle, which may be seen occupying the angle of junction of the roof and medial wall of the orbit (Fig. 20).

The **frontal nerve** is the largest of the three terminal branches of the **ophthalmic nerve.** It passes forward under the middle of the roof of the orbit, where it lies immediately above the levator palpebrae superioris muscle. About midway in its course through the orbit, the frontal nerve divides into a small **supratrochlear** and a larger **supraorbital branch.** The supratrochlear passes forward and medially to emerge onto the face at the superior margin of the orbit just above the trochlea for the superior oblique muscle. The supraorbital continues forward to turn upward onto the forehead at the **supraorbital notch or foramen;** it frequently divides into two or more branches before reaching the supraorbital notch.

The **lacrimal nerve** is the smallest of the three branches of the ophthalmic. It passes forward along the line of junction of the roof and the lateral wall of the orbit to end in minute twigs to the skin of the lateral part of the upper eyelid. It also gives a few small twigs to the lacrimal gland.

The **ophthalmic artery** enters the orbit at the optic foramen, where it lies below the optic nerve. Winding around the lateral side of the optic nerve and then crossing above it, it runs forward close to the medial wall of the orbit below the superior oblique muscle. It ends by dividing into two small branches, the **frontal** and the **dorsal nasal,** which emerge onto the face close to the infratrochlear nerve. In its course, the ophthalmic artery gives rise to

the upper eyelid behind the orbicularis oculi and in front of the palpebral conjunctiva.

Immediately below the levator palpebrae superioris is the **superior rectus muscle.** This is also a flat bandlike muscle, somewhat wider than the levator, which arises from the upper margin of the optic canal and is inserted into the sclera of the eyeball. The ocular muscles cannot all be exposed at present, but it is well to have a general idea of their arrangement and attachments before proceeding further with the dissection of the orbit. The **superior, medial, inferior,** and **lateral rectus muscles** are all flat bandlike muscles which arise at the apex of

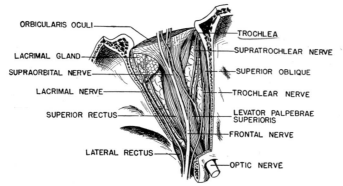

ORBICULARIS OCULI
LACRIMAL GLAND
SUPRAORBITAL NERVE
LACRIMAL NERVE
SUPERIOR RECTUS
LATERAL RECTUS

TROCHLEA
SUPRATROCHLEAR NERVE
SUPERIOR OBLIQUE
TROCHLEAR NERVE
LEVATOR PALPEBRAE SUPERIORIS
FRONTAL NERVE
OPTIC NERVE

FIG. 20. The left orbit, seen from above after removal of its roof.

lacrimal, supraorbital, posterior ethmoidal, and **anterior ethmoidal arteries,** which accompany the nerves of the same name. In addition to these branches, it supplies twigs to the ocular muscles and a group of small ciliary arteries which enter the eyeball.

The **lacrimal gland** is a small, oval, lobulated structure, which lies in the upper anterior lateral part of the orbit. Its secretion is poured into the upper part of the conjunctival sac through a number of minute ducts (Fig. 20).

Clean the **levator palpebrae superioris.** This narrow flat muscle arises at the upper margin of the optic canal and runs forward, just below the roof of the orbit, to be inserted into the superior tarsus. The **superior tarsus** is a thin but strong plate of fibrous tissue which lies in

the orbit from the **bony rim of** the **optic canal,** their origins thus encircling the optic nerve as it enters the orbit. Spreading forward through the orbit, they are all inserted into the **sclera** at points anterior to a plane which would divide the eyeball into anterior and posterior halves. The **superior oblique muscle,** which may now be cleaned, also arises from the margin of the optic canal, between the origins of the superior and medial recti. Its fibers pass forward to the **trochlea** at the upper medial angle of the orbital rim, and here the muscle turns downward, laterally, and posteriorly, passing under the superior rectus, to reach the sclera, where it is inserted on the lateral side posterior to the plane dividing the eyeball into anterior and posterior halves. The **inferior**

oblique muscle lies deeply in the anterior part of the orbit, where it will be seen in the final stages of the dissection.

Divide the frontal nerve a short distance in front of the optic canal and turn it forward. Divide the levator palpebrae superioris and the superior rectus at about the middle of the orbit and turn the anterior cut segments of the two muscles forward. Then turn the posterior cut segments backward. As this is done, the **superior division of** the **oculomotor nerve** will be found entering the deep surface of the superior rectus, which it supplies; a small branch of this nerve either pierces the superior rectus or winds around its medial border to supply the levator palpebrae superioris.

Reference to a macerated skull will show that the lateral rectus muscle, in passing from its origin to its insertion, must cross in front of the superior orbital fissure. The nerves already displayed near the roof of the orbit (i.e., the lacrimal, frontal, and trochlear) enter the upper part of the superior orbital fissure and pass above the lateral rectus. The nasociliary, oculomotor, and abducens nerves pass through the superior orbital fissure at a lower level and pierce the lateral rectus near its origin to enter the orbit more deeply.

The **nasociliary** is the third branch of the ophthalmic nerve. Passing forward and medially, it crosses above the optic nerve and ends near the upper anterior part of the medial wall of the orbit by dividing into **infratrochlear, anterior ethmoidal,** and **external nasal nerves.** Before its termination, it gives rise to the long root of the ciliary ganglion, the long ciliary nerves, and the posterior ethmoidal nerve. The **long root** of the **ciliary ganglion** is a small nerve which arises from the nasociliary far back in the orbit and passes forward along the lateral side of the optic nerve to reach the ciliary ganglion. The **long ciliary nerves** are three or four fine filaments which arise from the nasociliary as that nerve crosses above the

optic nerve and pass forward to pierce the posterior part of the sclera. The **posterior ethmoidal nerve** passes medially above the medial rectus and enters the posterior ethmoidal foramen to reach the mucosa of the ethmoidal air cells. The anterior ethmoidal is the largest branch of the nasociliary. It crosses above the medial rectus and enters the anterior ethmoidal foramen, eventually to reach the nasal cavity, where its distribution will be studied later. The **infratrochlear nerve** passes forward above the anterior part of the medial rectus and below the trochlea of the superior oblique to reach the skin of the face.

The **oculomotor nerve,** as it passes through the lateral rectus muscle, divides into a superior and an inferior division. The **superior division** turns upward, lateral to the optic nerve, to supply the superior rectus and the levator palpebrae superioris, as already observed. The **inferior division** runs forward for a short distance and then divides into three branches. Of these, one crosses below the optic nerve to supply the medial rectus; another sinks into the inferior rectus for the supply of that muscle; the third runs forward along the floor of the orbit to reach the inferior oblique muscle. From the branch to the inferior oblique, near its origin, arises the short root of the ciliary ganglion.

The **ciliary ganglion** is very small. It lies in the posterior part of the orbit at the lateral side of the optic nerve. It receives roots from the **nasociliary and** the **oculomotor nerves.** The branches which arise from it are the **short ciliary nerves.** These are numerous fine filaments which pass forward in close relation to the optic nerve to pierce the posterior part of the sclera (Fig. 21).

The **abducens nerve** enters the orbit deeply and passes forward directly into the lateral rectus muscle, which it supplies.

Separate the lids as widely as possible, or, if the contents of the orbit are dried, remove the lids and attempt to locate the insertions of the ocular muscles on the eyeball. By blunt dissection free the orbital contents from the lateral and inferior walls of the orbital cavity and reflect them medialward and upward. Identify the course of the **zygomatic nerve** in the lateral wall of the orbit. The **zygomaticotemporal** and **zygomaticofacial nerves** are branches of this nerve. Dissect the **inferior oblique muscle** from the front of the orbit. It arises from the maxilla at the anterior medial angle of the floor of the orbit and passes laterally and backward, below the inferior rectus, to be inserted into the

from sheep, pigs, or oxen. The dissection can be facilitated if the animal eyes are previously hardened in alcohol or formalin. Ideally, several eyes should be dissected: one in which the various coats can be stripped off the eyeball in succession, one bisected along the equator, and one bisected longitudinally on the long axis of the eyeball. But if a sufficient number of specimens cannot be obtained for this purpose, it is advisable to prepare an eyeball to be cut in half transversely at the equator of the eyeball, and then the anterior half should be bisected in the horizontal plane. This approach should

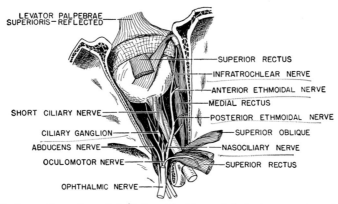

FIG. 21. Deep dissection of the left orbit. The ophthalmic artery is not shown.

lateral part of the sclera, posterior to a plane dividing the eyeball into anterior and posterior halves.

Eyeball

If the eyeballs of the cadaver are not dried, shrunken, and distorted, one of them should be removed from the orbit by cutting the muscles, vessels, and optic nerve, so that at least ½ in. of each of these structures is left attached to the eyeball. The connections of the ocular muscles to the eyeball and their relationship to the fascia bulbi should be noted and the muscles then reflected anteriorly towards the cornea. However, if the eyeballs of the cadaver are not suitable for study, then the following dissection should be done using eyes

show most of the structures to maximum advantage.

After observing the attachment of the ocular muscles to the eyeball and identifying the optic nerve, the ophthalmic vessels and nerves, the dissector should remove the conjunctiva, fascia bulbi, and the adnexa (muscles and vessels) from the eyeball. This can be accomplished by picking up with a forceps the conjunctiva and fascia bulbi close to the corneal margin and then making a cut through the fascia bulbi with a scissors and dividing this fascia from the underlying tissues around the corneal margin. These structures should then be dissected progressively backward toward the optic nerve. The **vorticose veins** will be found a little posterior to the equator of the eyeball, and a little further posteriorly, the **posterior ciliary arteries** and the **ciliary nerves** will be found piercing the sclera around the entrance of the optic nerve.

The dura mater, extending along the course of the optic nerve and surrounding it, should be cleaned and its attachment to the eyeball noted. If a fresh eye is being used, the central artery may be seen within the optic nerve, if that nerve is transected close to its entrance into the eyeball. Normally the eyeball occupies only the anterior half of the orbital cavity, the posterior half of the cavity being filled by the

paratus necessary for adjusting the focal length of the eye should be studied in one of the descriptive texts, and as many of these structures as possible should be seen in the subsequent dissection (Figs. 22 to 24).

Using a sharp scalpel, shave off thin slices of the sclera, which is greyish in color, from the region of the equator of the eyeball until the black choroid is exposed. Starting this dissection at a point ½ in. posterior to the attachment of either the medial or lateral rectus muscle to the eyeball, pass a blunt probe through the opening made in the sclera, and

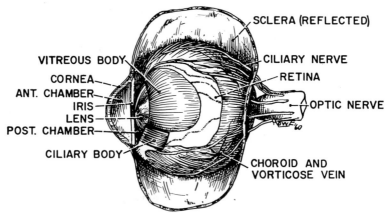

VITREOUS BODY
CORNEA
ANT. CHAMBER
IRIS
LENS
POST. CHAMBER
CILIARY BODY
SCLERA (REFLECTED)
CILIARY NERVE
RETINA
OPTIC NERVE
CHOROID AND VORTICOSE VEIN

Fig. 22. The coats and contents of the eyeball demonstrated by the reflection, or removal, of parts of the various coats. (*Modified from Wolff.*)

ocular muscles and the periorbital fat, which were removed from the eyeball.

The walls of the eyeball are made up of three concentric coats: (1) the outer coat consisting of the transparent **cornea** constitutes about one-sixth of the anterior outer coat, and the **sclera** makes up the posterior five-sixths; (2) the middle vascular coat is composed of the **choroid**, the **ciliary muscles** and the **ciliary process**, and the **iris**; (3) an inner **retinal coat** consists of an outer pigmented layer and an inner nervous layer. These three coats enclose three **transparent media: the aqueous humor,** the **lens,** and the **vitreous body.** The coats, the transparent media, and the ap-

gently detach the choroid from the undersurface of the sclera (Fig. 22). The point of a scissors can then be introduced into this opening and a cut made through all three layers around the circumference to bisect the eyeball. A second cut can then be made in the horizontal plane through the anterior half of the eyeball. This cut should be just above the central point of the cornea. The cephalic portion of the anterior half of the eyeball should then be elevated and the relation of the lens to the iris noted.

The contents of the eyeball should now be studied. The space behind the cornea is the **anterior chamber,** which is continuous through the **pupil** of the iris with the **posterior chamber.** The latter chamber is bordered by the pigmented **iris** anteriorly and the **lens** posteriorly. Both of these chambers contain **aqueous humor.** Behind the lens and within the confines of the retinal surface, note the **vitreous humor,** or vitreous body, within its transparent capsule, the **hyaloid membrane.**

Now study the coats of the eyeball, observing that the cornea is more convex than the sclera, and that it is thinner, particularly near the equator of the eyeball. These two layers

thelium of the anterior chamber. This chamber communicates with the **scleral sinus** through these spaces, and the sinus in turn communicates with the scleral veins. In the front of the ciliary body and in the peripheral part of the posterior chamber, a group of short, fingerlike folds, about 70, the **ciliary processes,** are present. These processes may extend to the outer border of the lens, and they are black, since the pigmented layer of the retina is attached to them.

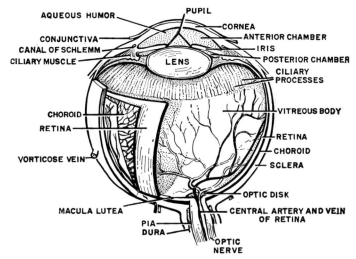

Fig. 23. Anatomy of the eyeball. (*By permission from Langley, Cheraskin, and Sleeper, "Dynamic Anatomy and Physiology," McGraw-Hill Book Company, Inc., Blakiston Division, New York, 1958.*)

the equator of the eyeball. These two layers of the outer coat become continuous at the **corneoscleral junction.** The **ciliary body,** which is continuous in front with the iris and behind with the choroid, is a whitish zone about 6 mm broad. Identify the **ciliary muscle,** which is firmly attached to the sclera at the corneoscleral junction. Note also the **iridocorneal angle,** the acute angle between the cornea and the iris. This angle is crossed by strands of connective tissue, the **pectinate ligament,** passing from the back of the corneal elastic membrane to the iris and sclera. The spaces, enclosed by this connective tissue, are lined with the meso-

The **lens** is surrounded by a **capsule,** and fibers extend from this capsule, the **suspensory ligament** of the lens, to the ciliary process. Between the two layers around the lens is the **zonular space.**

Locate the optic nerve and observe that it pierces the sclera as a bundle, about 3 mm to the nasal side of the posterior pole of the eyeball. At this point the sclera is thin. The optic nerve fibers next pierce the choroid and the outer layer of the retina, which is adherent to the choroid. These nerve fibers form a circle, the **optic disc** or papilla, which is the **blind spot.** The nerves then spread out as the inner layer of the retina. The central artery and vein each pass through the disc as two vessels which subdivide and supply the inner surface of the retina. About 3 mm lateral to the optic disc, note a yellowish, oval area, the **macula lutea,** in the center of which is a depression, the **fovea centralis.** This area is in the

it is reduced to two layers of cubical cells. The outer one of these layers is pigmented. The two layers do cover the ciliary body and iris to the margin of the pupil. Note that the curvature of the cornea is the chief focusing mechanism, while the lens is for finer adjustments. With advancing age, the lens hardens,

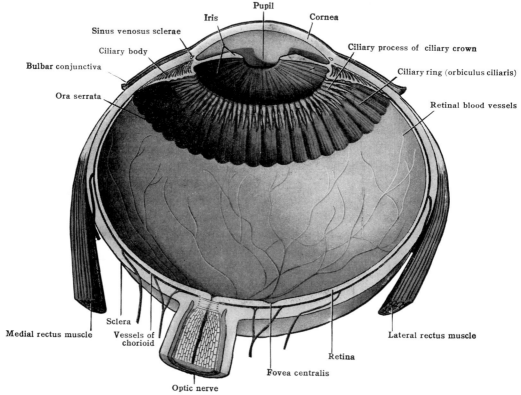

Fig. 24. Horizontal hemisection of the right eyeball viewed from above and behind. (*By permission from Schaeffer (ed.), "Morris' Human Anatomy,"* 11/e, *McGraw-Hill Book Company, Inc., Blakiston Division, New York, 1953.*)

direct axis of vision, and it is one of the most sensitive parts of the retina. Detach the choroid from the inner surface of the sclera and note the perichoroidal space.

A short distance behind the ciliary muscle the retina is thin and in the form of a wavy line, the **ora serrata.** Behind the ora serrata the true optic retina is found. In the front part, however, where light cannot strike the retina,

beginning at the center, and then accommodation for vision becomes increasingly difficult. If an animal's eye is used, the lens may be soft; however, when hardened, the lens may be split into concentric layers—similar to those of an onion. If an animal's eye has been used for this study, the **tapetum,** a part of the choroid layer posteriorly, will be seen as an area with a metallic sheen.

Prevertebral Region

With the cadaver lying on its back, make on each side of the skull a vertical cut with a saw, starting on the external surface about a ¼ in. posterior to the **mastoid process** and passing forward and medially, just posterior to the **jugular foramen.** Cut through the **dura** and **ligaments,** connecting the atlas to the occipital bone by a transverse incision through the

As the anterior part of the cranium, the pharynx, larger nerves, and vessels are retracted forward and downward, try to leave the **cervical sympathetic chain** and **ganglia** on the surface of the deep muscles attached to the cervical vertebrae. Clean the fascia from the posterior part of the pharynx. Remove the posterior part of the **jugular foramen** and **hypoglossal canal** with a chisel or bone forceps.

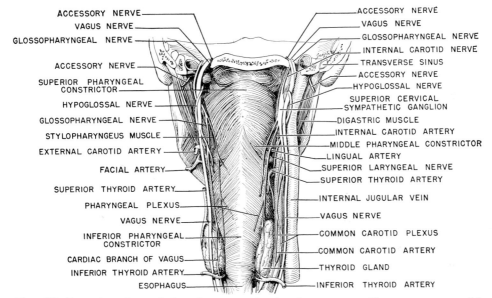

FIG. 25. Posterior view of the pharynx and related structures. The common carotid artery, most of the internal carotid artery, and the internal jugular vein have been removed from the left side. (*Modified from Sobatta-McMurrich.*)

foramen magnum. Insert a chisel through the foramen magnum between the **occipital condyle** and the **superior articular process of** the **atlas** on each side, or chisel through the occipital condyles if necessary. Pry and retract the anterior part of the cranium forward, cutting those cephalad parts of the sternomastoid, trapezius, or splenius muscles which may hinder protraction. Identify the insertions of the **longus capitis** and **rectus capitis anterior muscles** on the base of the skull and cut these muscles near their insertions to facilitate the dissection.

The course of the **glossopharyngeal, vagus, accessory,** and **hypoglossal nerves** can now be studied in their relationships to the pharynx and large vessels of the neck (Fig. 25).

Study the **cervical portion** of the **sympathetic trunk.** The trunk lies behind the carotid sheath in the fascia covering the anterior surfaces of the prevertebral muscles. It begins in front of the second cervical vertebra and descends to the neck of the first rib, in front of which it passes, to become continuous with the thoracic portion of the trunk. The cervical portion exhibits three ganglionic enlargements in its course. The largest of these is the **superior ganglion,** which lies in front of the second and third vertebrae and represents the highest part of the trunk. The **middle ganglion** is small, sometimes lacking, and lies in front of the sixth vertebra. The **inferior ganglion** lies just below the seventh vertebra; it is frequently fused with the first thoracic ganglion to form a large ganglionic mass in front of the neck of the first rib, which is known as the **stellate ganglion.** Note the nerve fibers connecting the middle and inferior cervical ganglia and those fibers which loop around the subclavian artery, the **ansa subclavia** (Fig. 27). From each of the cervical sympatheic ganglia there arises a **cardiac branch,** which descends into the thorax to join the cardiac plexus. In addition to these, communicating branches pass laterally to join the cervical nerves. The superior ganglion usually communicates with the first four cervical nerves, the middle ganglion with the fifth and sixth, and the inferior ganglion with the seventh and eighth. Above the superior ganglion, the trunk is continued as the internal carotid nerve, which accompanies the internal carotid artery into the carotid canal.

Review the positions of the jugular foramen, the hypoglossal foramen, and the external orifice of the carotid canal. In the **jugular foramen,** the internal jugular vein begins, and through it the **glossopharyngeal, vagus, and accessory nerves** leave the cranial cavity. The **hypoglossal nerve** leaves the cranial cavity at the **hypoglossal foramen.** As these structures descend in the neck, they all pass deep to the posterior belly of the digastric muscle. In order to expose their upper portions, the digastric should be elevated as far as possible from its attachment to the internal aspect of the mastoid process, and the course of the occipital artery reviewed.

Note the stylohyoid muscle and its origin on the styloid process. Observe that the **stylopharyngeus** and **styloglossus muscles** (Fig. 11)

as they run downward to reach the pharynx and the tongue, respectively, cross between the internal and the external carotid arteries, lying lateral to the internal and medial to the external carotid. Then clean and study the glossopharyngeal, vagus, accessory, and hypoglossal nerves as they emerge at the base of the skull (Fig. 26).

Observe that the glossopharyngeal, vagus, and accessory emerge from the medial end of the jugular foramen, lying medial and slightly anterior to the beginning of the internal jugular vein. The **glossopharyngeal nerve** descends vertically for a short distance and then turns forward to cross the lateral aspect of the internal carotid artery and wind laterally around the stylopharyngeus muscle. In the upper part of its course, the glossopharyngeal gives **branches to** the wall of the **pharynx.** As it winds around the **stylopharyngeus,** it gives a twig of supply to that muscle and continues forward to the posterior part of the tongue.

The vagus and accessory nerves are bound in fibrous sheaths in the jugular foramen. The **vagus** descends almost vertically, lying in the carotid sheath, where the greater part of its cervical course has already been exposed. Just below the jugular foramen it receives a communicating branch from the accessory. Slightly lower it exhibits an ovoid swelling, the **inferior ganglion (nodosum).** Just below the ganglion, the vagus gives off its **pharyngeal branch,** which runs forward, lateral to the internal carotid artery, to reach the wall of the pharynx, where it joins with the pharyngeal branches of the glossopharyngeal nerve to form the **pharyngeal plexus.** Somewhat below the origin of the pharyngeal branch, the vagus gives rise to a larger branch, the **superior laryngeal nerve.** This nerve runs downward and forward, passing deep to the internal carotid artery, and divides into the **internal** and **external laryngeal nerves,** which have already been exposed in the dissection of the carotid triangle.

The **accessory nerve,** below its communication with the vagus, bends laterally to cross either in front of or behind the internal jugular vein, and turns posteriorly and downward to pass deep to the posterior belly of the digastric and the occipital artery and reach the deep surface of the sternomastoid, from which point its further course has been studied.

The **hypoglossal nerve,** as it emerges from the hypoglossal foramen, lies medial to the arteries: the hypoglossal is lateral to both, the glossopharyngeal and pharyngeal branch of the vagus lie between the two, whereas the superior laryngeal branch of the vagus is medial to both (Fig. 26).

Attempt to display the three small arteries which supply the upper part of the wall of the **pharynx.** These are the **ascending pharyngeal,** the **ascending palatine,** and the **tonsillar arteries;** all three of these vessels are not usu-

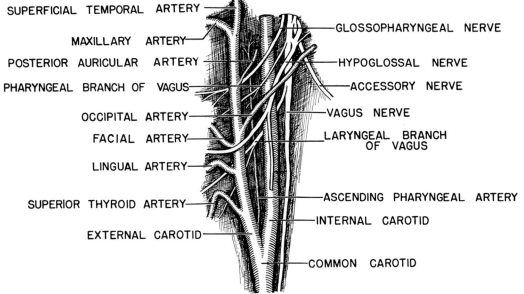

FIG. 26. Semidiagrammatic lateral view of the carotid arteries and the nerves associated with them on the left side of the neck.

vagus and accessory nerves. As it descends, it takes a spiral course around the vagus, passing first behind and then lateral to that nerve.

The **internal carotid artery** begins at about the level of the upper border of the thyroid cartilage as one of the terminal branches of the common carotid and ascends in front of the upper three cervical vertebrae to the base of the skull, where it enters the carotid canal. It has no branches in the neck. The internal carotid is in a medial relation to the pharyngeal wall. The nerves have the following relationships to the external and internal carotid

ally present in a single individual, however, the one which is lacking being replaced by branches from the other two. The ascending pharyngeal is usually the first branch of the **external carotid.** Arising from the medial aspect of that vessel, it ascends deeply on the wall of the pharynx, where it lies medial to the internal carotid artery. The ascending palatine and the tonsillar arteries are two small branches of the **facial artery,** which arise from that vessel as it lies deep to the digastric muscle. They ascend on the upper lateral part of the pharyngeal wall, the ascending palatine lying slightly posterior to the tonsillar. The ascending palatine passes deep to the styloglossus, whereas the tonsillar artery crosses it superficially (Fig. 11).

Review the attachments of the **scalenus anterior.** Then clean and study the **scalenus medius** and **scalenus posterior.** All three of these muscles originate from the transverse

continuous and cannot be entirely separated from one another.

Running upward from the upper border of the lateral part of the atlas to the basilar portion of the occipital bone are two small flat muscles, the **rectus capitis anterior** and the **rectus capitis lateralis.** The anterior primary division of the first cervical nerve emerges be-

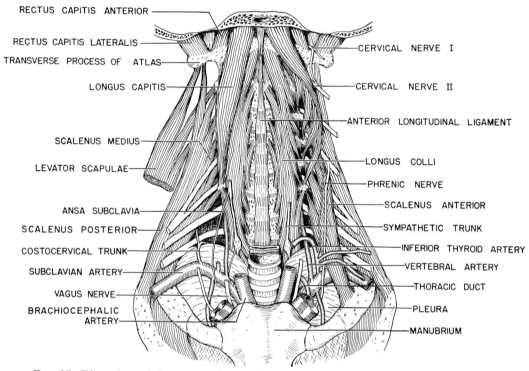

RECTUS CAPITIS ANTERIOR
RECTUS CAPITIS LATERALIS
TRANSVERSE PROCESS OF ATLAS
LONGUS CAPITIS
SCALENUS MEDIUS
LEVATOR SCAPULAE
ANSA SUBCLAVIA
SCALENUS POSTERIOR
COSTOCERVICAL TRUNK
SUBCLAVIAN ARTERY
VAGUS NERVE
BRACHIOCEPHALIC ARTERY

CERVICAL NERVE I
CERVICAL NERVE II
ANTERIOR LONGITUDINAL LIGAMENT
LONGUS COLLI
PHRENIC NERVE
SCALENUS ANTERIOR
SYMPATHETIC TRUNK
INFERIOR THYROID ARTERY
VERTEBRAL ARTERY
THORACIC DUCT
PLEURA
MANUBRIUM

Fig. 27. Dissection of the prevertebral region. The left longus capitis muscle has been everted laterally to display its slips of origin.

processes of the **cervical vertebrae.** The scalenus anterior and medius insert on the **first rib.** The scalenus posterior inserts on the **second rib.** The **longus capitis** arises from the anterior tubercles of the third through the sixth **cervical vertebrae** and has its insertion on the basilar part of the **occipital bone** (Fig. 27).

The **longus colli** is a complex muscle, which is usually regarded for convenience of description as consisting of three parts. It should be noted, however, that the three parts are

tween these two muscles to turn downward in front of the transverse process of the atlas.

The anterior aspects of the transverse processes of the successive cervical vertebrae are connected by a series of small **anterior intertransverse muscles.** No particular study of these muscles need be made, but they should be cut away to expose the course of the vertebral portion of the vertebral artery. The **vertebral artery** has already been seen to arise as a branch of the **subclavian** and to run upward in front of the transverse process of the seventh cervical vertebra to enter the costotransverse foramen of the sixth cervical vertebra. It continues its course vertically upward, passing through the **costotransverse foramina** of the upper six vertebrae. It then turns posteriorly and medially in the groove on the upper surface of the posterior arch of the atlas and enters the cranial cavity at the **foramen magnum.** It is surrounded by a plexus of small veins, which unite inferiorly to form the **vertebral vein.** In its upward passage through the neck, the vertebral gives rise to a series of small spinal branches which enter the vertebral canal at the intervertebral foramina.

Observe that the cervical nerves, as they emerge from the intervertebral foramina, pass behind the vertebral artery.

Fascial Spaces of Head and Neck

The fascial spaces of the head and neck have been described differently by various investigators. In some descriptions, every fascial envelope which encloses a muscle with its associated nerve and blood vessels is described as a fascial space. The intervals between the fascial-enclosed muscles or between the muscles and bones are also potential spaces which have been named in some instances. Of the many fascial spaces which may limit or aid in the spread of infections in the head and neck, a few of these spaces are usually involved in disease processes, and, in the strict sense of the term, only those spaces filled by loose connective tissue should be described as fascial spaces.

The concentric arrangement of the connective tissue around the structures in the neck forms three definite fascial areas. One beneath the skin, the superficial fascia which contains the platysma in the front and sides of the neck, may be instrumental in the spread of superficial infections from the face to the neck. The superficial muscles of the neck region, the

sternomastoid and the trapezius, are enclosed in a collar of deep fascia which splits into a pocketlike area just above the sternum, the **suprasternal space.** Deep to this layer, the underlying structures can be considered as being enclosed in two definite rings: one, around the cervical vertebrae and their associated muscles, the **prevertebral fascia;** and the other ring, more anteriorly located around the lower part of the pharynx, larynx, trachea, thyroid gland, and esophagus, the **visceral layer.** Since the cervical vertebrae and the cervical viscera can move independently of each other, there is a fascial space between the prevertebral and visceral layers, the **retropharyngeal space,** through which infections could travel from the region of the nasal or oral pharynx into the posterior mediastinum. This space can be studied by replacing the facial portion of the head on the cervical vertebrae and inserting fingers or an instrument into this space and tracing it downward into the posterior mediastinum. Potential spaces also exist around the esophagus, **paraesophageal,** and around the trachea, **paratracheal,** which also extend down into the posterior mediastinum.

Of the spaces around the facial portion of the skull, one of the more superficial ones is the **buccal space.** This space corresponds to the loose connective tissue which surrounds the buccal fat pad in the vicinity of the buccinator and masseter muscles. This space also extends backward to the pterygomandibular space and upward into the pretemporal space. The **pretemporal space,** along the superficial surface of the temporal muscle, extends beneath the zygomatic arch. It is limited superficially by the attachment of the temporal fascia to the zygomatic arch and superiorly by the attachment of this fascia to the outer surface of the temporal bone. Infections may extend from the mandible along this fascial space to the anterior part of the temporal region.

The parotid gland and the masseter muscle are enclosed in a fascial envelope, the **parotideomasseteric fascial space.** This space is important in limiting the spread of infections particularly from the parotid gland.

The fascia enclosing the masseter muscle, mandible, and the pterygoid muscles has been described differently, depending on which structures are to be enclosed in parts of this fascia. The **masseteric space** has been described as enclosing all three groups of structures listed above. Another subdivision of this fascial complex has been described as the **pterygomandibular space.** The latter space has as its lateral wall the inner surface of the mandible; its medial wall is formed by the medial pterygoid muscle; and its roof is the lateral pterygoid muscle. Within this space, the lingual nerve is located in front, and the inferior alveolar nerve more posteriorly. The inferior alveolar artery and veins are also found in this space.

After verifying the preceding fascial spaces, pass a probe through the lateral wall of the pharynx in the vicinity of the tonsils and note that as the pharyngeal constrictor is perforated, the tip of the probe enters a potential space, lateral to the constrictors, through which course the carotid artery, internal jugular vein, vagus nerve, and also the hypoglossal, glossopharyngeal, and spinal accessory nerves (Fig. 25). This space is the **parapharyngeal space.** Some investigators subdivide this space into a prestyloid and a retrostyloid area, using the styloid process as the anatomical dividing line.

The **submandibular space** is the potential space above the mylohyoid muscle inferiorly, the mucous membrane on the inferior lateral side of the tongue superiorly, and the geniohyoid and genioglossus muscles medially. An infection in the anterior part of this space, in front of the second molars will usually be confined to the floor of the mouth, but with spread of infections behind the last molars,

the infection will spread to the connective tissues of the neck.

The suprahyoid and infrahyoid muscles and the contents of the carotid sheath are sometimes described as each being in separate fascial spaces. These spaces, however, are seldom involved in the downward spread of infections from the region of the neck into the mediastinum.

An additional fascial layer, the **alar fascia,** is sometimes described between the prevertebral fascia posteriorly and the visceral fascia anteriorly. This alar fascia would subdivide the retropharyngeal space into two compartments.

Mouth

The interior of the mouth may be studied to better advantage in a living person than in the cadaver. The cavity of the mouth is partially divided into two parts, the vestibule and the mouth cavity proper. The **vestibule** is the narrow, cleftlike space which is bounded by the cheeks and lips externally and the teeth and gums internally. The **mouth cavity** proper is bounded anteriorly and laterally by the teeth and gums; posteriorly, it is continuous with the oral portion of the cavity of the pharynx. Both the vestibule and the mouth proper are lined with a layer of **mucous membrane,** which is interrupted only at the points where the teeth emerge from the gums. Anteriorly, this mucous membrane becomes continuous at the lips with the skin of the face. Posteriorly, it is continuous with the mucous membrane lining the pharynx. The **parotid duct** opens into the vestibule at the middle of the cheek.

The arched roof of the mouth is formed by the **hard** and **soft palates.** The actual boundary between the mouth and the pharynx is formed by the **glossopalatine arches,** which may be seen, if the mouth is opened wide and the tongue depressed, extending upward on each side from the side of the tongue to the undersurface of the soft palate. Farther posteriorly, in the side wall of the pharynx, the **pharyngopalatine arches** may be seen. The space enclosed between the glossopalatine and the pharyngopalatine arches is known as the **isthmus of** the **fauces** and is often spoken of as the passage of communication between the tongue to the floor of the mouth; this is the **frenulum linguae.** At each side of the base of the frenulum, the **opening** of the **submaxillary duct** may be seen at the summit of a small papilla. Extending posterolaterally along the floor of the mouth from the submaxillary opening is a low ridge, the **plica sublingualis,** caused

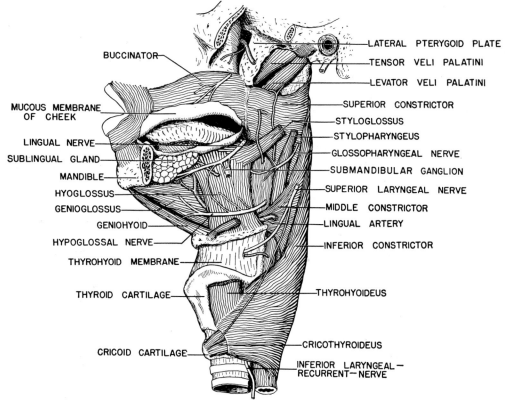

FIG. 28. Dissection to display the muscles of the pharyngeal wall, seen from the left side.

mouth and the pharynx, although it is itself actually a part of the pharynx. The **palatine tonsil** is lodged within the side wall of the isthmus.

Projecting from the floor of the mouth is the **tongue,** which is also covered by the **oral mucous membrane.** Observe a vertical fold of the mucous membrane running from the undersurface of the anterior free portion of the by the presence immediately below the mucous membrane of the sublingual gland. At the summit of the plica, the minute **orifices of** the **sublingual ducts** may sometimes be recognized.

Pharynx

The wall of the pharynx is composed of four layers. These are, from without inward, the **buccopharyngeal fascia,** the **muscular layer,** the

pharyngeal aponeurosis, and the **mucous membrane.** The buccopharyngeal fascia and with it the plexus of veins which it contains are to be removed in cleaning the muscles. The principal muscles comprising the muscular layer of the pharyngeal wall are the **superior, middle,** and **inferior pharyngeal constrictors.** The muscular layer is not entirely complete and, in regions where it is lacking, the pharyngeal aponeurosis is particularly dense. The constrictors arise anterolaterally and spread posteromedially around the wall of the pharynx to be inserted into a fibrous **median raphe** which represents a thickening of the pharyngeal aponeurosis along the posterior wall of the pharynx in the median line. Posteriorly, as they spread to their insertions, the constrictors overlap one another from below upward. It is therefore advisable to clean the inferior constrictor first.

The **inferior pharyngeal constrictor** is covered at its origin by the upper part of the sternothyroid muscle. It arises from the **thyroid cartilage** just behind the oblique line, from a **fibrous arch** bridging over the cricothyroid muscle between the thyroid and cricoid cartilages, and from the lateral surface of the **cricoid.** As it approaches its insertion in the **median raphe,** it spreads far superiorly, the upper fibers overlapping externally the insertion of the middle constrictor.

The **middle constrictor** arises from the upper border of the **greater cornu** and from the posterior border of the **lesser cornu** of the **hyoid bone;** it is overlapped at its origin by the hyoglossus. Its fibers radiate toward their insertion on the **median raphe,** this insertion being almost entirely under cover of the inferior constrictor.

The **superior constrictor** arises from the lower part of the posterior border of the **medial pterygoid plate,** from the **pterygomandibular raphe,** and from the highest part of the **mylohyoid line** on the inner surface of the mandible. The **pterygomandibular raphe** is a fibrous band running from the pterygoid hamulus to the inner surface of the mandible and serving to separate the fibers of the buccinator from those of the superior constrictor. The uppermost fibers of the superior constrictor reach as high as the **pharyngeal tubercle** of the occipital bone for their insertion; the remainder are inserted into the median raphe under cover of the insertion of the middle constrictor.

The **stylopharyngeus** has already been seen to arise from the **styloid** process. It reaches the wall of the pharynx at the upper border of the middle constrictor. Passing downward deep to that muscle, most of its fibers blend with the **constrictors,** although a few descend to gain an independent insertion on the **thyroid cartilage.**

Open the pharynx by a transverse incision in its posterior wall just below the base of the skull and a longitudinal incision along the line of the median raphe, and study the interior of the pharynx (Fig. 29).

Observe that the **wall of** the **pharynx** is complete laterally and posteriorly but that anteriorly it is very incomplete, since the pharynx communicates freely anteriorly with the nasal cavities, the mouth, and the larynx. The cavity of the pharynx is lined by a **mucous membrane** which is continuous anteriorly with the mucous membranes lining the nasal cavities, the mouth, and the larynx. The cavity of the pharynx is divisible from above downward into three parts. These are the nasal pharynx, the oral pharynx, and the laryngeal pharynx.

The **nasal portion of** the **pharynx** lies below the body of the sphenoid and the basal portion of the occipital bone and behind the nasal cavities, with which it communicates at the **choanae.** At the upper anterior part of the lateral wall of the nasopharynx on each side may be seen the opening of the **auditory tube.** This opening is bounded above and behind by a prominent ridge, the **torus tubarius.** A flexible probe introduced into this opening will pass laterally and backward into the **cavity of** the **middle ear.** Descending on the side wall of the pharynx from the torus tubarius is a slight fold of mucous membrane, which gradually disappears inferiorly; this is the **salpingopharyngeal fold.** Just behind the torus tubarius is a pocketlike depression in the lateral wall, the **pharyngeal recess.** In the posterior wall of the nasopharynx, between the two pharyngeal recesses, is a collection of lymphoid tissue known as the **pharyngeal tonsil.**

diffuse, aggregation of lymphoid tissue at the base of the tongue.

The **laryngeal portion of** the **pharynx** is a direct inferior continuation of the oral portion. In the upper part of its anterior wall is the **epiglottis;** below the epiglottis is the **superior aperture of** the **larynx;** below this aperture the anterior wall of the pharynx is formed by the mucous membrane in relation to the posterior aspect of the cricoid cartilage. The pharynx

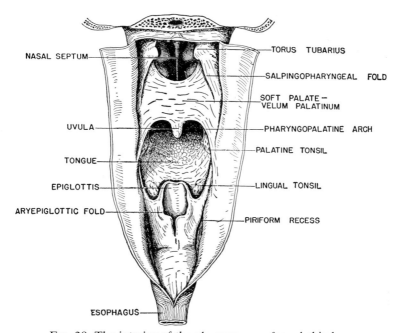

NASAL SEPTUM
TORUS TUBARIUS
SALPINGOPHARYNGEAL FOLD
SOFT PALATE – VELUM PALATINUM
UVULA
PHARYNGOPALATINE ARCH
PALATINE TONSIL
TONGUE
EPIGLOTTIS
LINGUAL TONSIL
ARYEPIGLOTTIC FOLD
PIRIFORM RECESS
ESOPHAGUS

FIG. 29. The interior of the pharynx, seen from behind.

The **soft palate** projects backward and downward into the pharynx, separating the nasal from the oral portion. Below the soft palate, the glossopalatine arches separate the mouth from the oral portion of the pharynx. Inferiorly, the posterior surface of the base of the **tongue** forms the anterior boundary of the oral pharynx. The pharyngopalatine arches appear as prominent folds on the lateral wall of the oral pharynx. Between the glossopalatine and pharyngopalatine folds on each side is an aggregation of lymphoid tissue, the **palatine tonsil.** The **lingual tonsil** is a similar, but more

ends inferiorly at the level of the lower border of the cricoid cartilage, where it becomes continuous with the esophagus. The **laryngeal aperture** (aditus laryngis) is bounded by the **aryepiglottic folds.** These are folds of the mucous membrane passing upward and forward from the arytenoid cartilages (which may be felt but not seen through the mucous membrane) to the lateral borders of the epiglottis. Lateral to the lower part of the aryepiglottic fold on each side is a deep pocket in the pharyngeal wall, the **recessus piriformis.**

Attention should next be directed to the **soft**

palate (velum palatinum). The soft palate is covered on both its superior and inferior surfaces by a layer of mucous membrane. Anteriorly, it is attached to the posterior border of the hard palate; posteriorly, it presents a free margin at the center of which is a conical projection, the **uvula;** laterally, on each side the soft palate joins the lateral wall of the pharynx. The main bulk of the substance of the soft palate consists of muscle fibers, most of which are inserted into the **palatal aponeurosis** —a sheet of fibrous tissue which extends posteriorly into the soft palate from the bony

muscle is lodged in the **pharyngopalatine fold.** It arises on each side from the posterior border of the **thyroid cartilage** and from the **pharyngeal aponeurosis** in close relation to the inner surface of the inferior constrictor. Running upward into the soft palate, its fibers are inserted into the **palatal aponeurosis** in two strata, the superior of which crosses above the levator and the inferior (and more anterior) below it.

The origin of the **levator veli palatini** is from the petrous part of the **temporal bone.** Sweeping downward and medially into the soft palate, most of its fibers are inserted into the **palatal**

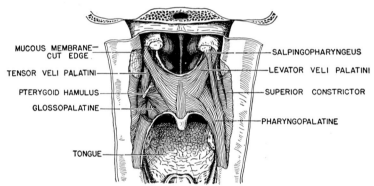

MUCOUS MEMBRANE— CUT EDGE

TENSOR VELI PALATINI—

PTERYGOID HAMULUS—

GLOSSOPALATINE—

TONGUE—

—SALPINGOPHARYNGEUS

—LEVATOR VELI PALATINI

—SUPERIOR CONSTRICTOR

—PHARYNGOPALATINE

FIG. 30. Dissection to display the muscles of the soft palate. The upper part of the pharyngopalatine muscle has been removed on the left side.

margin of the hard palate. In order to expose the muscles of the soft palate, it is necessary to remove carefully the mucous membrane from the superior surface of the soft palate and from the lateral wall of the nasal and oral portions of the pharynx.

The principal muscles of the soft palate are the tensor veli palatini and the levator veli palatini, which raise the palate, and the glossopalatine and pharyngopalatine muscles, which depress it. Nearest to the superior surface of the palate are the pharyngopalatine and the levator. These two muscles should therefore be cleaned first (Fig. 30) but they may be studied more easily after the facial part of the skull has been bisected.

The **pharyngopalatine (palatopharyngeus)**

aponeurosis near the median line; a few of them are continuous across the median line with fibers of the corresponding muscle of the opposite side.

The origin and upper portion of the **tensor veli palatini** is from the scaphoid fossa of the **sphenoid bone** and the inferior surface of the **auditory tube.** To expose its insertion, the palatal portions of the levator and the pharyngopalatine must be removed. Passing downward from its origin, the belly of the muscle lies just lateral to the medial pterygoid plate. At the hamulus it becomes tendinous; the tendon turns medially under the **hamulus** to enter the soft palate and spread out to be inserted directly into the **palatal aponeurosis** and the posterior border of the hard palate.

The **glossopalatine (palatoglossus) muscle** arises from the side of the posterior part of the **tongue.** Its fibers ascend, in the glossopalatine fold, to reach the undersurface of the **palatal aponeurosis,** into which they are inserted. It is the most inferior of the various muscular strata of the soft palate.

Nasal Cavities

The facial portion of the skull is to be divided into two parts. Cut through the soft palate with a scalpel in a sagittal plane slightly to the left of the median line. Starting at the left nostril, divide the fleshy and cartilaginous portions of the left side of the nose in the same plane. Then complete the division by a saw cut in the same plane through the roof of the left nasal cavity, the hard palate, and mental symphysis. Then using a scalpel bisect the tongue in the midsaggital plane.

Study the **nasal septum.** This is a bony and cartilaginous plate covered on each side by a layer of **mucous membrane.** It usually deviates somewhat to one side, most frequently to the right. The mucous membrane of the septum, and of the nasal cavities in general, is thick and spongy, containing numerous small mucous glands. Its upper third is designated as the **olfactory area,** since it contains the minute filaments of the olfactory nerves, which enter the nasal cavity through the small openings in the cribriform plate of the ethmoid bone. The olfactory mucosa is thinner and less rich in glands than is the mucosa of the lower two-thirds, or **respiratory area,** of the septum.

Strip the mucous membrane from the left side of the septum and observe the bony and cartilaginous framework of the latter. The bony portion of the septum is formed principally by the **vomer** and the **perpendicular plate of** the **ethmoid.** Anteriorly, the septum is completed by the **septal cartilage.** Anterosuperiorly, the septal cartilage joins the suture between the two **nasal bones.** Posterosuperiorly, it joins the

anterior border of the perpendicular plate of the ethmoid and, posteroinferiorly, the anterior border of the vomer.

With forceps, carefully remove, a bit at a time, the bony portion of the septum to expose the deep surface of the mucous membrane of the septum and the vessels and nerves which appear between the mucosa and the bone. In addition to the **olfactory nerve,** the septal mucosa receives nerves of general sensibility, which are derived from the **ophthalmic** and **maxillary nerves.** The anterior third of the septum is supplied by the medial nasal branch of the **anterior ethmoidal nerve,** which may be found descending on the deep surface of the anterior part of the septal mucosa, where it is accompanied by a small branch of the **anterior ethmoidal artery.** The posterior two-thirds of the septum is supplied by the **nasopalatine nerve.** This nerve is described as a branch of the pterygopalatine ganglion but is principally composed of afferent nerve fibers derived from the maxillary nerve. It reaches the upper posterior part of the septum by crossing the posterior portion of the roof of the nasal cavity and runs downward and forward between the mucosa and the bone of the septum to reach the **incisive canal,** through which it passes to terminate in the mucosa of the anterior portion of the hard palate. It is accompanied by a branch of the **sphenopalatine artery.**

Cut away the septal mucosa to expose the lateral wall of the nasal cavity. The lateral wall, like the septal wall, is covered by a thick, spongy mucous membrane, which shows the same subdivision into **olfactory** and **respiratory areas.** By means of the **superior, middle,** and **inferior nasal conchae,** which project from the lateral wall, the nasal cavity is partially subdivided into several regions. The portion of the cavity lying in front of the conchae and communicating with the exterior at the nostril is known as the **atrium.** The portion of the cavity lying below the superior concha and above the middle concha is the **superior meatus.** The **middle meatus** lies below the middle concha, and the **inferior meatus** below the inferior concha. The small portion of the cavity which lies above and behind the superior concha is known as the **sphenoethmoidal recess.** The uninterrupted medial portion of the nasal cavity, with which the atrium, the three meatuses, and the sphenoethmoidal recess are all in free communication, is known as the **common meatus.** Posteriorly, at the **choana,** the nasal cavity opens freely into the nasal portion of the pharynx.

When the conchae have been examined in position, they should be turned upward or broken away from the lateral wall with forceps to expose the various openings in the lateral wall which lie under cover of the conchae. In the lateral wall of the superior meatus will be seen one or more openings by which the more **posterior ethmoidal air cells** communicate with the nasal cavity. Through these openings, the nasal mucosa is continuous with the mucous membrane of the ethmoidal cells. The middle meatus is a considerably wider space than is the superior meatus. The portion of the middle meatus lying just below the anterior end of the middle concha leads upward into a closed passage known as the **infundibulum,** by which the **frontal sinus** communicates with the nasal cavity. Behind the infundibulum is a bulging prominence in the lateral wall known as the **ethmoidal bulla,** upon which the orifice connecting with the **middle ethmoidal air cells** will be seen. Running downward and backward from the infundibulum, below the ethmoidal bulla, is a curved groove, the **hiatus semilunaris.** In the hiatus will be seen the openings of the **anterior ethmoidal air cells** and the **maxillary sinus.** In the wall of the inferior meatus is the opening of the **nasolacrimal duct,** by which the tears are conveyed from the **conjunctival sac** into the nasal cavity. In the wall of the **sphenoethmoidal recess** is the orifice by which

the **sphenoidal sinus** communicates with the nasal cavity.

Observe that the sphenopalatine foramen, by which the nasal fossa communicates with the pterygopalatine fossa in a macerated skull, is not visible so long as the nasal mucosa is in place. The mucous membrane should now be stripped away carefully from the lateral wall of the nasal cavity to expose the **sphenopalatine foramen** and the vessels and nerves which pass through it.

The nerves which enter the nasal cavity at the sphenopalatine foramen are the nasopalatine nerve and the posterior superior nasal nerves. All are branches of the pterygopalatine ganglion. The **nasopalatine nerve,** as already observed, crosses the roof of the nasal cavity to reach the septum. The **posterior superior nasal nerves** are small twigs, usually very difficult to demonstrate, which are distributed to the posterior part of the lateral wall of the nasal cavity. The **sphenopalatine artery,** a branch of the third part of the maxillary artery, also enters the nasal cavity at the sphenopalatine foramen. Its branches accompany the nerves in their distribution to both the lateral wall and the septum.

The anterior part of the lateral wall of the nasal cavity is supplied by the **lateral nasal branch of** the **anterior ethmoidal nerve.** This nerve has already been seen to arise in the orbit as one of the terminal branches of the **nasociliary nerve.** Leaving the orbit by way of the anterior ethmoidal foramen, it enters the cranial cavity. Here, lying external to the dura, it crosses the cribriform plate of the ethmoid and enters the nasal cavity through a foramen at the side of the crista galli. Descending in a groove on the inner surface of the nasal bone, it divides into medial nasal, lateral nasal, and external nasal nerves. The **medial nasal branch** is distributed to the anterior part of the nasal septum, as already noted. The **lateral nasal** supplies the anterior part of the lateral wall of the nasal cavity. The **external nasal** emerges between the nasal bone and the nasal cartilage to reach the skin of the nose. The anterior ethmoidal nerve is accompanied in its distribution by the anterior ethmoidal branch of the ophthalmic artery.

Maxillary Nerve and Pterygopalatine Fossa

The sphenopalatine (pterygopalatine) ganglion may be located in either of two ways: first, by stripping the mucous membrane from the posterior lateral part of the hard palate and locating the palatine nerves and vessels. These can be traced craniad, by removing with a chisel or bone forceps the perpendicular part of the palatine bone, to the area of the pterygopalatine ganglion. In the other method, the approach is from the top downward and is accomplished by the following dissection. The superior orbital fissure may be opened more widely by the removal, with a saw, of a wedge-shaped piece of bone which will include the great wing of the sphenoid and the anterior part of the squamous part of the temporal bone. The apex of the wedge should reach the superior orbital fissure just above and in front of the foramen rotundum; attempt to preserve intact the bony rim of the **foramen rotundum.** Then remove the periosteum of the orbit and any structures which may still remain within it and trace out the course and distribution of the maxillary nerve.

Arising from the **semilunar ganglion,** the **maxillary nerve** passes forward in the lower part of the lateral wall of the cavernous sinus to the foramen rotundum. Here it leaves the cranial cavity and enters the upper part of the **pterygopalatine fossa.** Passing forward through the highest part of the pterygopalatine fossa, it bends laterally through the **pterygomaxillary fissure** to enter the infratemporal fossa, which it leaves almost at once by entering the posterior end of the **infraorbital canal.** From this point on, it is known as the **infraorbital nerve.**

The roof of the infraorbital canal should be removed with a chisel. Passing straight forward through the canal, which lies in the portion of the maxilla forming the floor of the orbit and the roof of the maxillary sinus, the infraorbital nerve emerges at the **infraorbital foramen** and breaks up, under cover of the quadratus labii superioris, into a number of cutaneous branches whose distribution has already been seen in the dissection of the face.

In the pterygopalatine fossa, the maxillary nerve gives rise to two short, thick **sphenopalatine branches** which descend to join the **pterygopalatine ganglion.**

In the short portion of its course which lies in the infratemporal fossa, the maxillary nerve gives rise to two branches, the zygomatic nerve and the posterior superior alveolar nerve. The **zygomatic nerve** passes upward through the inferior orbital fissure to reach the lateral wall of the orbit, external to the periosteum. Here it divides into **zygomaticofacial** and **zygomaticotemporal branches,** both of which enter canals in the zygomatic bone, through which they reach the face, where their distribution has already been seen. The **posterior superior alveolar nerve** usually divides into two branches, both of which descend on the infratemporal surface of the maxilla, where they enter small canals in the bone through which they are conveyed, in the lateral wall of the maxillary sinus to the roots of the upper molar teeth.

In its passage through the infraorbital canal, the infraorbital nerve gives rise to **anterior** and **middle superior alveolar nerves,** which pass through canals in the bony wall of the maxillary sinus to be distributed to the upper incisor, canine, and premolar teeth. The **superior alveolar nerves** also supply the mucous membrane of the upper gums.

The **pterygopalatine fossa** should now be studied. In addition to the maxillary nerve, which crosses its highest part, the pterygopalatine fossa contains the pterygopalatine ganglion and the terminal part of the maxillary artery.

The **pterygopalatine ganglion** lies below the **maxillary nerve** and lateral to the sphenopalatine foramen. It receives from the maxillary nerve the two **pterygopalatine nerves,** which are described as the sensory roots of the ganglion. Posteriorly, it receives the **nerve of** the **pterygoid canal,** described as its motor root. This nerve enters the fossa at the anterior end of the pterygoid canal. The principal branches which arise from the ganglion may be grouped as medial and descending branches.

The medial branches pass through the sphenopalatine foramen to enter the nasal cavity. They include the **posterior superior nasal nerves** and the **nasopalatine nerve,** whose distribution has already been seen in the dissection of the nasal cavity. The descending branches are the **palatine nerves.** These, of which there are usually three, descend in the pterygopalatine canal to reach the palate. The mucous membrane should be carefully stripped away from the hard palate to expose the distribution of these nerves. The largest of the palatine nerves is the **great or anterior palatine nerve.** Emerging at the greater palatine foramen, this nerve is distributed to the mucous membrane and glands of the hard palate. The **middle** and **posterior palatine nerves** are much smaller. Emerging at the lesser palatine foramina, they turn posteriorly into the soft palate.

The **third part of** the **maxillary** is very short. As it enters the pterygopalatine fossa, the vessel breaks up almost immediately into its four terminal branches. The **posterior superior alveolar artery** may arise from the second part of the maxillary. It accompanies the posterior superior alveolar nerve in its distribution. The **sphenopalatine artery** enters the nasal cavity at the sphenopalatine foramen and divides into branches whose distribution has already been observed. The **infraorbital artery** enters the infraorbital canal in company with the infraorbital nerve and gives rise to small branches

corresponding to the branches of that nerve. The **descending palatine artery** descends in the pterygopalatine canal where it gives rise to two small palatine arteries, beyond which point it is known as the great palatine artery. The latter accompanies the anterior palatine nerve into the hard palate; the small palatine arteries are distributed to the soft palate with the middle and posterior palatine nerves.

With bone forceps, attempt to open the pterygoid canal to expose the nerve which traverses it. The **nerve of** the **pterygoid canal** is formed at the posterior end of that canal (which is at the anterior wall of the foramen lacerum) by the junction of the **great superficial petrosal** and the **great deep petrosal nerves.** The former is a branch (nervus intermedius) of the facial nerve, which conveys preganglionic parasympathetic nerve fibers to the pterygopalatine ganglion. The great deep petrosal nerve is composed of postganglionic sympathetic fibers derived from the sympathetic trunk through the internal carotid plexus. It should be noted that the branches of the **pterygopalatine ganglion** consist very largely of **sensory fibers** derived from the **maxillary nerve** through its pterygopalatine branches, but that they also contain the **sympathetic postganglionics of** the **great deep petrosal nerve** and **parasympathetic postganglionics** derived from the **ganglion** itself.

Submandibular Region

Review the boundaries and contents of the digastric triangle and the attachments of the mylohyoid muscle. Cut the mucous membrane at the lateral inferior sides of the tongue and separate the tongue and adjacent structures from the mylohyoid muscle by retracting the tongue medially. By this means, the sublingual gland, the deep portion and duct of the submandibular gland, the terminal parts of the lingual and hypoglossal nerves, the submandibular ganglion, and the extrinsic muscles of the tongue will be exposed.

Clean the **sublingual gland.** This is a lobulated structure which is flattened from side to side. The superior surface is in relation to the mucous membrane on the floor of the mouth. The sublingual gland does not possess a single duct but a series of small, short ducts, which pass upward from its superior surface to open into the floor of the mouth. Observe that the **duct of** the **submandibular gland** runs forward and upward across the muscles of the tongue, passing deep to the lingual nerve and the sublingual gland, to open into the floor of the mouth near the anterior end of the sublingual gland.

The **lingual nerve** has already been traced from its origin to the point where it lies between the internal surface of the mandible and the mucous lining of the mouth in the region of the last molar. It should now be followed downward and forward across the muscles of the tongue to the deep surface of the sublingual gland, where it breaks up into its terminal branches. These branches are distributed to the mucous membrane of the tongue. The lingual is the **sensory nerve** of the anterior two-thirds of the tongue. It mediates impulses both of general sensibility and of the special sense of taste for this area. The former are carried through the **lingual branch** of the **mandibular;** the latter, through the **chorda tympani.**

Identify the **submandibular ganglion.** It is connected to the **lingual nerve** by two short communicating branches. It contains the cell bodies of **postganglionic neurons** of the **parasympathetic system. Preganglionic nerve fibers** reach it from the lingual nerve; these are derived from the **chorda tympani.** Of the postganglionic fibers which leave the ganglion, some pass directly into the submandibular gland for its supply, while others pass back into the lingual nerve to be distributed to the sublingual gland.

The **hypoglossal nerve** passes forward across the hyoglossus, where it gives branches to that muscle and to the styloglossus. Here it gives a branch to the geniohyoid and breaks up into terminal branches, which enter the substance of the tongue to supply the genioglossus and the intrinsic musculature of the tongue. It is usually connected, near the anterior border of the hyoglossus, by a connecting loop with the lingual nerve. The hypoglossal is the **motor nerve of** the **tongue,** supplying all of the extrinsic and intrinsic muscles of that organ.

The extrinsic muscles of the tongue should now be cleaned. They all have bony origins external to the tongue and are inserted into the fleshy mass of the tongue, where their fibers mingle with one another and with the fibers of the intrinsic muscles. The geniohyoid is not actually a muscle of the tongue but may best be considered with this group.

The **hyoglossus** is a thin quadrilateral sheet of muscle which arises from the lateral part of the **body** and the upper border of the **greater cornu of** the **hyoid bone.** Its fibers pass vertically upward into the **tongue** and interlace with the **intrinsic muscle fibers and** with the **styloglossus** (Fig. 11).

The **geniohyoid** is a flat, triangular muscle, which arises from the **mental spine** (genioid tubercle) on the internal aspect of the mandibular symphysis and is inserted on the upper border of the **body of** the **hyoid bone.** Immediately above it is the genioglossus, which also takes origin at the mental spine. From this origin, its fibers radiate upward and posteriorly into the **tongue,** the lower ones passing deep to the hyoglossus; a few of its lowest fibers are inserted on the hyoid bone.

The **styloglossus** is a slender muscle which arises from the tip of the **styloid process** and runs downward and forward to reach the side of the **tongue,** where its fibers interlace with those of the hyoglossus.

The **stylohyoid** muscle has already been cleaned. Observe now that it arises from the base of the **styloid process** and winds downward, forward, and laterally, to cross the external carotid artery externally. Arising from the styloid process between the origins of the stylohyoid and the styloglossus is a third slender muscle, whose upper portion should now be cleaned. This is the **stylopharyngeus;** it passes downward, forward, and medially to enter the wall of the **pharynx.** Running downward and forward across the external surface of the stylopharyngeus, the terminal part of the **glossopharyngeal nerve** may now be seen. This is the ninth cranial nerve, which provides the **sensory innervation of** the **posterior third of** the **tongue.** Near the posterior border of the hyoglossus it breaks up into terminal branches, which supply the mucous membrane of the posterior third of the tongue, mediating impulses both of general sensibility and of taste for this area.

The origin of the **lingual artery** as a branch of the external carotid has already been seen. The **first part** of the lingual artery extends from the external carotid to the posterior border of the hyoglossus. The **second part** extends transversely forward deep to the hyoglossus a short distance above the hyoid bone. Elevate the hyoglossus muscle to expose this portion of the vessel. Near the anterior border of the hyoglossus the **lingual artery** terminates by dividing into the sublingual and deep lingual arteries. From the second part of the lingual arise two or three **dorsal lingual branches** which ascend into the substance of the posterior part of the tongue. The **sublingual artery** runs forward and upward across the genioglossus to supply the sublingual gland and neighboring structures. The **deep lingual** runs upward on the genioglossus and bends forward into the free portion of the tongue, where it reaches as far as the tip.

Oral Cavity

The following material is presented for those students who require a more detailed knowl-

edge of the oral cavity than that given in the preceding pages (66 and 67).

Either use a mirror to study your own oral region or study that of one of your fellow students or the cadaver specimen to locate the **nasolabial groove** which separates the cheek from the upper lip on each side. This groove extends downward and laterally from the wing of the nose to a variable distance from the corners of the mouth. The **labiomental groove** should also be observed. This groove extends transversely, separating the chin from the lower lip (Fig. 31).

In addition to the facial muscles described previously, the upper and lower lips (**labia**) are composed of skin and subcutaneous tissue on the outer surface and **labial glands** covered by mucous membrane on the inside. The glands are of variable size, and the larger ones can be felt through the mucous membrane by moving the tip of the tongue against the inner surface of the lips, where they form an almost continuous layer in both the upper and lower lips.

Open the mouth and note that as the lips are separated the corners where the lips are connected, the **labial commissures,** are very thin, and they may be damaged by forcibly stretching the lips apart. The red zone of the lips is due to the thinness of the epithelium in this region; in the upper lip the red zone protrudes downward in the midline, the **tuberculum;** and a shallow depression in the skin of the upper lip, the **philtrum,** extends from just above the tuberculum to the nose.

With the mouth open, observe the boundaries of the **oral cavity.** The lips and the cheeks form the anterior and lateral boundaries, the palate forms the roof, and the tongue with the mucous membrane covering the subjacent muscles, forms the floor of this cavity. Its anterior opening is the **oral fissure,** the space between the two lips, and the posterior opening is the **oropharyngeal isthmus,** or the isthmus of the fauces, described previously.

The oral cavity is divided into the **oral vestibule,** the space between the teeth and alveolar processes centrally and the lips and cheeks peripherally, and the oral cavity proper, which contains the tongue and the subjacent

ward and note the fold of the mucous membrane in the midline, the **frenulum,** which extends from the gingiva to the lips. The frenulum is usually better developed in the upper than in the lower lip (Fig. 31).

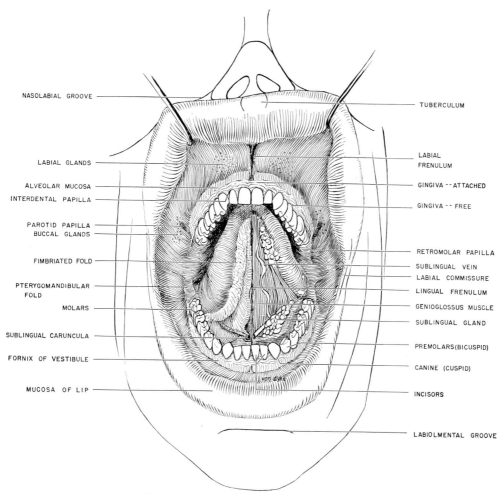

NASOLABIAL GROOVE

LABIAL GLANDS

ALVEOLAR MUCOSA
INTERDENTAL PAPILLA

PAROTID PAPILLA
BUCCAL GLANDS

FIMBRIATED FOLD

PTERYGOMANDIBULAR
FOLD

MOLARS

SUBLINGUAL CARUNCULA

FORNIX OF VESTIBULE

MUCOSA OF LIP

TUBERCULUM

LABIAL
FRENULUM

GINGIVA -- ATTACHED

GINGIVA -- FREE

RETROMOLAR PAPILLA
SUBLINGUAL VEIN
LABIAL COMMISSURE
LINGUAL FRENULUM
GENIOGLOSSUS MUSCLE
SUBLINGUAL GLAND

PREMOLARS (BICUSPID)

CANINE (CUSPID)

INCISORS

LABIOLMENTAL GROOVE

J. von dyke

FIG. 31. Diagram of the oral region. As drawn, the lips are retracted abnormally away from the jaws and the mandible is depressed beyond the usual range of movement, in order to illustrate the anatomical structures of this region. The tongue is elevated and the mucous membrane removed from one-half of its caudal surface.

sublingual groove around the front and the sides of the tongue. These structures can be studied by retracting the cheek laterally and by depressing the mandible and moving the tongue to one side. Also retract the lips out-

Next study the mucous membrane covering the inner surface of the cheek. This membrane lines the inner part of the buccinator muscle. Where this membrane is reflected onto the alveolar process, the point of reflection is referred to as the **fornix of the vestibule** or the **mucobuccal fold.** A tendinous slip, the **pterygomandibular raphe,** which extends between the pterygoid hamulus cephalad and the retromolar triangle caudad, produces a fold, the **pterygomandibular fold,** in the mucous membrane. **Buccal glands** are present in the submucous tissue of the cheek, and in the molar region they may be so numerous as to form a solid-appearing glandular body. Isolated sebaceous glands, which may become enlarged with age and visible (as yellowish bodies) through the mucous membrane, are found in the buccal mucosa just lateral to and behind the corners of the mouth.

Locate the **parotid papilla,** an elevation in the mucous membrane opposite the second upper molar, where the parotid duct opens into the oral vestibule. Using the bisected facial portion of the cadaver head, pass a flexible probe through the parotid papilla and note the course of the parotid duct. Then carefully strip the mucous membrane away from the inner side of the cheek and lips to see the buccal and labial glands and the muscles which form the peripheral borders of the oral cavity. While doing this, it will be noted that the mucous membrane covering the inner surface of the lips and cheeks is tightly attached to the labial and buccal muscles; whereas that part of the mucous membrane in the fornix of the vestibule is loosely attached to the submucous tissue to allow the lips and cheeks to be moved away from the jaws and teeth. Posteriorly, however, the mucous membrane is more firmly attached in the region of the molars.

Attention should now be directed to that part of the mucous membrane covering the jaws and the base of the teeth. If the cadaver specimen is edentulous or has only a few teeth remaining, the study of the **alveolar mucosa** and the **gingiva** (gums) should be made in a living subject. The **alveolar mucosa** is characterized by its thin texture, its dark-red color,

and its mobility. The **gingiva** is harder, very slightly movable, lighter in color, and is also stippled with prominent sulci, giving it an orange-peel appearance. The **marginal portion** of the gingiva is comparable to a collar extending around the cervical region of the tooth. This tapers to a sharp edge—the gingival margin or **free margin,** which is separated from the tooth surface by a shallow crevice. A shallow line or depression, the **gingival groove,** separates the marginal gingiva from the stippled, **attached gingiva.** Another line, the mucogingival junction, separates the attached gingiva from the alveolar mucosa. Also note that the mucous membrane may extend up between the teeth as **interdental papilla.** If some teeth are present in the cadaver, these various subdivisions of the mucous membrane should be determined by probing around the teeth and stripping the mucous membrane away from the teeth and jaws. As the mucous membrane is being stripped away, note that the **alveolar tubercle,** covered by gingiva, forms a round, large prominence on the posterior end of each upper alveolar process.

Also observe that behind the last molars, the gingiva may be elevated, forming the **retromolar papilla.** The **retroalveolar notch** is a groove varying in depth and extending from the junction of the maxilla and palatine bones to the lower end of the pterygoid process. The **retromolar pad** may also be apparent where the retromolar papilla of the lower jaw and the buccal glands (retromolar glands) are adjacent to one another and form an almost continuous pad.

Review the structure of the hard palate (bony part), the movable soft palate (muscular part), and the mucous membrane which covers them (Fig. 32). The posterior lateral part of this membrane was removed in tracing the course of the descending palatine nerves and vessels, but enough of it should be present to determine that the peripheral part of **this** mucous membrane is continuous with that of the vestibular gingiva. The **incisive** or **palatine papilla** should be noted immediately behind the upper central incisors, where this papilla covers the opening of the nasopalatine canal. Extending posteriorly from this papilla is a low ridge, the **palatine raphe,** running almost the entire length of the hard palate. Transverse **palatine folds** or **plicae** extend laterally across the anterior part of the hard palate. These folds are

amined, since they limit greatly the movement of the tissue covering the hard palate. The muscles of the soft palate have been studied in a previous part of the dissection.

Returning to the mucous membrane on the lateral side of oral cavity, reexamine the **pterygomandibular fold,** which covers the pterygomandibular raphe.

The mucous membrane on the lingual surface of the alveolar process is subdivided into

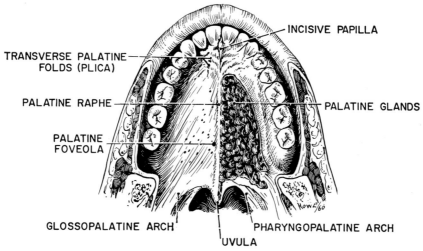

FIG. 32. Main anatomical landmarks on the caudal surface of the palate. The palatine glands on the left side have been exposed by the removal of the mucous membrane from this area.

much larger in certain animals where they play a role in mastication. Strip away the palatine mucous membrane and note that the submucosa contains fat, over the anterior part of the hard palate, and **palatine glands** mainly in the posterior part. These glands empty into the **palatine foveola,** which may be bilateral, or present only on one side of the midline (Fig. 32). In the molar region the connective tissue embedding the palatine vessels and nerves is usually thicker than in other areas of the palate. The connective tissue strands which extend from the periosteum of the hard palate to the mucous membrane should also be ex-

mandibular and alveolar mucosa. The submucosa (near the sublingual sulcus) is loose to allow for greater motility of the tongue. Elevate the tongue and observe the sickle-shaped fold of mucous membrane on the underside of the tongue, the **lingual frenum** or **frenulum** (Fig. 31), which extends from the mandibular process to the undersurface of the tongue. This frenum varies in length in different individuals. On each side of the lingual frenum the **sublingual glands** produce a prominence, the **sublingual eminence.** Fimbriated folds are extended from the end of the frenulum laterally and posteriorly. Large tortuous veins, the sublingual (ranine), are apparent on each side of the ventral surface of the tongue. Other veins accompany branches of the lingual artery.

Note the **sublingual fold** which contains the duct of the submandibular gland. This fold ends in a small papilla near the lingual frenulum, the **sublingual caruncula,** at which the submandibular duct and the larger duct of the sublingual gland open (Fig. 31). There are fifteen or more smaller ducts from the sublingual gland which open along the crest of the

the base, faces backward toward the pharynx. On the palatine surface of the tongue the V-shaped **terminal sulcus** separates the body from the base and marks fairly well the areas of the tongue supplied by the lingual nerve anteriorly and the glossopharyngeal nerve posteriorly. Where the two limbs of the terminal sulcus come together, a small depression, the **foramen cecum,** is located. This depression marks the point of embryological origin of the thyroid gland.

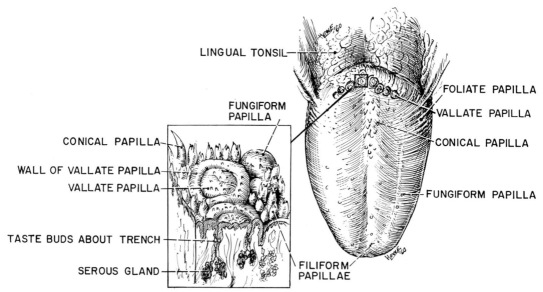

FIG. 33. (Right) Dorsal view of the tongue showing the types and locations of the papillae and (left) an enlarged view of the papillae. (*Modified from Braus.*)

sublingual plica. Strip the mucous membrane from the undersurface of the tongue to identify the sublingual gland, to locate the duct of the submandibular gland, and to observe the relationship of this duct to the lingual nerve. If possible pass a small probe or bristle into the duct of the submandibular gland and note the course of this duct in relationship to the mylohyoid muscle.

Next study the surface of the **tongue,** observing that the anterior two-thirds, the **body** and **tip,** have their oral surface turned up toward the hard palate, where the posterior one-third,

Just as the ridges on the palate are instrumental in mastication in some animals, the roughened tongue also serves a similar purpose, but in man this rough mucosa is merely in the form of several types of papillae. The larger **vallate (circumvallate) papillae,** 8 to 12 in number, are located just in front of the terminal sulcus, and they decrease in size from the midline laterally. These papillae have circular furrows around elevated prominences, with serous glands emptying into the deepest part of the furrows. In front of the vallate papillae, numerous hairlike **conical** and **fili-**

form papillae give the rest of the palatine surface of the tongue a velvety, grayish-pink color in the living individual. Between the filiform papillae are isolated, irregularly distributed **fungiform papillae.** They too are small mushroomlike elevations on the sides of which are located taste buds. The remains of food, mucus, etc., should be washed from, or gently scraped off, the lingual mucosa to identify these various types of papillae (Fig. 33).

Posterior to the terminal sulcus, the pharyngeal surface of the tongue is irregularly folded due to the presence of prominent accumulations of lymphatic tissue, the **lingual follicles.** The **lingual tonsil** is the term applied to the aggregate of the lingual follicles. The **lingual crypt,** a narrow depression, can be seen in the center of most of the follicles, where the ducts of small mixed glands, the **posterior lingual glands,** open. The muscles of the tongue and the relationship of the tongue to the epiglottis, which have been studied in a previous dissection, should be reviewed. The course and relationship of the lingual artery (p. 76) should also be reviewed.

Since the minute anatomy of the teeth forms a specialized part of dental training, it will have to suffice here merely to name the teeth. In the adult body, there are four incisors located in the anterior medial part of the maxilla and in the mandible. Lateral to these, on each side are strong, pointed teeth, the canines, and more lateral and posterior to the canines are two premolars on each side in each jaw and three molars (Fig. 31). The various anatomical subdivisions of the teeth and the structures which make up these subdivisions should be obtained from a complete text of dental anatomy.

With the loss of the teeth, the alveolar bone is resorbed, and the contours of the jaws become more rounded. If the central incisors are also missing, palpate the inner surface of the mandible for the **genial tubercles,** which may appear prominent under these conditions.

Review the relationships of the temporal and pterygoid muscles to that part of the mandible where a hypodermic needle would be inserted to inject an anesthetic around the inferior alveolar nerve.

If any of the maxillary molar teeth are present, study the relationship of their roots to the maxillary sinus and the distribution of the superior alveolar nerves to these teeth.

Internal Ear and Facial Nerve

Identify the **facial** and **statoacoustic nerves** entering the **internal auditory meatus.** Using a chisel, chip away the upper wall of this meatus and continue chipping away the bone carefully, following the course of the facial nerve laterally. Remove the **tegmen tympani** and expose the cavity of the middle ear. Note the location of the **geniculate ganglion** on the facial nerve. Examine the anterolateral surface of the temporal bone and identify the **greater** and **lesser superficial petrosal nerves.** Then turn the facial nerve upward and laterally and identify the **nervus intermedius** on its lower surface. Dissect the bone away from the statoacoustic nerve and note its division into the cochlear and vestibular nerves.

Follow the **cochlear nerve** forward and chip away part of the bone to identify the location of the **cochlea.** Similarly, carefully chip away the bone to identify the **vestibular nerve** and one or more of the **semicircular canals.**

Identify the **malleus, incus,** and **tympanic membrane** through the opening made in the tegmen tympani. Insert the handle of a probe into the external auditory meatus and, while gently pushing the probe inward, note the movement of the tympanic membrane.

Chip away the posterior part of the **mastoid** process and follow the course of the facial nerve inferiorly. Note the course of the chorda tympani in relation to the tympanic membrane, malleus, and incus. The **chorda tympani** is a continuation of the nervus intermedius. Attempt to locate the **stapes** and the **tensor tympani** muscle.

Middle Ear

The cavity of the middle ear should be exposed to permit study of its walls and the structures which are related to this cavity. To make this exposure, use a saw to cut caudad through the temporal bone. The plane of the cut should be made on a line extending from

The cavity of the middle ear or **tympanic cavity** is very irregular in shape, and it is compressed from the sides, resulting in the vertical being 2 to 3 times the transverse dimension. Using the tympanic membrane as a landmark, this cavity is divided into the **tympanic cavity proper** adjacent to the membrane and the **attic** or **epitympanic recess** above the level of the membrane. The tegmen tympani, the roof of this cavity, was removed in the preceding dissection.

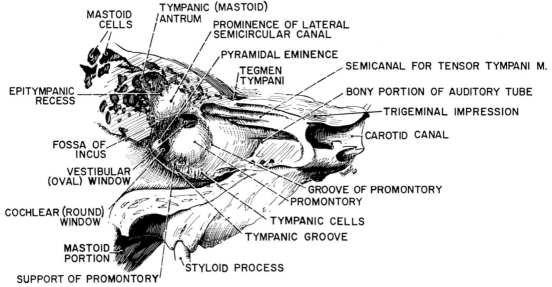

FIG. 34. Right temporal bone dissected to show the medial wall of the middle ear and the bony structures related to this area.

just lateral to the semicircular canals posteriorly to a point just lateral to the foramen lacerum anteriorly. The lateral part of the temporal bone can then be retracted downward, but it should be retained and replaced, to the medial segment of this bone for proper study of the structures related to the cavity of the middle ear.

Without the aid of magnification, only the more gross structures can be seen in the middle ear. The more detailed anatomy, particularly the smaller nerves of this region, should be obtained from one of the descriptive texts.

This cavity can be described as consisting of five walls. The **anterior or carotid wall** tapers, being wider above and narrower below. It is separated from the carotid canal by a thin plate of bone. Identify the **auditory tube,** which connects the pharynx with the cavity of the middle ear. The **tensor tympani muscle,** located in a semicanal above the auditory tube, should also be identified. This muscle might have been damaged in opening the cavity of the middle ear, but attempt to ascertain its connection to the malleus.

The **medial** or **labyrinthic wall** contains a

rounded prominence, formed over the first turn of the cochlea, the **promontory.** Using the promontory as a guide, locate on its superior-posterior edge the **fenestra vestibuli** (oval window) which usually contains the base of the stapes. A little below and posterior to the fenestra vestibuli, locate the **fenestra cochleae** (round window) which is closed by a membrane (Fig. 34).

The **posterior** or **mastoid wall** contains a variable number of **mastoid air cells,** particularly in the caudal part of the mastoid process. Above these cells is a cavity, the **mastoid antrum,** which communicates with the epitympanic recess. Also on the posterior wall will be found the **fossa incudis,** a small depression for the short crus of the incus, and the **pyramidal eminence.** This eminence is immediately posterior to the oval window and in front of the vertical portion of the facial canal. It contains the stapedius muscle.

The **lateral** or **membranous wall** consists mainly of the **tympanic membrane** and the ring of bone into which it is inserted. The malleus and the incus may be still attached to the tympanic membrane. If they are, review their attachments and the course of the chorda tympani nerve.

The **floor** or **jugular wall** is narrow, and it is separated from the jugular vein by a thin plate of bone.

The mucous membrane which lines the auditory tube is continued backward as the lining of the cavity of the middle ear and the structures which traverse this cavity. Note also that the mastoid air cells are lined by small outpouchings of this mucous membrane.

External Ear

The external ear should be studied next. Identify the **auricle** (pinna) and its subdivisions: the helix, anthelix, tragus, antitragus, lobule, concha, and auricular tubercle. Remove the skin from the auricle and attempt to identify some of the intrinsic and extrinsic muscles and ligaments of the auricle and the **auricular cartilage.** The cartilaginous and osseous portions of the **external auditory meatus** and its nerve supply should be reviewed from one of the standard descriptive texts.

Larynx ·

Before starting the dissection of the larynx, it is advisable to have a clear idea of its general plan of structure. A good model showing the laryngeal cartilages and their articulations is helpful in this. The cartilages which may be regarded as forming the skeleton of the larynx are the single thyroid and cricoid cartilages and the paired arytenoid cartilages. The **thyroid cartilage** consists of **two laminae,** which are joined in the midline anteriorly at the laryngeal prominence. It is deficient posteriorly; the free posterior margin of each lamina is prolonged superiorly and inferiorly as the **superior and inferior cornua,** respectively, of the thyroid cartilage. The **cricoid cartilage,** which lies below the thyroid and above the first ring of the trachea, forms a complete ring. This ring is relatively narrow anteriorly and laterally but is expanded posteriorly to form a broad plate, the lamina of the cricoid. The medial surface of the tip of the inferior cornu of the thyroid cartilage articulates with the lateral aspect of the cricoid. The **arytenoid cartilages** are small, pyramidal cartilages resting, one on each side, upon the upper border of the cricoid lamina, with which they articulate by true diarthrodial joints. Each arytenoid cartilage exhibits a lateral prolongation, the muscular process, and an anterior prolongation, the **vocal process.** At its pointed apex, or superior process, the arytenoid cartilage articulates with a small cartilaginous nodule, the **corniculate cartilage,** which lies within the aryepiglottic fold.

The cartilages of the larynx are connected with one another by means of ligaments and muscles. The most important of the ligaments is the **conus elasticus.** This is a membranous ligament whose inferior margin is attached to the upper border of the anterior and lateral parts of the cricoid cartilage; its superior margin is attached anteriorly to the inner surface of the thyroid and posteriorly to the vocal process of the arytenoid. Between these two attachments, the conus elasticus presents a free superior border, which is known as the **vocal ligament.** The vocal ligament lies internal to the lamina of the thyroid cartilage and is enclosed within the vocal fold of the laryngeal mucous membrane.

Clean the **thyrohyoid membrane.** This is a membranous ligament which extends from the upper border of the thyroid cartilage to the lower border of the body and greater cornu of the hyoid bone. The thyrohyoid membrane is pierced on each side by the **internal laryngeal nerve** and the **superior laryngeal artery.** It is strongest at its free posterolateral border, which runs from the superior cornu of the thyroid to the greater cornu of the hyoid, and in which a small cartilaginous nodule, the triticeate cartilage, is sometimes found.

Study the interior of the **larynx** as it may be seen through the superior laryngeal aperture. The larynx is clothed internally by a layer of mucous membrane which is continuous superiorly with the mucous membrane of the pharynx and inferiorly with that of the

trachea. The cavity of the larynx begins above at the **aryepiglottic folds.** From above downward, it is partially subdivided into three compartments by the presence of two pairs of transverse folds in its lateral walls. The upper of these folds are the ventricular folds, or **false vocal cords.** Below these are the vocal folds, or **true vocal cords,** which may be readily seen from above, since they project farther medially than do the ventricular folds. The highest compartment of the laryngeal cavity is known as the **vestibule of** the **larynx;** it lies behind the epiglottis and above the ventricular folds. The portion of the laryngeal cavity lying between the ventricular folds and the vocal folds is known as the **ventricle** of the larynx. The ventricle communicates below, by means of the **rima glottidis,** with the inferior compartment of the larynx. The rima glottidis is the narrow interval between the two vocal folds. The inferior compartment widens out inferiorly to become directly continuous with the trachea.

Attention should next be directed to the muscles of the larynx. By moving the arytenoid cartilages upon the cricoid cartilage or by changing the relative positions of the cricoid and thyroid cartilages, these muscles act to tense or relax, to approximate or separate, the vocal cords.

Clean first the **cricothyroid muscle.** This muscle arises from the anterolateral part of the arch of the **cricoid.** Running upward and backward, its fibers radiate slightly to be inserted on the lower border and inferior cornu of the **thyroid cartilage.** It is supplied by the external branch of the superior laryngeal nerve (Fig. 28).

Turn to the posterior aspect of the larynx and remove the mucous membrane forming the anterior wall of the pharynx below the superior laryngeal aperture. Then clean the posterior cricoarytenoid and the arytenoid muscles. As the mucous membrane is removed, identify and retain in position the **inferior** (recurrent) **laryngeal nerve,** which ascends on the posterior aspect of the larynx in close relation to the external surface of the pharyngeal mucosa.

The **posterior cricoarytenoid muscle** arises on each side from the posterior aspect of the **cricoid lamina.** Its fibers converge upward and

posterior aspect of the muscular process of the arytenoid cartilage and run upward and medially to cross the median line and reach the apex of the arytenoid cartilage of the opposite side. A few of them are prolonged forward within the aryepiglottic fold to the epiglottis as the **aryepiglottic muscle.**

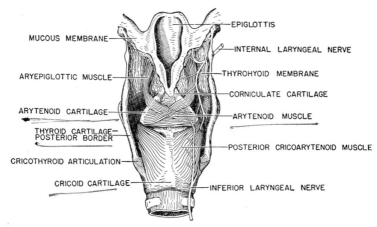

FIG. 35. Posterior aspect of the larynx after removal of the pharyngeal mucosa.

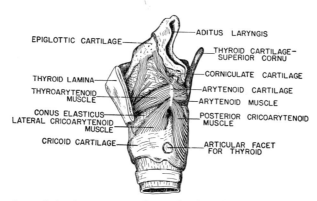

FIG. 36. Dissection of the larynx, seen from the left side. The greater part of the left lamina of the thyroid cartilage has been removed.

laterally to be inserted on the muscular process of the **arytenoid cartilage.** The **arytenoid muscle** is a single median muscle, whose fibers take origin on the posterior surface of one **arytenoid cartilage** and are inserted into the posterior surface of the other. It is roughly divisible into transverse and oblique portions. The oblique fibers of each side arise from the

Turn to the lateral aspect of the larynx. Sever the attachment of the thyrohyoid membrane to the thyroid cartilage on one side and disarticulate the inferior cornu of the thyroid from the cricoid. Detach the cricothyroid muscle from its origin on the cricoid cartilage. Then cut through the lamina of the thyroid cartilage vertically on the same side about $\frac{1}{4}$ in. posterolateral to the median line, and remove the lamina. Clean the lateral cricoarytenoid and the thyroarytenoid muscles (Fig. 36).

The **lateral cricoarytenoid muscle** arises from the upper border of the lateral part of the **cricoid arch.** Its fibers run upward and backward and converge to an insertion on the muscular process of the **arytenoid cartilage.** The **thyroarytenoid muscle** is variable in the extent of its development and frequently appears to be continuous with the upper border of the lateral cricoarytenoid. Its essential and constant portion is the **vocal muscle,** which extends from the inner surface of the angle of the **thyroid laminae** to the **arytenoid cartilage.** It lies within the vocal fold, just lateral to the vocal ligament.

The muscles of the larynx, with the exception of the cricothyroid, are supplied by the **inferior** (recurrent) **laryngeal nerve.** Ascending in the groove between the trachea and the esophagus, this nerve divides at the lower border of the cricoid cartilage into an anterior and a posterior branch. The **posterior branch** ascends on the posterior cricoarytenoid to supply that muscle and the arytenoid muscle. The **anterior branch** runs forward and upward to supply the lateral cricoarytenoid and the thyroarytenoid.

The **internal laryngeal nerve** is the sensory nerve of the larynx. Having pierced the thyrohyoid membrane, it reaches the deep surface of the laryngeal mucosa, in relation to which it ramifies (Fig. 35).

Carefully remove the lateral cricoarytenoid and the thyroarytenoid muscles and attempt to display the **conus elasticus,** which runs upward and medially, deep to these two muscles, from the upper border of the arch of the cricoid. Observe that its free upper border, the **vocal ligament,** lies within the vocal fold, where it is lateral to the mucous membrane and medial to the vocal muscle. The vocal ligament is attached anteriorly to the inner surface of the thyroid cartilage and posteriorly to the vocal process of the arytenoid cartilage.

Thorax •

Thoracic Wall

For the dissection of the thoracic wall and thoracic cavity, the body lies supine. Review the **medial** and the **lateral cutaneous branches of** the **intercostal nerves.** The latter emerge through the external intercostal muscles near the attachment of the digitations of the serratus anterior muscle and run downward and forward to be distributed to the skin on the lateral and anterolateral aspect of the trunk.

The bony wall of the thorax is made up of the **thoracic vertebrae,** the **sternum,** and the 12 pairs of **ribs** and their **costal cartilages.** The spaces between the ribs, known as the **intercostal spaces,** are filled by the external and in-ternal intercostal muscles. In these spaces also will be found the intercostal nerves and the intercostal blood vessels. For detailed study of the intercostal structures, the upper spaces will be found most favorable.

Study the **external intercostal muscles.** These are 11 pairs of thin muscular sheets whose fibers run downward and forward around the thoracic wall. Each takes origin from the **inferior border of a rib** and is inserted on the **superior border of** the next **rib below.** Posteriorly, the external intercostals begin at the tubercles of the ribs, but this fact cannot be well demonstrated now. Anteriorly, they extend only as far as the junctions of the ribs with their costal cartilages.

Between the cartilages, the muscle is replaced by a membranous layer, the **anterior intercostal membrane,** through which the fibers of the internal intercostal muscle are usually visible. Divide the external intercostal muscle and the anterior intercostal membrane along the upper border of the rib in several spaces and turn them upward to expose the internal intercostal muscle.

The **internal intercostal muscles** also occur in 11 pairs. Their fibers run downward and backward. Each takes origin from the **inner surface of a rib,** at the upper border of the costal groove when the groove is present, and is inserted at the **upper border of the next rib below,** close to the insertion of the corresponding external intercostal muscle. The costal groove is thus enclosed by the two layers of intercostal muscle. Posteriorly, the internal intercostals extend only to the angles of the ribs; anteriorly, they reach the lateral border of the sternum.

The **intercostal nerves and vessels** are situated for the greater part of their course in the costal grooves and, hence, under cover of the lower borders of the ribs. For their display, it is usually necessary to chip away the lower part of the rib, but this must be done with care to avoid injury to the nerves and vessels.

The **intercostal nerves** are the anterior primary divisions of the first 11 pairs of thoracic nerves. Their proximal segments will be seen in the dissection of the thoracic cavity. In the present dissection, several of them should be exposed in the costal groove as far posteriorly as can conveniently be reached and traced anteriorly. In the costal groove, the nerve lies between the internal intercostal and intercostal intima,* to each of which it gives twigs of supply. Each intercostal nerve gives rise to a rela-

---

* The intercostal vein, artery, and nerve in their course in the costal groove cause the deeper portion of the internal intercostal muscle to split off as a separate layer known as the **intercostal intima.**

tively large **lateral cutaneous branch,** which pierces the external intercostal muscle. As the trunk of the intercostal nerve is traced anteriorly, it will be found to enter the substance of the internal intercostal muscle a little in front of the midaxillary line. Near the junction of the rib and costal cartilage, it reaches the deep surface of the muscle. From this point, it runs forward between the internal intercostal muscle and the pleural membrane or the transversus thoracic muscle, which it also supplies; near the lateral border of the sternum, it bends anteriorly and pierces the internal intercostal muscle, the anterior intercostal membrane, and the pectoralis major muscle to end superficially as an **anterior cutaneous nerve of the chest.** This description holds good, as regards the terminal parts of the nerves, only for the upper five; the lower six intercostal nerves, after reaching the anterior ends of the intercostal spaces, run downward and forward into the anterior abdominal wall, where their distribution will be investigated when the abdominal wall is dissected.

The **intercostal arteries** occur in two paired groups, known as the anterior and the posterior intercostal arteries. The **posterior intercostal** arteries of the first two spaces are derived from the **superior intercostal artery,** a branch of the costocervical branch of the subclavian artery. The remaining nine pairs of posterior intercostals are direct branches of the **thoracic aorta.** These vessels will all be seen without difficulty in the final stages of the dissection of the thoracic cavity. In the lateral and anterior portions of the thoracic wall now under observation, they are, as noted above, usually impossible to demonstrate satisfactorily. They run forward in the costal groove, giving numerous small twigs for the supply of the intercostal muscles. The **anterior intercostal arteries** are small vessels, usually two to each space, which run posteriorly in the anterior parts of the intercostal spaces and end by anastomosing with the terminal twigs of the posterior intercostals. The anterior intercostals of the upper five spaces are branches of the **internal thoracic artery;** those of the lower six spaces are branches of the **musculophrenic artery.**

The **internal thoracic artery** should be exposed by removing the internal intercostal muscles in the upper five spaces for about 1 in. lateral to the sternum. This artery arises in the neck as a branch of the first part of the **subclavian artery.** It enters the thorax by passing downward behind the sternoclavicular joint and runs down in the anterior thoracic wall behind the first five costal cartilages, between which it may now be seen, usually accompanied by two veins. In the upper two spaces, it lies between the internal muscles and the pleura; lower down it is separated from the pleura by slips of the transversus thoracic muscle. The internal thoracic artery ends behind the sixth costal cartilage by dividing into the **superior epigastric** and the **musculophrenic arteries.**

The **transverse thoracic** is a small **muscle** of the anterior thoracic wall, of which only a very imperfect view can be obtained at present. It arises from the posterior surface of the lower half of the **body** and the **xiphoid process of** the **sternum.** From this origin, flat fibrous bands run upward and laterally to be inserted on the posterior surfaces of the **third** to **sixth costal cartilages.** It can be seen to best advantage when the sternum and costal cartilages are removed to open the thoracic cavity.

Thoracic Cavity

Before opening the **thoracic cavity,** it is well to have a clear idea of the general plan of its contents. The **thoracic wall,** which has already been studied, is made up of the 12 thoracic vertebrae, 12 pairs of ribs and their costal cartilages, the sternum, the external and internal intercostal, and the transverse thoracic muscles. In the wall are found also the intercostal vessels and nerves and, in close relation to the inner surface of the anterior part of the wall, the internal thoracic vessels.

Through the **superior thoracic aperture,** which is bounded by the upper border of the manubrium sterni, the first pair of ribs and their cartilages, and the upper border of the first thoracic vertebra, the thoracic cavity communicates freely with the root of the neck. Inferiorly, the thoracic cavity is separated from the **abdominal cavity** by a sheet of muscular and fibrous tissue, the **diaphragm.**

The **inferior thoracic aperture** is more irregular in outline and of much greater diameter than the superior aperture. It may be shown on the skeleton by a line beginning at the lower border of the twelfth thoracic vertebra and passing around on each side along the lower border of the twelfth rib, thence to the tip of the eleventh rib, the lowest part of the tenth costal cartilage, and along the continuous lower margins of the ninth, eighth, and seventh costal cartilages to the xiphoid process. This line will indicate approximately the line of origin of the muscle fibers which make up the peripheral portion of the diaphragm. The diaphragm does not, however, bridge across this aperture in a transverse plane but is dome-shaped, its central portion reaching a considerably higher level than its peripheral attachment, thus permitting the abdominal cavity to be enclosed within the lower part of the thoracic skeleton.

The contents of the thoracic cavity may be inclusively described as consisting of two pleural sacs, in each of which a lung is contained, and the mediastinum. The **pleural sacs** are **laterally** placed, lying internal to the ribs and intercostal muscles, while the **mediastinum** is the middle portion of the thoracic contents, lying between the two pleural sacs, in relation to the sternum anteriorly and the bodies of the vertebrae posteriorly.

Each **pleural sac** is a completely enclosed cavity which is almost entirely filled by the **lung.** The two pleural cavities are nowhere in communication with each other. Each pleural cavity is bounded by a serous membrane, the **pleura.** Each pleura is one continuous membrane, but from its relations to the lung and to the thoracic wall each pleura is regarded as consisting of two portions. These are the **visceral pleura,** that portion which forms the external covering of the lung itself, and the **parietal pleura,** that portion which forms the outer wall of the pleural cavity. These two portions are directly continuous with each other around the root of the lung.

It should be understood that the mediastinum is not a single anatomical entity. The term **mediastinum** is applied to the entire complex of **structures** which lie **between** the **right** and **left mediastinal pleurae,** extending from the superior thoracic aperture above to the diaphragm below, and from the posterior surface of the sternum to the anterior surfaces of the thoracic vertebral bodies.

If the musculature of the ventral abdominal wall has not been dissected before the thoracic cavity is opened, it is advisable to dissect free and reflect caudad those portions of the rectus abdominis and external oblique muscles which are attached to the lower ventral part of the thoracic cage above the level of the eighth rib and costal cartilages. The digitations of the serratus anterior muscle should be separated from each other, freed, and elevated from the subjacent ribs and external intercostal muscles as far dorsally as the level of the midaxillary line, from the level of the first to the eighth rib. In the removal of the intercostal muscles, described below, the parts of the origins of the pectoralis major and minor and serratus anterior muscles should be left attached to that portion of the thoracic cage which will be removed. This will facilitate future review of these muscles in their relation to the thoracic cage.

In the present dissection, the **thoracic cavity** is to be opened from the front by the removal of the anterior and lateral portions of its wall, without injury to the underlying **parietal pleura.** The **intercostal muscles** should be removed from the upper seven spaces on each side as far laterally as the midaxillary line. This must be done with care, as the pleura is separated from the internal surface of the internal intercostal muscles only by a very thin fibrous layer, the **endothoracic fascia.** The fingers may now be introduced between the ribs. A gentle pressure will suffice to separate the **pleura** from the internal surfaces of the ribs. The separation must be continued as far inferiorly as the eighth rib. The first rib should be left intact for the present, but the second through the sixth ribs on each side should be sectioned in the midaxillary line. The fingers should now be passed medially behind the costal cartilages and the sternum, first on one side and then on the other, and the pleura separated as completely as possible from this portion of the thoracic wall. The **internal thoracic artery** should be freed from the thoracic wall and left on the surface of the thoracic viscera.

The **manubrium sterni** should now be cut transversely with a saw, just below its junction with the **first costal cartilage.** Make another transverse cut through the lower part of the sternum, between its junction on each side with the sixth and the seventh costal cartilages, and then remove the portion of the sternum between the two cuts, together with the attached portions of the second through the sixth ribs. The xiphoid process and the sixth costal cartilages must be left in place in order not to injure the diaphragm. If the lower part of the neck has not yet been dissected, the upper part of the manubrium and the first costal cartilages must be left in place throughout the thoracic dissection. If, however, this dissection has been done, the first ribs may be cut at their junctions with their costal cartilages and the manubrium and attached portion of the second through the sixth ribs removed.

Pleura

The anterior lines of reflection of the right and left pleurae should next be observed. These are the lines along which the **costal** pleura of each side turns back to become the **mediastinal pleura.** In a subject with little fat, these lines may be at once apparent, but in an obese subject they will be hidden by a considerable amount of adipose tissue, which must be removed. In such a case, it will be found

margins diverge from each other. At about the level of the lower border of the manubrium, they approach each other and, indeed, frequently overlap to a slight extent in the midline. The right pleural margin passes vertically downward from this point, behind the middle

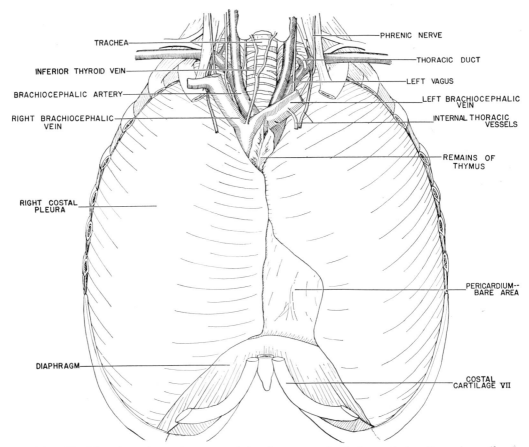

FIG. 37. The thoracic cavity, opened by the removal of the anterior thoracic wall, showing the anterior lines of pleural reflection.

helpful to make a small opening in the costal pleura 1 or 2 in. lateral to the midline. The handle of the scalpel may then be introduced through the opening and passed medially along the internal surface of the pleura. Its medial passage will be stopped when it reaches the line of reflection of the pleura. In the region of the **superior mediastinum,** which lies behind the manubrium sterni, the **two pleural**

of the sternum, to about the level of the sixth intercostal space, where it turns laterally and inferiorly across the **diaphragm** and can now be followed only as far as the junction of the eighth rib with its costal cartilage. Along this inferior part of the margin, the **costal pleura** becomes continuous with the **diaphragmatic pleura.** From the lower border of the manubrium, the left pleural margin passes vertically downward close to the right to about the level of the fourth costal cartilage; from this point, it diverges for a varying distance to the left. Inferiorly, it crosses the diaphragm in a manner similar to the right. Between the two pleural margins in the region where the left reflection diverges to the left, the anterior surface of the pericardium is exposed. This is known as the **bare area of the pericardium** and varies in its extent in different individuals (Fig. 37). The pericardium will be seen to be attached to the diaphragm inferiorly. Between the inferior divergent margins of the pleura and the lower border of the pericardium, a considerable portion of the **diaphragm,** which is covered by neither pleura nor pericardium, is now exposed. The origin of the muscle fibers which make up this part of the diaphragm from the xiphoid process and the seventh and eighth costal cartilages may now be seen.

Before proceeding to a study of the mediastinum, the **pleural sacs** should be opened. Make a longitudinal incision through the costal pleura from the level of the first to the seventh rib on each side. From each end of the longitudinal incisions, transverse incisions should be made laterally and medially, and the folds of pleura thus mapped out should be reflected to expose the pleural cavities and the lungs within them. During life, the lungs entirely fill the pleural sacs except for a very small interval, the pleural cavity, intervening between the external surface of the lung and the internal surface of the parietal pleural membrane which contains a small amount of fluid. In the cadaver the lungs may be shrunken and the relative size of the pleural cavity is thereby increased.

The embalmed **lungs** may now be seen within the cavities. They are usually a bluish grey in color with dark patches scattered over their surface. The external relations of the lungs may be understood by a study of the walls of the pleural cavities, which may now be explored with the fingers. In a perfectly normal and healthy pleural cavity, the **visceral pleura,** which is closely adherent to the outer surface of the lung and may be regarded as a part of the lung, is connected to the **parietal pleura** only by its continuity with the latter across the **root of** the **lung** and the **pulmonary ligament.** Perfectly healthy lungs are, however, relatively rare in the dissecting room, and numerous secondary adhesions between the visceral and parietal pleurae will usually be found. However, in many cases they may be readily broken down with the fingers.

The **costal portion of the pleura** is in intimate relation throughout with the inner surfaces of the **ribs** and **intercostal muscles.** Its most posterior extent is along the angles of the successive ribs, from which it is continued medially and forward across the lateral aspect of the bodies of the thoracic vertebrae, which may be readily felt through the pleura, to become continuous anteriorly with the **mediastinal pleura.** The uppermost portion of the pleura is dome-shaped and reaches up into the root of the neck some distance above the level of the first rib. This **apical,** or cervical, portion of the pleura is crossed anteriorly a short distance below its summit by the subclavian artery, which can usually be felt through the pleura. Along its inferior margin, the costal pleura is reflected upward onto the diaphragm as the diaphragmatic pleura. From the junction of the eighth rib with its costal cartilage, this pleural margin crosses the thoracic wall along a line slightly convex downward, which reaches approximately the level of the ninth rib in the midaxillary line and the eleventh in the scapular line. The lateral and posterior portions of the periphery of the diaphragm extend almost vertically upward from this line, so that the lowest portion of each pleural cavity is a pocketlike cleft between the lowest part of the costal pleura and the peripheral part of the diaphragmatic pleura, which is known as the **phrenicocostal sinus.** The narrow anteromedial prolongation of each pleural cavity to the midline, at the edge of which the costal pleura is reflected back to become the mediastinal pleura, is known as the **costomediastinal sinus.**

The **diaphragmatic pleura** is closely applied to the superior surface of the diaphragm, whose contour it follows exactly.

The contour and relations of the **mediastinal pleura** are not entirely alike on the two sides. On each side, however, the **root of** the **lung** will be seen connecting the lung to the posterior part of the mediastinum at about the level of the fifth to seventh thoracic vertebrae. The **visceral pleura** covering the lung is reflected across the root to become continuous with the **mediastinal pleura.** Anteriorly, superiorly, and posteriorly, the pleura is closely applied to the root of the lung, but inferiorly, the **pulmonary ligament,** a double fold of pleura, helps to hold the lung in place against the mediastinum. It consists of two layers of pleura with a small amount of fatty areolar tissue between them. These layers of pleura are continuous laterally with the visceral pleura on the inferior part of the mediastinal surface of the lung, superiorly with the pleura on the lung root, and medially with the mediastinal part of the parietal pleura. Inferiorly, they are continuous with each other and present a free margin stretching transversely across the pleural cavity a short distance above the diaphragm.

On the **right side,** in front of the root of the lung and the pulmonary ligament, the right lateral surface of the **heart** may be felt through the mediastinal pleura. This surface of the heart is composed almost entirely of the **right atrium,** which is here separated from the pleura only by the **pericardium.** Immediately above the diaphragm and in front of the lowest part of the pulmonary ligament, the **inferior vena cava** may be felt where it traverses the diaphragm to enter the right atrium of the heart. Running upward from the atrium in front of the upper part of the root, the **superior vena cava**

may be felt and directly continuous with this, running up to the superior thoracic aperture, the **right brachiocephalic vein.** The **arch of** the **azygos vein,** which opens into the posterior aspect of the upper part of the superior vena cava, may be felt immediately above the root of the lung. Above the azygos arch and behind the **right brachiocephalic vein,** the right mediastinal pleura is in contact with the **trachea.** Behind the trachea, the pleura is in relation to the **esophagus,** which here lies immediately in front of the vertebral column. A ridge caused by the presence of the **right phrenic nerve,** which traverses the mediastinum immediately subjacent to the mediastinal pleura, can usually be seen. The nerve is in relation above to the brachiocephalic vein and superior vena cava and below to the right atrium and the pericardium.

On the **left side** also, the mediastinal pleura is in relation below and anteriorly to the **heart** and **pericardium,** but it will be seen that the heart projects much farther toward the left than it does to the right, with the result that the capacity of the left pleural cavity is considerably less than is that of the right. The left surface of the heart is formed principally by the **left ventricle,** but its most superior and anterior part is formed by the **conus arteriosus** of the right ventricle, while the left atrium also contributes slightly to it. Above the root of the lung in a position similar to that of the **azygos arch** on the right side, the **arch of** the **aorta** can be easily felt through the pleura. Continuous with the posterior part of the arch and coursing vertically downward behind the root of the lung and the pulmonary ligament, the **descending aorta** will be felt. Running upward from the arch, the left **subclavian artery** is in relation to the pleura. The **esophagus** comes into relation with the **left mediastinal pleura** both near the trachea and again just before its passage through the diaphragm. The **left phrenic nerve** usually makes a low ridge in the left mediastinal pleura which crosses from above downward the brachiocephalic vein, the arch of the aorta, and the heart and pericardium.

When the pleural cavities have been thoroughly investigated, the **mediastinum** and its contents should be approached from the front. The subdivisions of the mediastinum are purely arbitrary and depend for their boundaries upon the extent of the **serous pericardium.** The serous pericardium, like each of the pleurae, is a single uninterrupted membrane which consists of visceral and parietal portions separated from each other by a narrow, enclosed space, the **pericardial cavity.** The **visceral portion of the serous pericardium** is closely applied to the external surface of the heart and is to be regarded as a part of that organ. From the surface of the heart, the visceral pericardium is prolonged for a short distance along the external surfaces of the vessels which join the heart and is then reflected from them to become the parietal pericardium. The **parietal pericardium,** which forms the external wall of the pericardial cavity, will appear as a considerably thicker and tougher membrane than the parietal pleura, due to the association with it of the fibrous pericardium. The **fibrous pericardium** is a layer of relatively dense fibrous tissue intimately blended with the external surface of the parietal serous pericardium, from which it cannot be separated as a definite membrane, and continuous through the fibrous sheaths of the vessels in the superior mediastinum with the **deep fascia of** the **neck.**

The parietal pericardium is firmly attached inferiorly to the central portion of the diaphragm. On each side, it is in relation to the right and left pleurae, from which it is separated only by a small amount of areolar tissue and the phrenic nerves. Anteriorly also, it is overlapped by the two pleurae, except for the small bare area which has already been seen. Posteriorly, it is loosely attached to the esoph-

agus and the descending aorta. The greatest superior extent of the pericardium is at the line of its reflection from the ascending aorta and the pulmonary artery. This is approximately at the level of a plane passing from the lower border of the manubrium sterni back to the lower border of the fourth thoracic vertebra, and, consequently, that plane has been chosen as the plane of separation of the **superior** from the **inferior mediastinum.**

Mediastinum

The **anterior mediastinum** is the portion of the **inferior mediastinum** which lies anterior to the **pericardium.** Superiorly, where the right and left pleurae are in contact with each other, it has virtually no existence. More inferiorly, it is as wide as is the bare area of the pericardium, but its anteroposterior extent is very slight and it contains no structures of importance. Occasionally, the remains of the thymus gland reach down into the upper part of the anterior mediastinum between the two pleurae (Fig. 37).

The **middle mediastinum** is the portion of the inferior mediastinum which contains the **pericardium.** The only important structures of the middle mediastinum which are not enclosed within the pericardium are the **two phrenic nerves** and the blood vessels which accompany them. These descend on each side immediately in front of the roots of the lungs between the mediastinal pleurae and the parietal pericardium. The middle mediastinum cannot be fully investigated until the pericardial cavity is opened. Attention should now be directed to the superior mediastinum.

The **superior mediastinum** lies above the pericardium and between the upper portions of the two mediastinal pleurae, extending from the manubrium sterni to the anterior surfaces of the upper four thoracic vertebrae. Through the superior thoracic aperture, it is in communication with the root of the neck, and the structures which connect the thoracic cavity with the neck will be found in this part of the mediastinum. To expose the anterior surface of the pericardium and to render the superior mediastinum accessible for study, the mediastinal pleura should now be separated from the mediastinum and turned laterally as far back as the roots of the lungs.

The most anterior structure of the superior mediastinum is the **thymus gland.** This is an elongated bilobed structure which lies behind the middle of the manubrium in relation posteriorly to the left brachiocephalic vein and the arch of the aorta. It varies considerably in its extent in different individuals and is usually represented in the adult by a mass of adipose tissue. After the position and extent of the thymus have been noted, it should be removed.

Define the upper limit of the anterior extent of the pericardium. This is the line along which the parietal pericardium is reflected inward and down onto the pulmonary artery, aorta, and superior vena cava as the visceral pericardium of these vessels. In an obese subject, this line of reflection is obscured by adipose tissue. Make a short transverse incision through the anterior exposed part of the pericardium. The handle of the scalpel can then be introduced through this opening and passed upward in the pericardial cavity between the anterior surface of the heart and the inner surface of the pericardium. The upward passage of the knife will be stopped at the line of reflection between visceral and parietal pericardium.

The large vessels of the superior mediastinum should now be cleaned and studied. Since the first rib and the upper part of the manubrium are left in place for their relationship to the subjacent structures, these bones may prevent study of the structures in the superior mediastinum. If the first rib on each side is held down by pressure applied to the costochondral junction, and the lower part of the manubrium pulled up, the ribs may be frac-

tured so that the manubrium can be retracted and elevated to facilitate study of the structures in the mediastinum. Most anteriorly will be found the brachiocephalic veins and the upper part of the superior vena cava. The **right brachiocephalic vein,** which begins behind the right sternoclavicular articulation, is formed by the union of the **right internal jugular** and **subclavian veins.** From here, it courses downward behind the right border of the manubrium, where it joins the left brachiocephalic at about the level of the lower border of the first costal cartilage. The **left brachiocephalic vein** begins at the union of the **left internal jugular** and **subclavian veins** behind the left sternoclavicular articulation. From here it runs downward and to the right to join the right brachiocephalic. In addition to the two large tributaries which form it, each brachiocephalic vein receives the **internal thoracic vein** of its own side. The **inferior thyroid veins,** which descend from the neck in front of the trachea, usually join the left brachiocephalic vein, either singly or by a common trunk. The **left superior intercostal vein** should also be identified. This vessel drains the upper two or three left intercostal spaces. Its terminal portion will be found crossing the left side of the arch of the aorta to enter the inferior aspect of the left brachiocephalic vein.

The **superior vena cava** is formed by the union of the two brachiocephalic veins behind the lower border of the first right costal cartilage. From here it runs vertically downward to enter the **right atrium of the heart.** Its terminal portion is in the middle mediastinum, enclosed by the pericardium. Its upper portion is in the superior mediastinum. In addition to the brachiocephalic veins, it receives the **azygos vein.** The arched terminal portion of this vessel will be found crossing above the root of the right lung to enter the posterior aspect of the superior vena cava.

The **thoracic portion of** the **aorta** is divided

for descriptive purposes into three parts, each of which is in a different subdivision of the mediastinum. The first part, or **ascending aorta**, is in the middle mediastinum, enclosed by the pericardium. The second part, the **arch of** the **descending aorta**, which passes downward through the **posterior mediastinum.**

Study of the **aortic arch** and its branches will be facilitated by sectioning the left brachiocephalic vein near its origin and reflecting it to

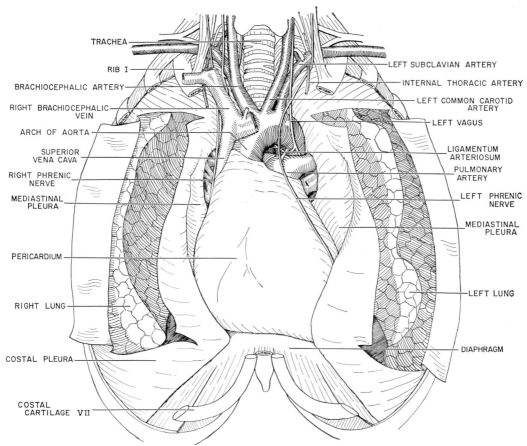

FIG. 38. Contents of the thoracic cavity. The pleural sacs have been opened and the mediastinal pleura stripped laterally on each side to expose the pericardium and the structures of the superior mediastinum.

aorta, is in the superior mediastinum and should now be studied. It begins behind the lower border of the manubrium sterni, slightly to the right of the midline, and takes an arched course upward, backward, to the left, and downward to become continuous at the left side of the fibrocartilaginous disc between the fourth and fifth thoracic vertebrae with the

the right. If this is done, the left superior intercostal vein should also be cut where it enters the brachiocephalic and retained in position.

To the left, the arch of the aorta is in contact with the mediastinal pleura above the root of the left lung. Crossing the left side of the arch from above downward, and separating it from the pleura, will be found the **left phrenic nerve** and, more posteriorly, the **left vagus.** If the dissection is carefully done, two much smaller nerves may be found running downward across the arch between the phrenic and the vagus. These are the **superior cervical cardiac branch of the left sympathetic trunk** and the **inferior cervical cardiac branch of** the **left vagus,** both of which join the cardiac plexus.

The nerve supply of the heart and lungs is derived from the **cardiac** and **pulmonary plexuses,** which belong to the autonomic part of the nervous system. In the ordinary dissection, which must be done in considerable haste by an inexperienced dissector, a complete display of these plexuses and their branches of origin and distribution is not practical. They are, however, of the greatest physiological importance, and it is well to have a general knowledge of their location so that any portions of them which are met as the dissection proceeds may be recognized. The **cardiac plexus** is formed by branches from both sympathetic trunks and from both vagus nerves. The **cervical portions of** the **sympathetic trunks** usually each contribute three small branches to the plexus, which arise in the neck and enter the superior mediastinum through the superior thoracic aperture. Numerous small twigs are also given to the plexus from the **thoracic portions of** the **sympathetic trunk.** In addition to these nerves, two branches arise from each **vagus** in the neck and run down to join the plexus, while other branches leave the vagi in the upper part of the thorax. The cardiac plexus consists of two parts, superficial and deep, which are, however, intimately connected with each other. The **superficial cardiac plexus** lies just under the arch of the aorta. It receives the superior cervical cardiac branch of the left sympathetic and the inferior cervical and thoracic branches of the left vagus. The remaining cardiac branches of the left vagus and sympathetic and all the cardiac branches of the right go to the **deep cardiac plexus,** which lies be-

hind the arch, in front and at the sides of the terminal part of the trachea. From the cardiac plexuses, small autonomic nerve filaments pass along the vessels to form the pulmonary and coronary plexuses. The **pulmonary plexuses** constitute the nerve supply of the lungs. There are on each side an anterior and a posterior pulmonary plexus, which lie respectively anterior and posterior to the pulmonary artery at the root of the lung. From the pulmonary plexuses, autonomic nerves pass into the substance of the lung. The coronary plexuses supply the heart, branches of distribution accompanying the coronary arteries.

Under the arch of the aorta and slightly to the left of it, the large **pulmonary artery** will be found emerging from the pericardium. Its extrapericardial course is very short; the pulmonary trunk terminates under the left side of the arch by dividing into right and left branches. The **short left branch** goes horizontally to the left to enter the root of the left lung. The **longer right branch** passes horizontally to the right under the arch of the aorta and then behind the superior vena cava and under the arch of the azygos vein to reach the root of the right lung. Connecting the undersurface of the arch of the aorta with the upper and anterior aspect of the pulmonary trunk, a thick, cordlike structure will be found. This is the **ligamentum arteriosum,** the remnant in the adult of the **ductus arteriosus** of the fetus. In the adult it is solid, but during fetal life the ductus arteriosus is an open channel which permits blood to pass from the pulmonary trunk directly into the aorta. Crossing the undersurface of the arch behind the ligamentum arteriosum, the **inferior laryngeal** or recurrent **branch of** the **left vagus** will be found. This nerve leaves the vagus as the latter crosses the left side of the arch and turns medially and posteriorly beneath the arch to run upward through the superior mediastinum into the neck in relation to the trachea and esophagus. Under the arch of the aorta, it usually gives a few small twigs to the **superficial cardiac plexus.** Behind the pulmonary artery, the **left bronchus** runs to the left and downward under the arch of the aorta to enter the root of the left lung.

Superiorly, the principal structures in relation to the arch are its own three large branches, which should now be cleaned and examined.

The first is the **brachiocephalic artery.** This vessel arises behind the middle of the manubrium and passes upward, backward, and to the right to end at the level of the right sternoclavicular articulation by dividing into the **right subclavian** and the **right common carotid arteries.** The **right vagus nerve** will be found running downward and posteriorly between the artery and the right brachiocephalic vein (Fig. 38).

The second branch of the aortic arch is the **left common carotid artery.** It arises just to the left of the brachiocephalic artery and runs upward, to the left, and backward to enter the neck behind the left sternoclavicular articulation.

The **left subclavian artery** arises from the posterior part of the arch and runs upward to the level of the left sternoclavicular articulation, from which it arches to the left across the front of the dome of the left pleura. The **left vagus nerve** descends between the left subclavian and left common carotid arteries to reach the left side of the arch of the aorta.

A fourth, much smaller, branch is occasionally found arising from the arch of the aorta between the brachiocephalic and the left common carotid. This is the a. thyreoidea ima, or **lowest thyroid artery,** which runs up into the neck in front of the trachea. Rarely, it may arise from the lowest part of the brachiocephalic artery instead of the aortic arch. In about 90 per cent of cases, it is entirely lacking.

The entire thoracic course of the two phrenic nerves may now be studied. Each **phrenic nerve** enters the thorax through the superior thoracic aperture by crossing the medial border of the **anterior scalene muscle.** As it leaves the anterior scalene, it lies anterior to the subclavian artery and immediately comes into relation with the internal thoracic artery. The **right phrenic nerve** runs down along the lateral side of the right brachiocephalic vein, then along the lateral side of the superior vena cava, and, finally, along the right lateral surface of the pericardium to reach the diaphragm. The **left phrenic** descends between the left subclavian and left common carotid arteries, crossing in front of the left vagus nerve, then across the left side of the arch of the aorta in front of the root of the left lung, and, finally, along the left lateral surface of the pericardium to reach the diaphragm. Small **pericardiacophrenic blood vessels** will be found accompanying the nerves. The arteries are branches of the internal thoracic arteries; the veins drain either into the internal thoracic veins or into the brachiocephalics.

Pericardium

Attention should now be directed to the **middle mediastinum.** Make a transverse incision clear across the middle of the exposed anterior surface of the pericardium. From each end of this transverse incision, longitudinal incisions must be carried downward to the diaphragm and upward almost to the upper limit of the pericardium. The two flaps so marked out may then be turned downward and upward respectively, thus opening the pericardial cavity and exposing the anterior surface of the heart (Fig. 39).

The **pericardial cavity** will appear as a narrow interval between the **external surface** of the **heart** and the internal surface of the **parietal pericardium.** In the cadaver, this cavity is sometimes partially obliterated by pathological adhesions between the heart and the parietal pericardium, or it may be filled with a coagulation of fluid present before death or with an effusion of the substance used to inject the arteries after death. If any such material is present, it should be removed. Anteriorly, inferiorly, and at each side, the heart normally lies quite free in the pericardial cavity, and there is no connection here between the **parietal pericardium** and the **visceral pericardium** which forms the thin outermost layer of the

side. On each side, two **pulmonary veins** enter the upper posterior part of the heart. Within the pericardial cavity, these vessels are all covered by prolongations of the serous pericardium.

In connection with the pericardial reflections, two small subdivisions of the pericardial cavity should be noted. These are the transverse sinus and the oblique sinus. The **trans-**

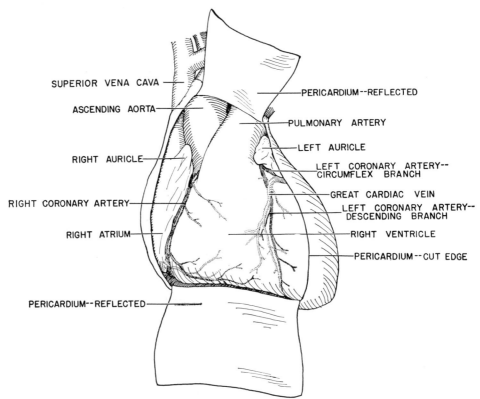

SUPERIOR VENA CAVA

ASCENDING AORTA

RIGHT AURICLE

RIGHT CORONARY ARTERY

RIGHT ATRIUM

PERICARDIUM--REFLECTED

PERICARDIUM--REFLECTED

PULMONARY ARTERY

LEFT AURICLE

LEFT CORONARY ARTERY--CIRCUMFLEX BRANCH

GREAT CARDIAC VEIN

LEFT CORONARY ARTERY--DESCENDING BRANCH

RIGHT VENTRICLE

PERICARDIUM--CUT EDGE

FIG. 39. The sternocostal surface of the heart, exposed by reflection of the pericardium.

heart wall. The vessels joining the base of the heart should now be identified.

Most anterior is the **pulmonary artery,** which joins the upper left portion of the anterior surface of the heart. To the right of the pulmonary artery and somewhat overlapped by it is the aorta. Still farther to the right and more posterior is the intrapericardial portion of the **superior vena cava.** The **inferior vena cava** will be found piercing the diaphragm to enter the lower posterior part of the heart at the right

verse sinus of the pericardium is a tunnellike passageway lying behind the ascending aorta and the pulmonary artery and connecting at each side with the general pericardial cavity. If the finger or a blunt instrument is introduced behind the pulmonary artery from the left side and pushed transversely to the right, it will traverse the transverse sinus and emerge behind the right side of the ascending aorta and in front of the superior vena cava.

The **oblique sinus** is a pocketlike subdivision

of the pericardial cavity which lies behind the base of the heart. It can be reached by pulling the lower free portion of the heart forward, upward, and to the right. Inferiorly and to the left, the oblique sinus communicates freely with the general pericardial cavity. Its posterior wall is formed by the parietal pericardium which lies in front of the esophagus and the descending aorta. Its anterior wall is formed by the visceral pericardium on the posterior surface of the left atrium. The right border is formed

of the pericardial cavity at the two ends, the venous end, through which blood enters the tube, and the arterial end, through which blood leaves it. The **venous portion of** the tubular **embryonic heart** is represented in the adult by the **two atria** and the **veins** which join them; the **arterial portion** is represented by the **two ventricles** and the **arteries** which leave them. Each of the lines of pericardial reflection of the adult marks the position of one of the two ends of the embryonic heart tube. These lines

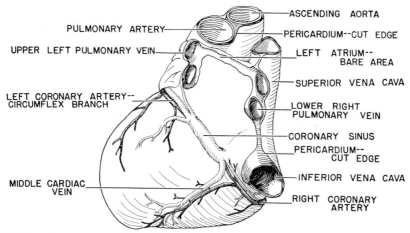

FIG. 40. Posterior aspect of the heart, after removal from the body. The vessels have been cut along the lines of pericardial reflection.

by the reflection from the parietal to the visceral pericardium across the left side of the right pulmonary veins and the inferior vena cava; its left border is formed by a line of pericardial reflection across the right side of the left pulmonary veins. The superior border is the line of junction of the visceral and parietal pericardium along the upper posterior border of the left atrium. The oblique sinus is bounded entirely by the venous reflection of the pericardium.

Although eight large vessels traverse the pericardial cavity to reach the heart, there are only two lines of pericardial reflection. This results from the embryonic development of the heart as a simple tube connected to the wall

of pericardial reflection should now be studied (Fig. 40).

The **arterial reflection** can be easily seen at the upper anterior part of the pericardial cavity, where the **aorta** and the **pulmonary artery** are ensheathed in a common pericardial covering which is reflected from their external surfaces to become continuous with the parietal pericardium along a line encircling the vessels. The other line of reflection is more complex and encircles all six of the veins which enter the heart. Starting at the right side of the **superior vena cava,** where that vessel enters the pericardial cavity, the line along which the visceral and parietal pericardium are continuous runs downward along the right side of the **right pul-**

Coronary Sulcus — Rt. atrium from Rt. Ventricle, Lf. atrium from Lf. Ventricle
Ant. Longitudinal Sulcus — Lf. Ventricle from Rt. Ventricle
Post. Longitudinal Sulcus — Lf. Ventricle from Rt. Ventricle

100   *Manual of Human Dissection*

monary veins and the **inferior vena cava,** across in front of the latter and up along its left side and the left side of the **right pulmonary veins,** then across the posterior aspect of the upper part of the **left atrium,** down on the right side of the **left pulmonary veins,** upward again along their left side, then to the right along the posterior wall of the **transverse sinus,** and, finally, across the front of the superior vena cava to reach the starting point. It should be noticed that the transverse sinus lies between the two pericardial reflections and marks the site of the obliterated **dorsal mesocardium** or dorsal mesentery of the embryonic heart.

Heart

Attention should now be directed to the anterior or **sternocostal surface of the heart.** This surface is formed principally by the **right ventricle,** but all four chambers of the heart contribute to it. Its right margin is formed by the **right atrium,** the auricle of which will be seen as a pointed appendage projecting upward and farther to the left than does the main part of the atrium. The **right atrium** is separated from the **right ventricle** by the **coronary sulcus,** which crosses the anterior surface of the heart, running downward and slightly to the right.

The **sulci** on the external surface of the heart are grooves or furrows in the muscular wall of the organ. In the undissected heart, however, they do not ordinarily appear as grooves since they may be so filled by **epicardial fat** that the visceral pericardium covering them is not indented. Usually they may be readily recognized by the presence of this fat and by the fact that the **coronary arteries** and their larger branches are lodged in them.

The **right ventricle** forms about two-thirds of the **sternocostal surface** of the heart. It is widest below, just above the diaphragm. Superiorly, it narrows and becomes continuous with the **pulmonary artery.** The left extremity of the anterior surface is formed by the **left**

ventricle. This is separated from the right ventricle by the **anterior longitudinal sulcus,** which runs downward and to the left. At the left of the base of the pulmonary artery, the **auricle of** the **left atrium** forms a small part of the sternocostal surface.

The relation of the anterior surface of the **heart** to the **anterior thoracic wall** is of importance and can be studied by replacing the portion of the sternum and its attached ribs previously removed. The exact outline of the heart as projected against the chest wall varies somewhat in individual cases but on the average is about as follows. Beginning at a point corresponding to the lower border of the second left costal cartilage about ½ in. to the left of the edge of the sternum, the left border follows a line somewhat convex to the left, running down to the fifth intercostal space about 3½ in. from the midline. From here, the inferior border follows a nearly straight line across to the sixth right costal cartilage about ½ in. from the junction of this cartilage with the sternum. From here, the right margin, somewhat convex to the right, runs upward to the upper border of the third right costal cartilage about ½ in. from the sternum. The upper border, which corresponds to the junction of the superior vena cava with the right atrium and the junction of the right ventricle with the pulmonary artery, lies behind a line running from the upper border of the third right cartilage about ½ in. to the right of the sternum to the lower border of the second left cartilage about ½ in. to the left of the sternum.

The heart may be moved about in the pericardial cavity for observation of its other surfaces. The right lateral surface is formed entirely by the **right atrium** and is in relation through the parietal pericardium with the right phrenic nerve and the right mediastinal pleura. The inferior or diaphragmatic surface is separated from the sternocostal surface by the sharp inferior border or **margo acutus.** This

Sternocostal surface — Rt. Ventricle, Lf. Ventricle
Rt. Lateral   "   — Rt. Atrium
Lf.   "   "   — Lf. Ventricle
Post.   "   — Lf. Atrium

Thorax   101

surface rests against the diaphragm, from which it is separated only by the diaphragmatic portion of the parietal pericardium. It is crossed by the inferior or **posterior longitudinal sulcus,** which meets the **anterior longitudinal sulcus** at the margo acutus. This sulcus separates the **right ventricle** from the **left ventricle,** each of which forms about half of the diaphragmatic surface.

The **coronary sulcus** completely encircles the heart, separating the two **atria** from the two **ventricles.** The **anterior** and **posterior** (or inferior) **longitudinal sulci,** which separate the two ventricles, begin at the **coronary sulcus** and meet near the left extremity of the **margo acutus.**

The left side has a more rounded border, **margo obtusus,** which is formed entirely by the **left ventricle** and is interposed between the sternocostal and diaphragmatic surfaces. The heart projects farthest to the left and inferiorly at its apex, which is also formed entirely by the left ventricle.

The posterior surface corresponds to the **base of** the **heart,** to which the vessels are attached. Its only free portion is the surface of the left atrium which forms the anterior wall of the **oblique sinus.**

For the most part, the interior of the heart can be studied to best advantage after the organ has been removed from the body. It is advisable, however, to open the **right atrium** while the heart is still in situ. Before doing this, it will probably be necessary to open the pericardial cavity more widely on the right side than has previously been done. This can be accomplished by carrying a transverse incision backward through the right portion of the parietal pericardium. The right atrium should then be opened by three incisions. Make a longitudinal incision through the wall of the atrium beginning slightly below the tip of the auricle and runnning down to the inferior border of the atrium a little to the right of the

coronary sulcus. From each end of this longitudinal incision, carry a transverse incision backward to the posterior border of the atrium. The upper incision will cross the atrium just below the termination of the superior vena cava and the lower just above the termination of the inferior vena cava. The flap thus marked out can then be turned to the right and backward and the interior of the atrium exposed. The cavity is usually filled with coagulated blood. This should be removed and the wall of the atrium cleaned as thoroughly as possible

The inner surface of the right atrium, as of all the chambers of the heart, is lined with thin smooth epithelium, the **endocardium,** which is continuous with the **endothelium** of the blood vessels and through which the muscular layer or **myocardium,** which forms the main thickness of the atrial wall, can be seen. The myocardium of the posterior part of the wall of the right atrium, into which the veins open, is smooth. This portion of the atrium is known as the **sinus venarum.** It is marked off from the roughened anterior part by the **crista terminalis.** The latter will be seen as a longitudinal muscular ridge running from the inferior vena cava to the superior vena cava on the inner surface of the right wall of the atrium. Running forward from the crista terminalis on the inner surface of the atrial wall are smaller transverse muscular ridges, the **musculi pectinati.** These are particularly well developed in the auricle.

The **superior vena cava** opens into the highest part of the **sinus venarum.** Its opening has no valve. Below and posteriorly is the large opening of the inferior vena cava. Running across in front and to the left side of this opening is an endocardial fold, the **valve of** the **inferior vena cava** or Eustachian valve. To the left of the caval orifice is another opening in the lower posterior wall of the atrium for the **coronary sinus,** a vein which is lodged in the posterior part of the coronary sulcus. This opening also is guarded by a rudimentary valvular fold. Anteriorly, inferiorly, and toward the left, the right atrium communicates with the right ventricle through the very large **tricuspid or right atrioventricular orifice.** The position of this opening corresponds to that of the lower and right portion of the coronary sulcus on the exterior of the heart. It lies behind the body of the sternum at about the level of the fourth intercostal space. It is guarded by the **tricuspid valve.** Other minute orifices may be seen scattered over the atrial wall. These

vena cava. In many cases, a valvular passageway through the atrial septum persists in the adult, running from the upper part of the fossa ovalis behind the limbus to open into the left atrium.

When study of the right atrium is completed, the heart should be removed from the body. An excellent opportunity is now afforded for a review of the lines of **pericardial reflection,** since the heart is to be removed by cutting through the vessels along the lines of reflection

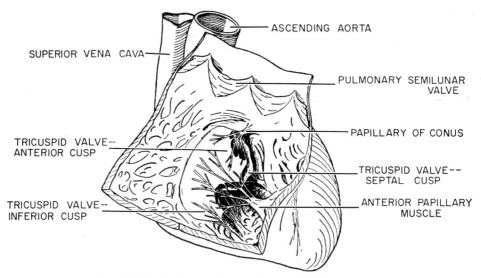

FIG. 41. The interior of the right ventricle of the heart.

are the openings of the **venae cordis minimae,** small veins which carry blood from the heart wall.

The posteromedial wall of the right atrium is formed by the **atrial septum,** which separates it from the left atrium. On this wall a shallow oval depression will be seen. This is the **fossa ovalis** and indicates the position of the **foramen ovale** through which blood passed in the fetal heart from the right atrium directly into the left atrium. The fossa ovalis is bounded superiorly and anteriorly by a low semicircular ridge, the **limbus fossae ovalis,** which is usually continuous below with the valve of the inferior

of the pericardium. First cut through the ascending aorta and the pulmonary artery just below the level at which the pericardium is reflected from them. By pulling these cut vessels forward, the **transverse sinus** can now be opened up and the continuity of the **coronary sulcus** along its lower border demonstrated. Next, cut the superior vena cava transversely just below its entrance into the pericardial cavity, the inferior vena cava just above the diaphragm, and the four pulmonary veins near their entrance into the heart. The **visceral pericardium** covering these veins will necessarily be cut at the same time as the vessels, and, if the knife is also carried through the pericardium along the line of reflection connecting the veins, the heart will be freed from the pericardial wall and can be removed from the body. It should be observed that the only portion of the external surface of the heart which is devoid of a visceral pericardial covering is a narrow area running transversely across the upper posterior aspect of the organ between the **upper right pulmonary vein** and the **upper left pulmonary vein.** This area, which lies between the transverse sinus and the upper end of the oblique sinus, is formed by the upper border of the left atrium. When the heart is in position, it is in direct relation to the inferior surface of the right branch of the pulmonary artery (Fig. 40).

The **ascending aorta** takes origin from the **left ventricle** behind the left side of the sternum at the level of the third intercostal space. Behind the right side of the junction of the manubrium and body of the sternum, it becomes continuous with the arch of the aorta. At its beginning, it is overlapped anteriorly and to the left by the pulmonary artery, which should be separated from it to expose the aortic sinuses. The **aortic sinuses** are three swellings or dilatations of the **ascending aorta** at its base. They correspond in position to the **aortic semilunar valves,** which lie within the ascending aorta and which will be seen somewhat later. The names used to describe the sinuses and the valves do not correspond to their actual position in the body. The terms used are right, left, and posterior. It should be observed that the **right aortic sinus** is actually anterior in position, the **left sinus** lies posteriorly and to the left, and the **posterior sinus** is posterior and to the right.

The only branches of the ascending aorta are the right and left **coronary arteries.** These are the arteries which supply the heart itself with blood and should now be cleaned and studied. The coronary arteries and their larger branches

are lodged in fat which may fill the sulci on the external surface of the heart. Cleaning them involves the removal of much of this fat. The **cardiac veins,** which carry blood back to the right atrium from the heart wall, will be met at the same time, and the larger of these should also be studied. Nerve filaments will be found in association with the vessels; these belong to the **coronary plexus** of nerves and represent branches of distribution of the **cardiac plexus.** They should be noted but may be removed to faciliate cleaning of the vessels (Figs. 39 and 40).

The **right coronary artery** arises from the **right aortic sinus** behind the right border of the pulmonary artery. It runs downward and to the right in the **coronary sulcus** and then backward in the posterior part of the coronary sulcus where it terminates by anastomosing with the **left coronary.** At the upper end of the posterior longitudinal sulcus, it gives a large **posterior descending (interventricular) branch** which runs in that sulcus. Throughout its course, it gives branches which run downward over the wall of the ventricle and smaller branches which run upward in the wall of the right atrium. A large **right marginal branch** usually arises from it near the margo acutus. The **right coronary artery** carries blood mainly to the walls of the right atrium and right ventricle and, through its posterior interventricular branch, to the posterior half of the interventricular septum.

The **left coronary artery** arises from the left aortic sinus and passes to the left, behind the pulmonary artery in that portion of the coronary sulcus which lies in the **transverse sinus** of the **pericardium.** As it emerges from the left end of the transverse sinus, it is overlapped by the auricle of the left atrium and here divides into its two main branches, the anterior descending branch and the circumflex. The **anterior descending (interventricular) branch** runs downward and forward in the **anterior longitudinal sulcus,** giving numerous smaller branches to the sternocostal surface of the heart. The **circumflex branch** passes to the left and posteriorly in the **coronary sulcus** to anastomose with the terminal part of the right coronary. From it arise numerous branches to the left atrium and left ventricle and a **left marginal branch** of considerable size which follows the margo obtusus. The left coronary artery supplies most of the walls of the left atrium and left ventricle and the anterior half of the interventricular septum.

The **cardiac veins** return to the right atrium the blood carried to the heart wall by the coronary arteries. The largest of them is the **coronary sinus,** which is lodged in the posterior part of the coronary sulcus. It runs downward and to the right to terminate in the right atrium at the orifice which has already been seen in the interior of the atrium. The **great cardiac vein** runs upward in the **anterior longitudinal sulcus** and then around the left margin of the heart in the coronary sulcus to terminate in the coronary sinus, which may be regarded as its direct continuation. The **middle cardiac vein** ascends in the posterior longitudinal sulcus to join the coronary sinus near the termination of the latter; it is sometimes larger than the great cardiac vein. The **small cardiac vein** winds around the right margin of the heart in the coronary sulcus, to join the coronary sinus near its termination. The **anterior cardiac veins** are small veins which run upward on the right side of the anterior surface of the right ventricle. They may join the small cardiac vein or enter the right atrium directly. The **oblique vein** of the left atrium is a small channel which runs downward and to the right on the posterior surface of the left atrium to join the coronary sinus. It cannot always be demonstrated. It is of interest because it represents a remnant of the left superior vena cava of the embryo.

When study of the blood vessels supplying the heart wall is completed, the **right ventricle** should be opened. Make an incision beginning at the cut edge of the pulmonary artery and running downward through the anterior wall of the pulmonary artery and the right ventricle to the margo acutus; this incision should run parallel to the anterior longitudinal sulcus and about $\frac{1}{2}$ in. to its right side. From the lower end of this incision carry another incision to the right, parallel to and just above the margo acutus, to within $\frac{1}{4}$ in. of the coronary sulcus. By this means the right ventricle and the pulmonary artery together will be widely opened. Any blood which fills them should be washed out.

The walls of the **right ventricle** are anterior, inferior, and medial. The **anterior wall** corresponds to the sternocostal surface of the heart and the **inferior wall** to the diaphragmatic surface. The **medial wall,** which is actually posteromedial in position, is formed by the interventricular septum and separates the right ventricle from the left. This wall bulges forward and to the right, giving the cavity of the right ventricle a semilunar shape in transverse section. Almost the entire inner surface of the ventricle is thrown into irregular muscular ridges and bands, the **trabeculae carneae.** The cavity of the right ventricle narrows superiorly to become continuous with the **pulmonary artery.** The narrow superior portion of the right ventricle just below the pulmonary artery is known as the **conus arteriosus.** The conus, which is relatively free from trabeculae carneae, is marked off from the main ventricular cavity by a transverse muscular ridge on the septal wall of the ventricle, the **supraventricular crest.**

Posteriorly and to the right, the ventricle communicates with the right atrium. The **atrioventricular orifice** is surrounded by a ring of fibrous tissue, the **right anulus fibrosus.** The muscle fibers in the wall of the atrium are not continuous through this ring with the muscle fibers of the ventricular wall, but this fact cannot be demonstrated very well in the ordinary dissection. To the inner margin of the anulus fibrosus the **tricuspid** or **right atrioventricular valve** is attached.

The **tricuspid valve** is an annular sheet of fibrous tissue, covered on each of its surfaces by a layer of endocardium; it is attached peripherally to the **anulus fibrosus** and has a free margin projecting into the cavity of the ventricle. It is incompletely divided into **three flaps** or **cusps** by three notches in the free margin. The position of the cusps is usually as follows: the **anterior cusp** is in relation to the anterior sternocostal wall of the ventricle; the **posterior (inferior) cusp,** to the diaphragmatic wall; the **medial or septal cusp** is in relation to the medial wall. It should be observed that all three cusps are continuous with one another toward the anulus fibrosus and show a separation only near the free margin. Occasionally four cusps may be present.

Small fibrous strands will be seen running from the wall of the ventricle to attach to the free margin and to the ventricular surface of the tricuspid valve. These are the **chordae tendineae,** which serve to keep the cusps of the tricuspid valve from being forced back into the atrium when the ventricle contracts. Their attachment to the ventricular wall is at the **papillary muscles.** The papillary muscles are conical projections of the ventricular myocardium. The position of the papillary muscles of the right ventricle is not entirely constant. There is usually one large **anterior papillary** projecting into the ventricle from the anterior wall. From it, **chordae tendineae** run to the adjacent margins of the anterior and posterior cusps of the valve. There is usually a single, small **papillary muscle on** the **posterior wall of** the **conus arteriosus** just to the left of the supraventricular crest. This is known as the papillary of the conus and gives chordae tendineae to the anterior and septal cusps. Sometimes a large **posterior papillary muscle** is found projecting from the diaphragmatic wall, but more frequently this is represented by a group of

smaller posterior papillaries, from which chordae tendineae run to the septal and posterior cusps of the valve. The tricuspid valve serves to prevent the backflow of blood from the ventricle into the right atrium. Where blood enters the ventricle from the atrium, the valve is forced against the ventricular wall, leaving a wide opening. If, however, blood attempts to flow back through this opening, the pressure forces the free edges of the three cusps together into the lumen of the ventricle closing the atrioventricular orifice.

The orifice which leads from the conus arteriosus of the right ventricle into the pulmonary artery lies behind the edge of the sternum at about the level of the upper border of the third costal cartilage. It is guarded by the pulmonary semilunar valves, which should now be examined. These three valves are described as the **anterior, right,** and **left pulmonary semilunar valves,** and together they completely surround the pulmonary orifice internally. It should be observed that the anterior valve actually lies anteriorly and to the left and the right valve anteriorly and to the right, while the left valve is posterior in position. The anterior valve will probably have been injured when the ventricle was opened, but the structure of all three is similar. Each consists of a semilunar fold of fibrous tissue covered on both surfaces by an endothelial layer. One margin of each is attached to the wall of the pulmonary artery along a line convex toward the cavity of the ventricle. The other margin is free and projects into the lumen of the artery. When blood flows from the ventricle into the artery, the valves are forced against the walls of the vessel. If blood attempts to flow from the artery into the ventricle, the valves bulge into the lumen and the three free margins meet, closing the orifice. At the middle of each free margin is a small fibrocartilaginous body, the **nodulus.** When the valve is closed, the three noduli meet at the center of the lumen.

The **left atrium** may next be opened. This should be done by two incisions in the posterior wall of the atrium. The first should run from side to side across the posterior wall parallel to and just above the coronary sulcus. The other incision should be carried upward from the middle of the first to the upper border of the atrium; it will cut the posterior wall of the atrium longitudinally about halfway between the right and the left pulmonary veins. If it seems desirable to open the atrium still more widely, a third incision may be made transversely across the upper border of the atrium between the two upper pulmonary veins. The cavity of the atrium should be cleaned.

The wall of the left atrium is smooth throughout, except in the auricle, where muscular ridges and strands are apparent. The auricle communicates with the main cavity of the atrium at its upper left side, just in front of the opening of the upper left pulmonary vein. The four **pulmonary veins** open directly into the atrium without valves. Below and to the left, the atrium communicates with the left ventricle by the **left atrioventricular or mitral orifice,** which is somewhat smaller than the tricuspid orifice.

To the right and anteriorly, the wall of the left atrium is formed by the **atrial septum.** At the anterior part of this wall, a shallow semilunar depression will be seen, bounded posteriorly by a low ridge which corresponds in position to the **fossa ovalis** in the right atrium. An attempt should now be made to pass a blunt probe from the fossa ovalis of the right atrium forward and to the left through the atrial septum into the left atrium. In about 25 per cent of cases, a narrow passageway remains patent in this location in the adult, a remnant of the **foramen ovale** of the fetus. Such a passage is not necessarily attended by any symptoms of disease during life, since the pressure of the blood in the two atria keeps its walls in apposition.

The **left ventricle** is next to be studied. It and the ascending aorta can be opened together by a single incision. Enter the scalpel just below the coronary sulcus and carry it downward through the wall of the left ventricle along a line lying slightly to the left of the anterior longitudinal sulcus to the apex of the heart. The same incision should then be continued upward from the point at which it was begun, through the coronary sulcus and the wall of the ascending aorta. This incision will cut the circumflex branch of the left coronary artery near its origin, where that vessel lies in the coronary sulcus; it will pass upward through the base of the ascending aorta just behind the origin of the left coronary artery and then straight upward to the cut end of the aorta. The ascending aorta and the left ventricle may then be spread open, cleaned of blood, and studied.

It will be observed that the **wall of** the **left ventricle,** except at the apex, is much thicker than is that of the right. The cavity of the ventricle is roughly conical in outline, the apex of the cone being represented by the apex of the heart, and its base by the atrioventricular and aortic orifices together, the latter lying in front and slightly to the right of the former. The **ventricular wall** is covered throughout by **trabeculae carneae,** except in its upper anterior part, which leads to the aortic orifice and is known as the **aortic vestibule.** The anterior and right portion of the wall is formed by the interventricular septum, so that the left ventricle lies not only to the left of, but also behind, the right ventricle.

The **left atrioventricular orifice** lies behind the left side of the sternum at about the level of the fourth costal cartilage. Like the right orifice, it is surrounded by a fibrous ring, the **left anulus fibrosus,** through which there is no continuity between the atrial and the ventricular musculature. The orifice is guarded by the **mitral or biscuspid valve** which is essentially similar to the tricuspid valve in structure, with the difference that it ordinarily has only two cusps. These **cusps are anterior and posterior in position.** Like the cusps of the tricuspid valve, they are prevented from being forced into the atrium by **chordae tendineae,** which run from the papillary muscles to the free margins and ventricular surfaces of the cusps. In most cases, two very large papillary muscles will be found in the left ventricle. One of these springs from the lower part of the septal wall of the ventricle and the other from the dia-

lunar valves already examined, but it should be observed that they are much stronger. In position they correspond to the aortic sinuses and are similarly named. One of the valves may have been cut in opening the ventricle. Above the **right valve** on the inner wall of the aorta will be seen the orifice of the right coronary artery; above the **left valve** is the orifice of the left coronary artery. The **posterior valve** is in close relation to the anterior cusp of the mitral valve (Fig. 42).

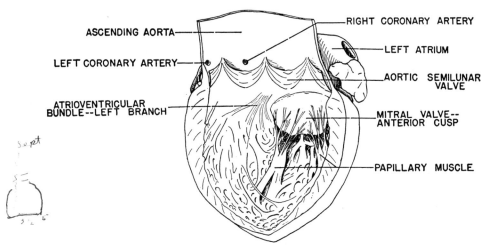

ASCENDING AORTA

LEFT CORONARY ARTERY

ATRIOVENTRICULAR BUNDLE--LEFT BRANCH

RIGHT CORONARY ARTERY

LEFT ATRIUM

AORTIC SEMILUNAR VALVE

MITRAL VALVE-- ANTERIOR CUSP

PAPILLARY MUSCLE

FIG. 42. The interior of the left ventricle of the heart.

phragmatic wall; from each of them chordae tendineae pass to both cusps of the valve. It should be noted that while a considerable portion of the right ventricular cavity intervenes between the tricuspid and pulmonary orifices, the only structure separating the mitral orifice from the aortic orifice is the **anterior cusp of** the **mitral valve.**

The **aortic orifice** lies behind the left side of the sternum at about the level of the third intercostal space. It leads from the upper anterior part of the **left ventricle** into the **ascending aorta** and is posterior to the conus arteriosus of the right ventricle. It is guarded by the three **aortic semilunar valves.** In details of structure, these valves are similar to the pulmonary semi-

Certain features of the **interventricular septum** deserve particular attention. It will be observed that the septum is for the most part **thick and muscular.** A small portion of it, however, is thin in character, the **membranous part** of the **interventricular septum.** This is the upper posterior part of the septum and, in the left ventricle, lies just below and between the right and the posterior aortic semilunar valves. If the septum is held up to strong light, the extreme thinness of this part of it can be very easily demonstrated. It should be noted further that the membranous part of the septum is not entirely interventricular. Inferiorly it separates the left and right ventricles, but its highest part lies between the left ventricle and the right atrium, since the peripheral attachment of the septal cusp of the tricuspid valve crosses its right side.

It has been observed that the myocardium of the atria is not continuous with that of the ventricles but is interrupted by the anuli fibrosi. Conduction of impulses from the atrial musculature to the ventricular musculature is accomplished by the **atrioventricular bundle,** a branched bundle of **specialized cardiac muscle.** The **central point** or **node** of this bundle lies just behind the membranous part of the interventricular septum, in the region where the left and right anuli fibrosi meet. It receives strands of **specialized muscle fibers from the walls of both atria** and gives a **branch to each ventricle.** The bundle as a whole cannot be satisfactorily demonstrated in the ordinary cadaver heart, but the left branch can frequently be seen without dissection, spreading downward over the septal wall of the left ventricle, immediately subjacent to the endocardium, through which it is often plainly visible. Individual strands from this branch, covered only by a layer of endocardium, sometimes bridge across the lower part of the cavity of the ventricle to reach the posterior papillary muscle. They have been called the **false chordae tendineae,** since they resemble the chordae in appearance, though not in structure or function.

Trachea, Bronchi, and Lungs

The next step in the dissection is the study of the **trachea** and the removal of the lower part of the trachea, the two **lungs,** and the **pleurae** from the body. First strip the remains of the pericardium from the cut ends of the aorta, the pulmonary artery, and the superior vena cava; it is well to remove completely all the pericardium above the level of the upper pulmonary veins. The superior vena cava should then be turned laterally to the right, and the arch of the aorta turned laterally to the left. To do this, it will be necessary to cut the

brachiocephalic artery slightly above its origin; the brachiocephalic may then be left in place against the trachea and the arch of the aorta, with the left common carotid and left subclavian arteries still attached, swung over to the left side, thus exposing the lower part of the trachea and the right pulmonary artery (Fig. 43).

The **trachea** divides into the **right** and **left bronchi** at the carina, about the level of the fifth thoracic vertebra, each bronchus then passing downward and laterally into the root of the corresponding lung. The **pulmonary artery** divides into **right** and **left branches** in front of the **left bronchus.** By replacing the aortic arch in position, it can be demonstrated that the left bronchus and the right branch of the pulmonary artery lie under the arch. The **deep cardiac plexus** will be found in front of the lowest part of the trachea between that structure and the right pulmonary artery. In cleaning the lower part of the trachea and the bronchi, groups of large **tracheal** and **bronchial lymph nodes** will be met. These are usually blackened by the deposition in them of carbon particles removed from the air in the lungs. When their position has been noted, they should be removed. Observe that the **left bronchus** makes a sharper angle with the trachea than does the right. The right pulmonary artery may be cut through near its origin from the main trunk if the extrapulmonary portions of the bronchi cannot be satisfactorily cleaned while the pulmonary artery is intact.

Attempt to identify the **bronchial vessels** before the lungs and trachea are removed. The origin, course, and distribution of these vessels are described subsequently.

The two lungs, together with the lower part of the trachea, the pulmonary artery and its branches, the pulmonary veins, and the remnants of the pleura are now to be removed together. First cut through the **ligamentum**

arteriosum, which connects the pulmonary trunk to the undersurface of the arch of the aorta. The **recurrent branch of the left vagus** turns upward behind this ligament on the inner surface of the aortic arch to reach the groove between the trachea and esophagus; care should be taken not to injure it. Cut through the

dium from them or by cutting through each of the veins again just external to the pericardium. Next, separate the parietal pleura completely from the thoracic wall wherever it may still be attached by introducing the hand between the external surface of the pleura and the thoracic wall. In most cases, it will strip off very readily

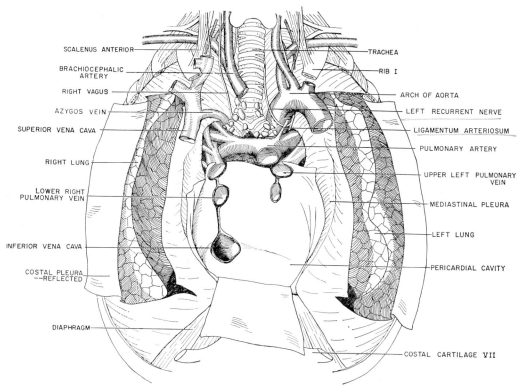

FIG. 43. Dissection of the thoracic cavity, after removal of the heart. The arch of the aorta has been turned to the left and the superior vena cava to the right.

trachea, transversely, about 2 in. above its bifurcation. The **esophagus** lies immediately behind the trachea, to which it is loosely attached by areolar tissue. Consequently, some care is necessary to avoid cutting the esophagus at the same time as the trachea. Pull the lower cut portion of the trachea forward and separate its posterior surface from the anterior surface of the esophagus. Next, free the cut ends of the **pulmonary veins** from the pericardium. This may be done either by stripping the pericar-

except in the case of the diaphragmatic pleura. This may be left in place and the remainder of the parietal pleura cut away from it with the knife. The trachea, bronchi, lungs, pulmonary artery and veins, and pleurae are held in place only by a little areolar tissue, and the whole complex of structures should be removed together from the body. In separating the **left bronchus** from the posterior part of the arch and the beginning of the descending aorta, be careful not to injure the **left vagus nerve,** which runs downward behind the bronchus to come into relation with the esophagus. Behind the **right bronchus, the right vagus** and the **azygos vein** are apt to be injured if care is not taken. Cut the left bronchus and pulmonary vessels transversely to separate the lungs.

The lungs may now be studied outside the body. The remains of the parietal pleura should be cut away along the lines of reflection between visceral and parietal pleurae and discarded. The surfaces of each lung are **costal, mediastinal,** and **diaphragmatic**. A sharp **inferior border** (margin) separates the diaphragmatic surface from the costal and mediastinal surfaces. Anteriorly, the costal and mediastinal surfaces are separated from each other by a sharp **anterior border** (margin). Posteriorly, there is not so distinct a border separating the mediastinal from the costal surface. The portion of the costal surface which lies immediately posterior to the mediastinal surface is in relation, not to the ribs, but to the sides, of the bodies of the vertebrae. The remainder of the costal surface is in relation to the ribs and intercostal spaces; it is very extensive and convex. The greatest posterior extent of the lung, as well as its greatest convexity, is on this surface along a line corresponding to the angles of the successive ribs. The mediastinal surface is related through the mediastinal pleura with the various structures of the mediastinum, and the mediastinal surface of each lung shows characteristic grooves and ridges corresponding to the mediastinal structures adjacent to it. The anterior margin of the left lung is indented by a wide **cardiac notch** (incisura) corresponding to the protrusion of the apex of the heart to the left side. Each lung is marked anteriorly a little below its apex by a **groove** (sulcus) caused **by the subclavian artery.**

The **lungs** are divided into **lobes** by **interlobar fissures.** These fissures cut through the substance of the lung from the periphery almost to the root. Unfortunately, they are often

difficult to demonstrate in the cadaver, since adhesions between the opposing surfaces of the lobes, partially or wholly obliterating the fissures, are very frequent. The **primary fissure** of each lung lies in an oblique plane running downward and anteriorly from the posterior aspect a little below the apex to the anterior part of the diaphragmatic surface. The **left lung** has only **two lobes, upper** and **lower,** separated by this fissure. In the **right lung,** there is a **second fissure** running nearly horizontally backward and laterally from the anterior border at about the level of the fourth chondrosternal junction to meet the main fissure. The **right lung** thus possesses **upper, middle,** and **lower lobes,** the upper and middle lobes together corresponding to the upper lobe of the left lung.

The **hilus of** each **lung** is the region on its mediastinal aspect where the structures comprising the **root of** the **lung** enter it. The principal structures entering the hilus of each lung are the **bronchus,** the **pulmonary artery,** and the **pulmonary veins.** Observe that the pulmonary veins are the most anterior in position and the bronchus is most posterior. The bronchi and the vessels should be followed into the lungs by dissecting away the lung substance.

Each **bronchus** is continued downward and laterally to the base of the lungs as the **stem bronchus.** From the stem bronchus arise a series of branches which are distributed to the various lobes and from the lobar bronchi, segmental bronchi for the various bronchopulmonary segments. The names and locations of the **bronchopulmonary segments** should be reviewed in one of the standard anatomical texts, since they are of importance in diagnosis and surgery of various diseases of the lungs. Near the hilus, the pulmonary artery crosses the bronchus anteriorly to reach a position posterolateral to the stem bronchus, which position it retains throughout the rest of its course. The first branch of the **right bronchus** is known as the **eparterial bronchus,** since it arises above the point at which the right pulmonary artery crosses the bronchus. The eparterial bronchus is distributed to the **upper lobe of** the **right lung** and is accompanied by a branch of the right pulmonary artery and a tributary of the right superior pulmonary vein. The remaining branches of the right bronchus are known as **hyparterial bronchi,** since they arise below the crossing of the pulmonary artery. The larger ones run anteriorly (ventrally) or posteriorly (dorsally) from the stem bronchus, and the ventral and dorsal branches usually arise alternately. The **first hyparterial bronchus** is ventral and is distributed to the **middle lobe;** it is accompanied by a branch of the artery and a tributary of the upper right pulmonary vein. The **remaining hyparterial branches** are distributed to the **lower lobe** and are accompanied by branches of the artery and tributaries of the lower vein.

There is no eparterial bronchus in the **left lung.** The first hyparterial bronchus is quite large; it is distributed to the **upper lobe** and is accompanied by a branch of the left pulmonary artery and the upper left pulmonary vein. The remaining branches of the stem bronchus are distributed to the **lower lobe,** accompanied by branches of the artery and tributaries of the lower left vein.

The **pulmonary artery** carries **venous blood** to the lungs for aeration, after which it is returned to the heart by the **pulmonary veins.** The function of the **bronchial arteries** is to supply **arterial blood** to the lung substance itself. They should be looked for on the posterior aspect of the bronchi, the ramifications of which they follow in their distribution to the lungs. There are usually **two bronchial arteries in** the **left lung** and **one in** the **right.** The origin of the bronchial arteries will, of course, have been torn away in the removal of the lungs. The **left** ones arise from the upper part of the **descending aorta;** the **right** may

arise from the **descending aorta** or from one of its **upper right intercostal branches,** or the **subclavian** or **internal thoracic** arteries.

Posterior Mediastinum

The **posterior mediastinum** and the deeper structures of the superior mediastinum should now be studied. Cut through the azygos vein at its termination in the superior vena cava and remove the remnants of the superior vena cava and the brachiocephalic veins. Remove any remnants of the parietal pleura which may remain adhering to the thoracic wall, with the exception that the diaphragmatic pleura may be left on the diaphragm. All of the pericardium except its diaphragmatic portion should also be removed. The removal of the portion of the parietal pericardium which formed the posterior wall of the oblique sinus will expose the lower part of the esophagus. The **esophagus** should be cleaned and studied. In cleaning the esophagus expose but do not injure the **esophageal plexus;** this is a plexus of nerves derived from the **two vagi** which is in intimate relation to the external surface of the esophagus (Fig. 44).

The **esophagus** is flattened to present anterior and posterior surfaces. It enters the thorax through the **superior thoracic aperture.** In the superior mediastinum, it lies behind the trachea and in front of the bodies of the vertebrae. In the upper part of the posterior mediastinum, the descending aorta lies to its left side and slightly posterior to it. More inferiorly, the esophagus inclines slightly forward and toward the left so that it comes to lie in front of the aorta; it leaves the thoracic cavity by passing through an aperture in the **muscular part of** the **diaphragm** at about the level of the tenth thoracic vertebra.

The course of the two vagi in the posterior mediastinum should now be traced. After descending behind the left bronchus, the **left vagus** crosses in front of the descending aorta to reach the anterior surface of the esophagus, where it breaks up to form the **anterior part of** the **esophageal plexus.** The **right vagus** passes downward across the medial aspect of the arch of the azygos vein to reach the posterior surface of the esophagus, where it breaks up to

anterior wall of the esophagus and observe that the lumen appears in section as a slitlike aperture, corresponding to the anteroposterior flattening of the organ.

Then free and elevate the esophagus from the underlying structures.

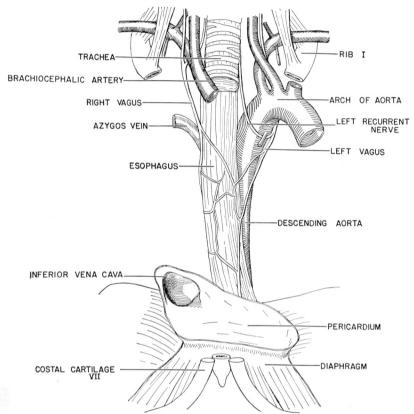

FIG. 44. Semidiagrammatic representation of the more anterior structures of the posterior mediastinum. The arch of the aorta has been turned to the left.

form the **posterior part of** the **esophageal plexus.** The anterior and posterior parts of the plexus communicate freely with each other around the borders of the esophagus. A short distance above the diaphragm the plexus is usually resolved again into the **main trunks of** the **two vagi.** As they pass through the **esophageal hiatus of** the **diaphragm,** the left vagus lies on the anterior aspect of the esophagus and the right vagus on its posterior aspect.

Make a longitudinal incision through the

Clean and study the **descending aorta.** It begins at the left side of the fibrocartilage between the fourth and fifth thoracic vertebrae as a continuation of the arch of the aorta and lies entirely in the **posterior mediastinum.** In its descent through the posterior mediastinum, it inclines slightly forward and to the right and leaves the thorax through the **aortic orifice of** the **diaphragm** (hiatus aorticus) which lies in the median plane in front of the first lumbar vertebra. The only branches arising from its

Ant. = bron.
media.
esoph.

anterior aspect are the **bronchial arteries**, of which mention has already been made, and a variable number of small **esophageal** and **mediastinal branches**. If the descending aorta is pulled forward, a series of **paired aortic intercostal branches** will be seen arising from its

common carotid, left subclavian arteries, and the arch of the aorta. Then clean the sympathetic trunks (Fig. 45).

Each **sympathetic trunk** begins in the **neck** and is continued through the **thorax** into the **abdomen** and **pelvis**. It will be found passing

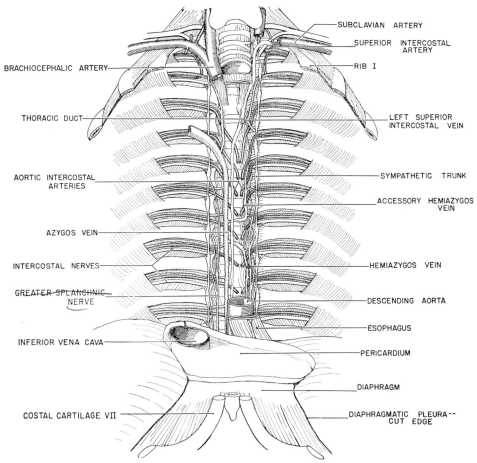

FIG. 45. Dissection of the posterior thoracic wall, showing the deeper structures of the posterior mediastinum.

posterior aspect. There are usually nine pairs of aortic intercostals, one for each pair of intercostal spaces beginning with the third.

The posterior intercostal arteries, the azygos system of veins, the proximal portions of the intercostal nerves, and the thoracic portions of the sympathetic nerve trunks should now be studied together. Free and elevate the left

through the superior thoracic aperture in front of the head of the first rib and running downward through the thorax in front of the heads of the ribs in the areolar tissue just external to the parietal pleura. In the lower part of the thorax, it inclines slightly forward, coming to lie against the sides of the bodies of the vertebrae. It leaves the thorax by passing behind the diaphragm. A series of **ganglionic enlargements** occur along its course. These ganglia generally lie against the heads of the ribs; the first thoracic ganglion is sometimes fused with the lowest cervical ganglion to form a **large stellate ganglion.** Identify the **greater splanchnic nerve.** This large nerve arises from the sympathetic trunk by a series of roots, usually three but frequently more, which pass forward and downward along the sides of the vertebrae. The roots join to form the greater splanchnic nerve, which passes downward through the posterior muscular part of the diaphragm. The **lesser splanchnic nerve** runs forward and downward from the sympathetic trunk at a lower level; it also passes through the diaphragm slightly posterior to the greater splanchnic nerve. Each of the **thoracic ganglia** usually communicates with the corresponding **intercostal nerve** by two small posteriorly directed branches, the **grey** and **white rami communicantes.**

The **intercostal nerves** are the anterior primary divisions of the first 11 pairs of thoracic spinal nerves; one will be found in each **intercostal space** emerging from the posterior aspect of the bodies of the vertebrae between the heads of the adjacent ribs. They should be followed laterally in the intercostal spaces, where it will be observed that they lie on the internal surfaces of the external intercostal muscles, which extend as far medially as the heads of the ribs. It should be noted that the **internal intercostal muscles** extend medially only as far as the angles of the ribs and here the intercostal nerves pass out of sight by continuing laterally between the internal and intima intercostal muscles. Each intercostal nerve is accompanied by an **intercostal vein** and an **intercostal artery** throughout its course; the nerve is usually the most inferior in position and the vein the most superior of the three structures.

The **posterior intercostal arteries** of the first two intercostal spaces are usually derived from the **costocervical branch of** the **subclavian.** The superior intercostal branch of the costocervical trunk will be found descending in front of the neck of the first rib; it gives a branch to the first intercostal space and usually continues downward over the neck of the second rib to end as the intercostal artery of the second space. The posterior intercostal arteries of the lower spaces are branches of the **descending aorta.** Observe that the upper aortic intercostals run upward as well as laterally across the bodies of the vertebrae to reach the spaces they supply. As they cross the bodies of the vertebrae and the heads of the ribs, the right aortic intercostals cross the posterior or external aspects of the thoracic duct, azygos vein, and right sympathetic trunk; the left aortic intercostals have a similar relation to the hemiazygos or accessory hemiazygos vein and the left sympathetic trunk.

The thoracic duct and azygos system of veins should be studied next. Dissect the descending aorta free from the surrounding connective tissue and then retract it outward, cutting, if necessary, some of the aortic intercostal arteries to facilitate the retraction of the aorta. Then clean the thoracic duct.

The **thoracic duct,** which drains all the lymph from the inferior extremities, pelvis, abdomen, thorax, left upper extremity, and left side of the head, is a small, very thin-walled vessel, usually white or grey in color. It enters the thorax through the **aortic orifice of** the **diaphragm,** in which it lies behind and to the right of the aorta, and ascends in the midline through the **posterior mediastinum,** where it lies in front of the bodies of the vertebrae and right aortic intercostal arteries and behind the esophagus. In the **superior mediastinum,** it bends to the left, emerging from behind the left side of the esophagus to come into relation with the left pleura; it continues upward into the root of the neck, where it arches across the dome of the pleura to terminate in the origin of the **left brachiocephalic vein** or the termination of the **left subclavian** or **left internal jugular vein.**

The azygos system of veins consists of the azygos, hemiazygos, and accessory hemiazygos veins, the longitudinal channels into which most of the intercostal veins are drained. The **azygos vein** is a continuation of the **right ascending lumbar vein** of the abdomen; it enters the thorax through the **hiatus aorticus,** where it lies to the right of and behind the aorta and to the right of the thoracic duct. It ascends through the **posterior mediastinum** along the right side of the fronts of the bodies of the vertebrae to about the level of the fourth thoracic vertebra, where it arches forward over the root of the right lung to enter the **superior vena cava.** It receives all the right intercostal veins except the first. The veins from the second, third, and fourth spaces, however, usually do not enter the azygos directly but unite to form a common trunk known as the right superior intercostal vein, which descends along the bodies of the upper vertebrae to reach the azygos. The intercostal vein of the first space usually drains into the brachiocephalic vein of its own side or into one of the tributaries of the brachiocephalic.

The drainage of the intercostal spaces of the left side is subject to a great deal of minor variation, and no precise description can be given to fit all cases. In the majority of cases, the left superior intercostal vein, the terminal part of which was seen at an earlier stage of the dissection crossing the left side of the arch of the aorta to terminate in the left brachiocephalic vein, receives the intercostal veins of the second, third, and fourth spaces. The **hemiazygos vein** is a continuation of the **left ascending lumbar vein;** it enters the thorax by passing through the **muscular substance of** the **diaphragm** and will be found ascending in the **posterior mediastinum** in front of the left sides of the lower thoracic vertebrae and behind the left side of the aorta to about the level of the eighth vertebra. Here it turns to the right behind the aorta and thoracic duct to enter the **azygos;** it receives the intercostal veins of the lower four or five spaces. The veins from the spaces between those drained by the **hemiazygos** and those drained by the **left superior intercostal vein** are drained by the **accessory hemiazygos.** This is a longitudinal channel in line with the hemiazygos but at a higher level. Superiorly, it frequently communicates with the **left superior intercostal vein;** inferiorly, it may join the **hemiazygos** or may cross the vertebral column to join the **azygos** independently of the hemiazygos.

Abdomen ·

Abdominal Wall

Before starting the dissection of the anterior abdominal wall, the surface landmarks should be observed. A glance at a skeleton will make it apparent that the **bony wall of** the **abdominal** cavity is much less complete than is that of the thoracic cavity. Superiorly, due to the dome-like shape of the diaphragm, the abdominal cavity is protected by the **lower ribs,** and inferiorly the **coxal (hip) bones** help to form its wall, but, in the region between, the only skeletal support of the abdominal wall is contributed by the **lumbar vertebrae.**

The **costal arch,** corresponding to the lower borders of the seventh to tenth costal cartilages on each side, can usually be seen and felt from the surface. At the apex of the arch, a depression is found on the surface of the body, corresponding to the **xiphoid process of** the **sternum.** Below, on each side, the **anterior superior iliac spine** should be identified. Running backward and somewhat upward from the spine, the **iliac crest** can be readily palpated. In the midline below, the **pubic symphysis** can be felt, usually through a fairly heavy covering of fat; a little distance lateral to it on each side a sharp bony projection, the **pubic tubercle,** should be located. Stretching between the pubic tubercle and the anterior superior iliac spine and separating the abdomen from the thigh, a curved linear depression is usually apparent. This corresponds to the line of the **inguinal ligament.** Another linear depression stretches downward in the midline from the xiphoid process toward the pubis. This corresponds to the **linea alba.** On this line, nearer to the pubis than to the sternum, is the **umbilicus** or navel. In well-developed subjects, another depressed line can be seen on each side, 3 or 4 in. lateral to the linea alba and parallel to it above but turning medially below. This indicates the position of the **linea semilunaris,** the lateral border of the rectus abdominis muscle.

When these points have been identified, the following incisions should be made through the skin: (1) in the midline, from the junction of the body with the xiphoid process of the sternum downward to the pubic symphysis (This incision must encircle the edge of the umbilicus.), (2) from the upper end of the first incision, laterally and slightly downward across the body wall to the posterior axillary line, (3) from the lower end of the first incision, laterally along the pubic crest to the pubic tubercle

and then laterally and upward along the line of the inguinal ligament and for about 2 in. along the line of the iliac crest. The large quadrilateral flap of skin thus mapped out should now be reflected laterally on each side to expose the superficial fascia of the abdominal wall.

On its external aspect, the **superficial fascia** of the anterior abdominal wall does not differ appreciably from the same layer in other parts of the body, with the exception that in obese subjects it is extremely thick. Identify and dissect the **superficial epigastric, superficial circumflex iliac, umbilical, and thoracoepigastric veins** within the superficial fascia. Some or all of these veins become enlarged, if the main venous channels within the abdomen are occluded, to serve as collateral pathways for the return of venous blood around the site of occlusion. The size and course of these superficial veins may vary, but, as a general rule, they connect the superficial veins of the inguinal region with those around the umbilicus or with the intercostal or axillary veins.

Cut through the entire thickness of the superficial fascia in a straight line running transversely from one anterior superior iliac spine to the other. In making this incision, be careful not to cut through the **aponeurosis of** the **external oblique muscle** or the **sheath of** the **rectus muscle,** which lie immediately subjacent to the superficial fascia; when these have been reached, they may be recognized by their light, glistening appearance. All the superficial fascia above this transverse incision should now be entirely removed to expose the upper part of the rectus sheath and the external oblique muscle. As the fascia is being removed, watch for the cutaneous nerves and vessels of the anterior abdominal wall. The **anterior cutaneous nerves and vessels,** which are the terminal portions of the lower intercostal nerves and vessels, pierce the rectus sheath in series from above downward 1 in. or so lateral to the

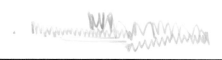

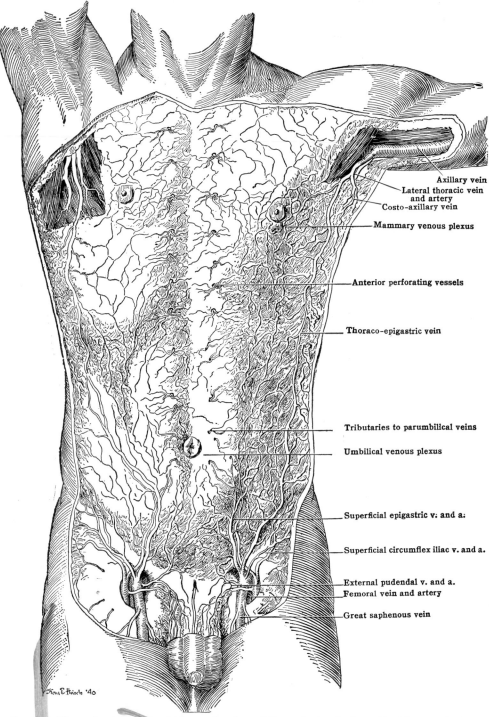

Axillary vein
Lateral thoracic vein
and artery
Costo-axillary vein

Mammary venous plexus

Anterior perforating vessels

Thoraco-epigastric vein

Tributaries to parumbilical veins

Umbilical venous plexus

Superficial epigastric v. and a.

Superficial circumflex iliac v. and a.

External pudendal v. and a.
Femoral vein and artery

Great saphenous vein

Fig. 46. The subcutaneous arteries and veins of the anterior body wall. (*By permission from Schaeffer (ed.), "Morris' Human Anatomy," 11/e, McGraw-Hill Book Company, Inc., Blakiston Division, New York, 1953.*)

linea alba; running downward and forward over the lateral part of the external oblique muscle will be found the **lateral cutaneous branches** of the same nerves and vessels.

The superficial fascia on the lower part of the anterior abdominal wall, where it still remains in place, is peculiar in that it may be separated into a superficial and a deep layer artificially by dissection. Microscopic sections of the subcutaneous tissue in this area show that it is similar in structure to the subcutaneous tissue in other parts of the body, which is known to consist of only one layer.* Present evidence also indicates that Camper and Scarpa did not describe the layers with which their names are now associated. Since the old concepts of Camper's and Scarpa's fasciae are still taught by many anatomists and clinicians, an attempt should be made to identify what these layers were considered to be. The **superficial layer,** known as the **fascia of Camper,** is much the thicker; it exhibits the usual characteristics of the panniculus adiposus and is directly continuous below the line of the inguinal ligament with the superficial fascia of the thigh. The **deeper layer, the fascia of Scarpa,** which lies just external to the lower part of the aponeurosis of the external oblique muscle, is more **membranous** in character and ends immediately below the inguinal ligament by fusing with the deep fascia (fascia lata) of the thigh. Medial to the pubic tubercle it is continued downward over the scrotum, of which it forms the dartos layer, and posteriorly over the urogenital triangle of the perineum.

Make a median vertical incision as far down as the pubic symphysis, through the superficial fascia on the lower part of the abdominal wall. The triangular flaps of fascia thus marked out should be reflected downward and laterally on each side toward the inguinal ligament. Scarpa's and Camper's fasciae should be re-

* Based on the observations of Tobin and Benjamin (*Surg. Gynec. & Obst.,* **88:** 545, 1949).

flected together as a single layer. Scarpa's fascia was formerly described as the membranous stratum, usually reddish in color, on the deep surface of the reflected flap. The reflection can be continued only a very short distance beyond the inguinal ligament, because this fascia here blends with the fascia lata. With removal of the fascia, the **external oblique muscle** and the **rectus sheath** will be completely exposed. At the same time, the **subcutaneous (superficial) inguinal ring** and a portion of the **spermatic cord** (round ligament in the female) will be uncovered. In series with the cutaneous nerves already exposed on the upper part of the abdominal wall, look for the terminal **cutaneous portions of** the **iliohypogastric** and the **ilioinguinal nerves,** which are derived from the first lumbar nerve. The former pierces the aponeurosis of the external oblique, often as two separate branches, a short distance above the inguinal ligament; the latter emerges through the superficial inguinal ring with the spermatic cord. In dissecting the ilioinguinal nerves, try not to destroy the external spermatic fascia.

Observe the **linea alba.** This is a dense aponeurotic band, running from the **xiphoid process** to the **pubic symphysis** and intervening between the two recti muscles. The recti cannot be seen at present, as each is hidden by the thick anterior layer of its aponeurotic sheath. The **linea semilunaris** is the line which marks the **lateral border of** the **rectus muscle** and the line along which the sheath becomes continuous with the aponeuroses of the three muscles which make up the lateral part of the anterior abdominal wall. The most superficial of these, the external oblique, should now be studied.

The **external oblique muscle** arises by eight fleshy slips from the outer surfaces of the **lower eight ribs** just lateral to their junctions with their costal cartilages. The upper slips are closely related to the serratus anterior and the lower to the latissimus dorsi. The fibers arising from the lower two or three ribs run downward to be inserted into the anterior third of the **outer lip of** the **iliac crest.** The remaining fibers are not inserted into bone but run downward and forward to end in a broad sheet of fascia known as the aponeurosis of the external oblique. Medial to the linea semilunaris the **aponeurosis of** the **external oblique** is continued to the **linea alba** as one of the constituents of the **anterior layer of** the **sheath of** the **rectus abdominis muscle.** Between the **anterior superior spine of** the **ilium** and the **pubic tubercle,** the inferior border of the aponeurosis is thickened to form the **inguinal ligament.**

Define and observe the **superficial inguinal ring.** This is an opening in the aponeurosis of the external oblique just above the medial end of the inguinal ligament; through it the **spermatic cord** (round ligament in the female) emerges from the inguinal canal. The edges of the superficial inguinal ring are fairly thick and are known as the **superior (medial) crus** and the **inferior (lateral) crus.** A short distance cephalad to these crura, note some fibers running at about a right angle to the course of the fibers in the aponeurosis of the external oblique. These are the **intercrural** fibers (Fig. 47). The **inguinal canal** is an oblique passageway through the lower part of the anterior abdominal wall; through this canal, the spermatic cord passes in its course from the interior of the **abdominal cavity to** the **scrotum.**

The superficial inguinal ring is not an actual opening in the aponeurosis of the external oblique until it is made so by dissecting away the **external spermatic fascia.** This fascia is the **outermost covering of** the **spermatic cord** and may be regarded as an extension over the cord, downward into the scrotum, of the external oblique aponeurosis. It is a much thinner layer than the aponeurosis, with which it is continuous around the lips of the superficial inguinal ring (Fig. 47).

The rectus abdominis muscle should now

be studied. To open the rectus sheath, make a longitudinal incision through its exposed anterior portion, parallel and just lateral to the linea alba, from a point just below the xiphoid process of the sternum to a point just above the pubic symphysis. From each end of this incision carry a transverse incision laterally to the linea semilunaris. Observe that above the upper transverse incision the anterior part of the rectus sheath becomes much thinner and blends with the fascia of the pectoralis major muscle. The thin portion of the sheath above the upper transverse incision should be removed and the flap marked out by the three incisions turned laterally to expose the anterior surface of the rectus muscle.

First observe whether or not the **pyramidalis muscle** is present. This small triangular muscle, which is totally lacking in about one-fifth of all cases, lies in front of the lower part of the rectus. It arises from the upper border of the **body of** the **pubis*** and is inserted into the **linea alba** for a varying distance between the symphysis and umbilicus. Next study the rectus. The **rectus abdominis is** a broad flat muscle enclosed in an aponeurotic fascial sheath. It arises from the upper border of the **body of** the **pubis** and the **anterior surface of** the **symphysis** and is inserted upon the anterior surfaces of the fifth, sixth, and seventh **costal cartilages** and the **xiphoid process** of the sternum. Observe its **tendinous inscriptions.** These are irregular transverse tendinous bands, usually three in number, which cross the muscle, and are quite firmly attached to the anterior part of the sheath.

Detach the rectus from the linea alba; elevate and transect this muscle by a transverse incision at the level of the umbilicus, and turn the muscle lateralward to expose the posterior layer of its sheath. This must be done

---

* The term **body of** the **pubis** refers to that part of the pubic bone near the symphysis rather than that part related to the acetabulum.

with care, since there are other structures enclosed within the posterior part of the sheath that must be cleaned and studied as the muscle is being reflected. These are the terminal parts of the lower intercostal nerves and the superior

the rectus, which muscle they supply, and branches of them finally pierce the anterior layer of the sheath, where they have already been seen as the **anterior cutaneous nerves of** the **abdominal wall.**

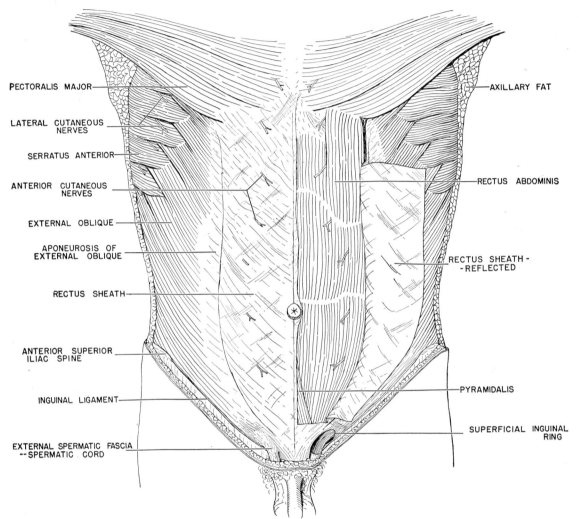

PECTORALIS MAJOR

LATERAL CUTANEOUS NERVES

SERRATUS ANTERIOR

ANTERIOR CUTANEOUS NERVES

EXTERNAL OBLIQUE

APONEUROSIS OF EXTERNAL OBLIQUE

RECTUS SHEATH

ANTERIOR SUPERIOR ILIAC SPINE

INGUINAL LIGAMENT

EXTERNAL SPERMATIC FASCIA --SPERMATIC CORD

AXILLARY FAT

RECTUS ABDOMINIS

RECTUS SHEATH - -REFLECTED

PYRAMIDALIS

SUPERFICIAL INGUINAL RING

FIG. 47. Superficial dissection of abdominal wall. Anterior sheath has been reflected to expose the rectus abdominis, and the external spermatic fascia removed to show the borders, medial and lateral crura, of the superficial inguinal ring on one side. Note the intercrural fibers cephalad to the superficial ring.

and inferior epigastric arteries. The **lower** five **intercostal nerves** pierce the posterior layer of the rectus sheath in longitudinal series near its lateral margin. They enter the deep surface of

The **superior epigastric artery** is one of the terminal branches of the **internal thoracic.** It enters the rectus sheath by passing downward behind the seventh costal cartilage. It enters the deep surface of the muscle. The **inferior epigastric artery** is a branch of the **external iliac artery.** Its origin will be seen somewhat later in the dissection. It enters the lower lateral part of the rectus sheath and runs upward between the muscle and the posterior layer of the sheath, finally entering the muscle to anastomose with the superior epigastric. Occasionally a continuous anastomosing channel may be found connecting the two epigastric arteries on the deep surface of the rectus. Both arteries are accompanied by veins.

Observe that the **posterior layer of** the **rectus sheath** is **thicker** and tougher **above** than below. In many cases, a **sharp inferior margin** may be seen about halfway between the umbilicus and the pubis, at which the posterior layer of the sheath appears to stop. This is the **linea semicircularis** (arcuate line). Below the arcuate line, the rectus muscle rests posteriorly against the **transversalis fascia,** a thin fascial layer which lies just external to the extraperitoneal fat in the lower anterior abdominal wall. More frequently a distinct arcuate line is not discernible, the posterior layer of the sheath merely becoming gradually thinner in this region. The thinning of the posterior part of the sheath inferiorly is caused by the fibers forming it (which are the medial continuations of the aponeuroses of the internal oblique and transversus muscles) passing in this region in front of the rectus to join the anterior layer of the sheath.

The further dissection of the anterior abdominal wall for the display of the internal oblique and transversus muscles should be done completely only on one side. On the other side, the anterior abdominal wall should be retained undisturbed below a transverse line at the level of the anterior superior iliac spine for subsequent study of the inguinal canal and its relation to inguinal hernia, from the interior of the abdominal cavity.

The external oblique muscle should now be reflected to expose the internal oblique. Care is necessary here, since the layers of muscle in the anterolateral part of the abdominal wall are thin and separated from each other only by thin layers of fascia. Detach the upper four slips of origin of the external oblique from the fifth to eighth ribs. Then make a longitudinal incision through the muscle, running from the interval between its fourth and fifth slips of origin downward to the iliac crest. From the lower end of this incision, carry a transverse incision through the muscle and its aponeurosis medially to the linea semilunaris. From the medial end of the transverse incision, make a third incision running downward through the aponeurosis to reach the upper border of the superficial inguinal ring. By these incisions, the external oblique muscle and its aponeurosis will be cut into three portions. First reflect the large upper medial segment forward and medially to the linea semilunaris. Observe that at this line the **external oblique aponeurosis** joins the **anterior layer of** the **rectus sheath.** Then turn the smaller triangular lower medial segment downward and forward to the inguinal ligament (Fig. 48).

The reflection of the external oblique muscle and its aponeurosis will expose the internal oblique muscle and will also open up the medial portion of the inguinal canal. Clean and study the **internal oblique.** This muscle arises from the fused portion of the **lumbodorsal fascia** lateral to the sacrospinalis, from the intermediate lip of the anterior two-thirds of the **iliac crest,** and from the **fascia of** the **iliopsoas muscle,** being attached only by loose areolar tissue to the **inguinal ligament.** * The highest fibers are inserted upon the lower borders of

* This concept is based on work by McVay and Anson (*Surg. Gynes. & Obst.,* **74:** 746, 1942) and is the basis for one of the standard repairs for inguinal hernia, in which the muscles and fascia are sutured to the ligament (Cooper's) on the superior ramus of the pubis rather than to the inguinal ligament.

the **lower** three or four **ribs.** The remaining fibers, as they approach the linea semilunaris, pass into an **aponeurosis** which joins the **rectus sheath; inferiorly,** however, the **entire** aponeurosis splits into **two parts,** some fibers joining the **anterior** and some the **posterior layer of**

The **inguinal canal** has been partially opened by the reflection of the external oblique aponeurosis. This canal is an oblique passageway through the anterior abdominal wall, and it lies just above the medial third of the inguinal ligament. Its **anterior wall** is formed throughout

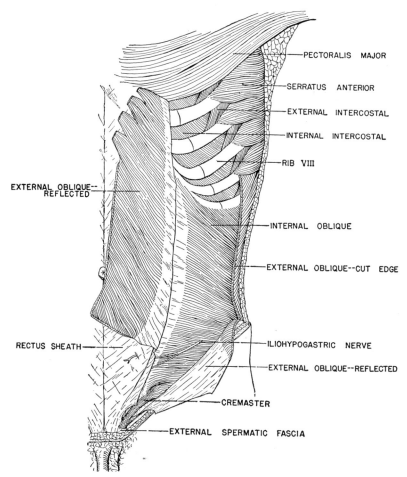

PECTORALIS MAJOR

SERRATUS ANTERIOR

EXTERNAL INTERCOSTAL

INTERNAL INTERCOSTAL

RIB VIII

EXTERNAL OBLIQUE-- REFLECTED

INTERNAL OBLIQUE

EXTERNAL OBLIQUE--CUT EDGE

RECTUS SHEATH

ILIOHYPOGASTRIC NERVE

EXTERNAL OBLIQUE--REFLECTED

CREMASTER

EXTERNAL SPERMATIC FASCIA

Fig. 48. The left side of the anterior abdominal wall after reflection of the external oblique muscle.

the **sheath; inferiorly,** however, the **entire aponeurosis** of the internal oblique passes **in front of** the **rectus.**

The **iliohypogastric nerve,** whose terminal part was already seen piercing the external oblique, should now be traced back to the point at which it pierces the lower portion of the internal oblique.

by the **aponeurosis of** the **external oblique.** Laterally, however, the **lower fibers of** the **internal oblique muscle** aid the external oblique aponeurosis in forming the anterior wall of the inguinal canal. Consequently, only the medial portion of the canal is at present open for inspection. Observe that the **spermatic cord,** as it emerges into this part of the inguinal canal from behind the lower part of the internal oblique muscle, receives a covering known as the **cremasteric fascia** and **muscle.**

The **cremaster muscle** is a thin layer of muscle fibers which run downward upon the **spermatic cord.** When the scrotum is dissected, it will be found that some of these muscle fibers are prolonged along the cord as far as the **testis,** which they encircle. After the cord has emerged through the superficial inguinal ring, the cremaster layer is covered externally by the external spermatic fascia. The **cremaster muscle** may be regarded as a prolongation over the spermatic cord of the lowermost fibers of the **internal oblique** and **transversus abdominis muscles.**

Observe the **lacunar ligament,** which stretches across from the medial end of the **inguinal ligament** to the **pecten of** the **pubis.** For about ½ in. of its course immediately internal to the superficial inguinal ring, the spermatic cord rests inferiorly upon the superior surface of the lacunar ligament. Consequently, this ligament is said to form the **floor of** the most **medial part of** the **inguinal canal.**

The internal oblique muscle should now be reflected. In cutting through the internal oblique, be careful not to cut the lower intercostal nerves, which cross its deep surface, in the narrow interval between the internal oblique and transversus muscles. Make a longitudinal incision through the internal oblique in the same line as that of the longitudinal incision previously made in the external oblique. Medial to this incision, the internal oblique should be detached above from any attachment it may have to the ribs and below from its attachment to the iliac crest and the inguinal ligament. The broad, flat medial portion of the muscle may then be reflected forward and medially to the linea semilunaris. This will expose the external surface of the transversus abdominis muscle and the vessels and nerves which lie between the transversus and the internal

oblique (Fig. 49). Elevate the dorsal part of the internal oblique and note its connections to the lumbodorsal fascia.

The **lower five intercostal** and the **subcostal** (twelfth thoracic) **nerves** run downward and forward across the external surface of the transversus muscle, giving twigs of supply to the transversus and the internal and external oblique muscles. At the linea semilunaris, they enter the rectus sheath, from which point their further distribution has already been seen. The **iliohypogastric** and **ilioinguinal nerves,** branches of the anterior primary division of the first lumbar nerve, have a similar course across the lower part of the transversus. They do not, however, enter the rectus sheath. The iliohypogastric has already been seen to pierce the internal oblique. The **ilioinguinal nerve** will be found crossing the transversus just above the lateral part of the inguinal ligament to enter the **inguinal canal,** through which it accompanies the spermatic cord to the superficial inguinal ring.

Clean the exposed portion of the **deep circumflex iliac artery.** At present it may be found piercing the transversus a short distance medial to the anterior superior iliac spine and running posteriorly **along** the **iliac crest** between the transversus and the internal oblique. Just in front of the anterior superior spine, it gives off a large branch which ascends on the transversus.

The **transversus abdominis** has a continuous origin from the inner surfaces of the **lower** six **costal cartilages,** the **lumbodorsal fascia,** the internal lip of the **iliac crest,** and the **fascia of** the **iliopsoas,** being attached only by areolar tissue to the **inguinal ligament.***   Its fibers cross the abdominal wall horizontally to end near the linea semilunaris in an **aponeurosis** which joins the **rectus sheath.** Throughout most of its extent, the aponeurosis of the transversus joins the **posterior layer of** the **rectus sheath; in-**

* See footnote on p. 121.

feriorly, however, it passes into the **anterior layer of** the **sheath.** Observe that the **lowest portion of** the **aponeurosis** does not reach the rectus sheath at all but passes downward, lateral to the narrow inferior portion of the sheath, to be attached directly to the **pecten of** the **pubis.** This portion of the aponeurosis of

transversalis fascia, the deepest layer of the anterior abdominal wall, is exposed. This layer forms the **posterior wall of** the **inguinal canal** throughout the length of the canal. Medially, however, the posterior wall of the inguinal canal is reenforced by the falx inguinalis, as has been seen.

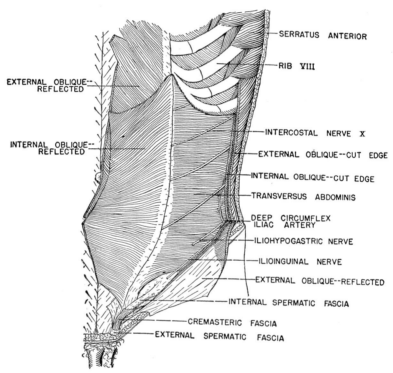

EXTERNAL OBLIQUE-- REFLECTED

INTERNAL OBLIQUE-- REFLECTED

SERRATUS ANTERIOR

RIB VIII

INTERCOSTAL NERVE X

EXTERNAL OBLIQUE--CUT EDGE

INTERNAL OBLIQUE--CUT EDGE

TRANSVERSUS ABDOMINIS

DEEP CIRCUMFLEX ILIAC ARTERY

ILIOHYPOGASTRIC NERVE

ILIOINGUINAL NERVE

EXTERNAL OBLIQUE--REFLECTED

INTERNAL SPERMATIC FASCIA

CREMASTERIC FASCIA

EXTERNAL SPERMATIC FASCIA

Fig. 49. The left side of the anterior abdominal wall, after reflection of both the external and the internal oblique muscles.

the transversus is known as the **falx inguinalis.** It is sometimes referred to as the **conjoined tendon** because it also receives a few of the lowermost fibers of the internal oblique. Observe that the falx inguinalis lies immediately behind the portion of the spermatic cord that rests inferiorly upon the lacunar ligament. Consequently, it is one of the constituents of the **posterior wall of** the **inguinal canal.**

Arching across from the lateral part of the inguinal ligament to the falx inguinalis, the

By reflection of the external and internal oblique muscles, the entire anterior wall of the inguinal canal has been removed. The internal opening, or inlet, of the canal is thus exposed from the outside. This inlet, known as the **deep inguinal ring,** lies just above the middle of the inguinal ligament. It is described as an opening in the transversalis fascia, but as seen from the outside it does not appear so, since the transversalis fascia is prolonged outward along the spermatic cord (Fig. 49).

Penis, Scrotum, and Testes · · · · · · · · · · · · · · · · ·

Attention should next be directed, in the male body, to the penis and scrotum. Make a longitudinal incision through the skin of the penis running downward from the pubic symphysis to the tip. Then reflect the skin laterally to each side. Observe that the skin at the end of the **penis** forms a free fold, the **prepuce,** which covers the **glans penis,** the rounded extremity of the penis. The inner surface of the prepuce is covered with a layer of the epithelium which is continuous around the margin of the glans with the epithelium covering the glans. The prepuce should be cut away from the margin of the glans penis as the skin is removed.

The **root of** the **penis** is situated **in** the **perineum,** firmly attached to the bone and fascia of that region. The **free portion** of the organ, now under observation, is suspended from the pubic symphysis. Define the **suspensory ligament of** the **penis.** This is a fibrous band which runs downward from the **symphysis pubis** to divide into two parts which are attached to the **deep fascia** on each side of the **body of** the **penis.**

Clean the vessels and nerves on the dorsum of the penis (anterior surface of the dependent organ). Most superficially, in the midline, is the **superficial dorsal vein,** which should be dissected free from the surrounding connective tissue and reflected laterally with the superficial fascia. In the **deep fascia** (Buck's fascia) on the dorsum of the penis will be found the deep dorsal vein and the dorsal arteries and nerves, all of which enter the present area of dissection by passing between the two parts of the suspensory ligament. The **deep dorsal vein** is in the midline. On each side of it are the **dorsal arteries,** and lateral to the artery on each side is the **dorsal nerve.** Numerous small branches arise from the artery and nerve as they approach the glans.

Attempt to separate by dissection the two main parts of which the **body of** the **penis** is composed. These are the **corpus cavernosum penis** and the **corpus cavernosum** (spongiosum) **urethrae.** Observe that the **glans penis** is the expanded end of the corpus cavernosum urethrae.

The **scrotum** is a sac of **skin** and **fascia** which contains the lower ends of the **spermatic cords** and the **testes and their coverings.** The coverings of the testis are prolongations of the fascial coverings of the spermatic cord, which are successively given to the cord, as has already been observed, in its passage through the inguinal canal. In addition to these, the testis has as its innermost covering, a serous layer, the **tunica vaginalis,** which was originally continuous with the peritoneal membrane of the abdominal cavity and its adjacent layer of extraperitoneal connective tissue and fat.

On both sides, make a longitudinal incision through the skin of the scrotum from the region of the superficial inguinal ring down to the lower end of the scrotum; then reflect the skin from the anterior aspect of the scrotum. Observe that this skin is thin and is rather firmly attached to the underlying superficial fascia.

The **superficial fascia of** the **scrotum** is known as the **dartos tunic.** It is devoid of fat and usually dark red in color, due to the presence in it of **smooth muscle fibers.** In the midline, it is prolonged backward to form a **median septum** which divides the scrotal sac into two parts. Reflect the dartos tunic from the anterior aspect of the testis and free the spermatic cord and testis, together with their coverings, entirely from the scrotum. Then study the spermatic cord between the superficial inguinal ring and the testis.

The individual reflection of the **fascial coverings of** the **spermatic cord** is extremely difficult of achievement in most cases, but it should be

125

attempted. These coverings are, from without inward, the **external spermatic fascia,** the **cremasteric muscle and fascia,** and the **internal spermatic fascia.** When they have been opened, the various constituents of the spermatic cord proper will be exposed and should be identified within a layer of connective tissue which is continuous with the extraperitoneal tissue of the abdomen through the inguinal canal.

The **ductus deferens** can always be recognized by its hard cordlike feeling. Through it the spermatozoa pass from the **testis to** the **urethra.** It is usually the most posterior of the structures in the spermatic cord. Its small artery may be seen on its external surface. The **internal spermatic (testicular) artery** is the principal artery of supply for the testis. It is surrounded by the **pampiniform plexus of veins,** which returns blood from the testis. The **genital nerve** is a small nerve which supplies the **cremaster muscle.** It arises in the abdominal cavity as a branch of the genitofemoral branch of the lumbar plexus.

The **tunica vaginalis** of the testis is a serous membrane which forms a completely enclosed sac. It is invaginated by the **testis and epididymis** so that it presents visceral and parietal portions. The **visceral tunica vaginalis** is closely applied to the superior, inferior, anterior, medial, and lateral aspects of the testis and epididymis. Posteriorly, the testis is not covered by the tunica vaginalis, whose visceral portion is here reflected at each side to become continuous with the **parietal tunica vaginalis.** Between the visceral and parietal portions is a narrow cavity filled by a small amount of **serous fluid.** Open this cavity by making a longitudinal incision through the anterior part of the parietal tunica vaginalis. This will expose the testis and epididymis, covered by the visceral tunica vaginalis. It should be observed, however, that diseased testes with complete or partial obliteration of the cavity of the tunica vaginalis are fairly common in cadavers.

The **testis** is an oval body, somewhat flattened at the sides. It normally lies free in the cavity of the tunica vaginalis except posteriorly, where it is attached to the scrotal wall and to the epididymis. The **epididymis** is a curved, elongated structure applied to the posterolateral aspect of the testis. The lower end or **tail of** the **epididymis** (cauda epididymidis) is held to the lower end of the testis by the visceral tunica vaginalis. Its enlarged upper end or **head** (caput epididymidis) surmounts the upper end of the testis. The intervening portion or **body** (corpus epididymidis) is partially separated from the testis by an inpocketing of the lateral part of the cavity of the tunica vaginalis. This cleftlike portion of the cavity is known as the **sinus of** the **epididymis.**

Free the body and tail of the epididymis from the testis by cutting through the tunica vaginalis along each side of the epididymis. Observe that the **ductus deferens** begins at the **tail of** the **epididymis,** to run upward into the spermatic cord. Cut carefully through the visceral tunica vaginalis along its line of reflection from the upper end of the testis onto the head of the epididymis to demonstrate the **efferent ducts** of the testis. These ducts (ductuli efferentes) are 15 to 20 small ducts which carry the spermatozoa from the upper end of the testis into the head of the epididymis. In the epididymis, these ducts eventually all unite to form a single duct, the **ductus epididymidis.** The body and tail of the epididymis consist of this single duct very greatly coiled upon itself. At the lower end of the tail, it widens out to form the ductus deferens.

Observe that the arteries and veins of the testis enter and leave its posterior border, where it is not covered by the tunica vaginalis. Section the **testis** transversely at about its middle to see its structure in the cut surface. Immediately internal to the tunica vaginalis is a heavy fibrous layer, the **tunica albuginea.** Along the posterior border, where the vessels enter, this layer is thickened to form the **mediastinum testis.** From the mediastinum, fibrous partitions or septules radiate through the gland, dividing it into **lobules.** The **seminiferous tubules** are contained within the lobules.

Inguinal Region—Inguinal Hernia ·········

Make a transverse incision through the entire anterior abdominal wall, including the peritoneum, from a point a little above the anterior superior iliac spine on one side to the same point on the other side. Then draw the lower segment of the divided wall as far forward as possible and observe the disposition of the peritoneum on the inner surface of the lower part of the abdominal wall. The peritoneum does not form a perfectly smooth internal covering for the abdominal wall but projects backward into the abdominal cavity in the form of five ridges on the internal surface of the wall.

In the midline, running upward from the pubic symphysis to the umbilicus, is a ridge caused by the presence of the **middle (median) umbilical ligament, or urachus,** which ascends from the apex of the bladder. Starting at the lower part of the anterior abdominal wall a short distance lateral to the midline on either side and running upward and medially to the umbilicus is another peritoneal ridge, caused by the presence of the **lateral (medial) umbilical ligament,** a fibrous cord which represents the obliterated portion of the **fetal hypogastric artery.** Still farther lateral is another peritoneal ridge caused by the **inferior epigastric artery,** which runs upward and medially in the lower part of the anterior abdominal wall to enter the sheath of the rectus muscle. The latter ridge is often not very well marked. By means of these peritoneal ridges, the peritoneum clothing the inner surface of the lower anterior wall is divided into three pairs of peritoneal fossae or pouches, which represent partial subdivisions of the general peritoneal cavity. Between the middle and the lateral umbilical ligaments on each side is the **supravesical fossa;** between the lateral ligament and the inferior epigastric artery is the **medial inguinal fossa;** lateral to the inferior epigastric artery is the **lateral inguinal fossa.** The relative width of the supravesical and medial inguinal fossae is subject to a good deal of variation and often differs on the two sides of the same body.

From the transverse incision already made in the anterior abdominal wall, carry a longitudinal incision down to the pubis. This incision should lie just to the side of the midline. Then approach the intact inguinal canal from the interior of the abdominal cavity (Fig. 50).

Carefully remove a roughly circular piece of peritoneum and the subjacent extraperitoneal tissue, about 2 in. in diameter, from the internal abdominal wall, with the deep inguinal ring as the center of the circle. The position of the **deep inguinal ring** can often be readily recognized while the peritoneum is still in place from the fact that the peritoneum dimples into it for a short distance. If this is not the case, its approximate location can be determined by comparison with the side where the ring has already been exposed from the exterior.

The **transversalis fascia** stretches upward from the inguinal ligament. As seen from the inside, the deep inguinal ring appears as an opening in this fascia just above the middle of the inguinal ligament. Observe that the **ductus deferens** enters the abdominal cavity at the **deep inguinal ring.** At the inguinal ligament, it turns downward and medially and crosses in front of the external iliac vessels to run toward the brim of the pelvis immediately external to the peritoneum. In the **female,** its place is taken by the **round ligament** of the **uterus.**

The **external iliac artery and vein** are large vessels which run downward across the medial side of the present area of dissection to disap-

the ductus deferens and that it runs upward in the anterior abdominal wall to pierce the transversalis fascia and enter the **rectus sheath.** In some cases, another branch will be seen arising from the external iliac in common with the inferior epigastric but turning medially to cross the external iliac vein and run to the pelvic brim. This is the **obturator artery,** which in the majority of the cases arises within the pelvis as a branch of the hypogastric (internal iliac) artery.

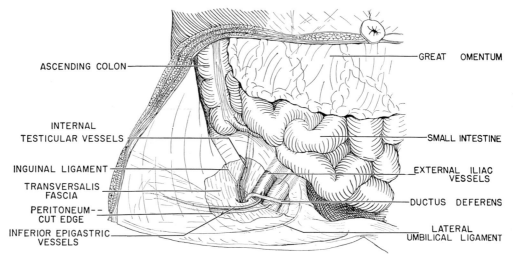

INTERNAL
TESTICULAR VESSELS

ASCENDING COLON

GREAT   OMENTUM

INGUINAL LIGAMENT

TRANSVERSALIS
FASCIA

PERITONEUM--
CUT EDGE

INFERIOR EPIGASTRIC
VESSELS

SMALL INTESTINE

EXTERNAL   ILIAC
VESSELS

DUCTUS   DEFERENS

LATERAL
UMBILICAL LIGAMENT

FIG. 50. Dissection to expose the right deep inguinal ring from the inner surface of the abdominal wall.

pear behind the inguinal ligament. The artery is lateral to the vein. Lateral to the artery, above and behind the inguinal ligament, is a layer of fascia known as the **iliac fascia,** which covers the **psoas major and iliacus muscles.** Running downward on the iliac fascia a short distance lateral to the external iliac artery to reach the deep inguinal ring will be found in the male the **testicular artery and vein** and the **external spermatic (genital) nerve.**

Clean the **inferior epigastric artery.** Observe that it arises from the **external iliac** just before the latter passes behind the inguinal ligament, that it is crossed internally near its origin by

An **inguinal hernia** is the protrusion of a portion of the **abdominal contents,** usually a loop of intestine, **into** the **inguinal canal.** Two principal types of inguinal hernia may occur. An **indirect,** or oblique, **inguinal hernia** is one in which the loop of intestine enters at the **deep ring,** traverses the entire length of the **inguinal canal,** and emerges at the **superficial ring.** A **direct inguinal hernia** is one which pushes through the posterior wall of the canal at some point **medial to the deep ring,** traverses the **medial end of** the **canal,** and emerges at the **superficial ring.** Any inguinal hernia will push before it, as the most internal of its coverings, a layer of peritoneum, but its outer coverings will differ according to the point at which it enters the canal.

If the little finger is introduced into the deep ring from the interior of the abdominal cavity and pushed through the inguinal canal to the superficial ring, the coverings of an indirect hernia may be readily demonstrated. It will be found that they are the same as the normal coverings of the spermatic cord. As the finger emerges through the superficial ring it is covered externally by internal spermatic, cremasteric, and external spermatic fascia. If such a hernia reaches as far as the scrotum, it will appear there in the interval between internal spermatic fascia and parietal tunica vaginalis.

Observe that the **coverings of a direct inguinal hernia** will not be the same in all cases. A direct hernia which enters the posterior wall of the canal just **medial to** the **deep ring** will push before it a covering of transversalis fascia, which will take the place of the internal spermatic fascia and will appear **in the scrotum**

in the interval **between internal spermatic and cremasteric fascia.** A direct hernia, however, which enters the inguinal canal by pushing through the **medial end of its posterior wall,** will receive neither internal spermatic fascia nor cremasteric fascia but in place of them coverings derived from the transversalis fascia and the falx inguinalis respectively. As the hernia passes through the superficial ring, it will lie internal to the external spermatic fascia and will appear **in** the **scrotum,** covered by peritoneum, transversalis fascia, and falx inguinalis, in the **interval between external spermatic and cremasteric fascia.**

Femoral hernia may occur through the **femoral canal.** Insert a finger into the pelvic opening of this canal and identify its boundaries by palpation. It is bounded by the **lacunar ligament** medially, the **inguinal ligament** superiorly, the **femoral vein** and its fascial covering laterally, and the **superior ramus of** the **pubis,** covered by the pectineal fascia, inferiorly.

Abdominal Cavity ·

The abdominal cavity has already been partially opened by a transverse and a lower longitudinal incision. Completely open the cavity by making a second longitudinal incision through the entire thickness of the wall, running upward from the transverse incision to the costal arch immediately to the left of the median line. By this means, the **peritoneal cavity,** which is contained within the abdominal cavity, will be widely opened from the front.

Topographical Regions

The **abdominal cavity** is arbitrarily divided for purposes of reference into nine regions by

two transverse and two longitudinal planes. The upper transverse plane passes transversely through the abdominal cavity at the level of the lowest portions of the tenth costal cartilages; the lower transverse plane is at the level of the anterior superior iliac spines. The longitudinal planes pass through the cavity on each side in the line of the linea semilunaris, the lateral border of the rectus abdominis muscle. The subdivisions of the cavity made by these planes are, above the upper horizontal plane, a **right and left hypochondriac** and a **median epigastric region;** between the two transverse planes, a **right and left lumbar** and an **umbilical** region; below the lower transverse plane, a **right and left inguinal,** or iliac, and a **hypogastric region** (Fig. 51).

The **peritoneum** is the great **serous membrane** of the abdominal cavity. In the **male,** it forms a completely **closed sac,** the peritoneal cavity. In the **female,** the peritoneum is pierced by **two small openings,** the **mouths of** the **uterine tubes,** but elsewhere completely encloses the peritoneal cavity.

the right side about 1 in. parallel and lateral to the xiphoid process and extending the cut into the anterior part of the diaphragm. Then retract the two parts of the lower thoracic cage laterally to each side.

Inspection of Viscera

The **liver** is a large, solid, brownish-red organ occupying the right hypochondriac and

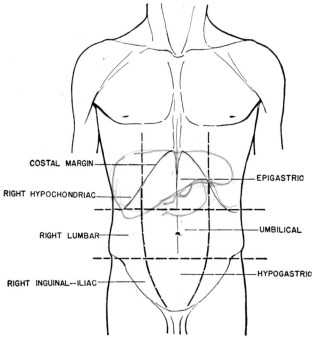

COSTAL MARGIN

RIGHT HYPOCHONDRIAC

RIGHT LUMBAR

RIGHT INGUINAL--ILIAC

EPIGASTRIC

UMBILICAL

HYPOGASTRIC

FIG. 51. Diagram to illustrate the planes of subdivision of the abdominal cavity as projected on the surface of the body.

closes the peritoneal cavity. The peritoneum is an extremely complex membrane, because it is invaginated by numerous abdominal organs whose outer serous coat it forms. Before proceeding to a detailed study of the peritoneum, identify the various abdominal organs which project into the peritoneal cavity.

If the lower ribs, costal cartilages, and xiphoid process prevent examination of the liver and the adjacent viscera, their study can be facilitated by cutting the costal cartilages on

parts of the epigastric and left hypochondriac regions. The **stomach** is continuous with the esophagus just below the diaphragm; it is to be found in the epigastric and left hypochondriac regions, partially overlapped anteriorly by the liver. The appearance of the stomach varies greatly in different subjects. Its walls are often completely collapsed and contracted, so that its characteristic outline does not appear. Behind the upper part of the stomach and just below the diaphragm in the left hypochondriac

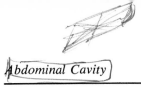

region is the **spleen,** a solid organ similar in color to the liver. At its right extremity, behind the liver, the stomach narrows to become continuous with the **duodenum,** the **first part of** the **small intestine.** Only the beginning of the duodenum can now be seen, passing to the right behind the liver to disappear in the posterior wall of the peritoneal cavity. If it is advisable to inflate the stomach, air may be pumped into the esophagus through the mouth; or, if the thorax has been dissected, it may be introduced into the esophagus just above the diaphragm. The esophagus should then be ligatured to prevent escape of the air. It may be necessary also to ligature the first part of the duodenum to prevent the air from passing into the small intestine. Usually, the stomach can be studied without inflating it.

When the **stomach** is full, observe that its broad convex anterior surface (which is actually anterosuperior in position) is covered by the liver above but is in contact with the lower anterior part of the diaphragm and the anterior abdominal wall below. The curved right and upper border of this surface is known as **the lesser curvature** of the stomach; the much longer curved border formed by the left and inferior margin is known as the **greater curvature.**

Descending from the lower part of the greater curvature is the **great omentum,** a broad **free fold of peritoneum** containing a considerable quantity of fat. The extent of the great omentum below the greater curvature varies in different subjects; in some cases it extends well into the hypogastric region, completely covering anteriorly the coils of small intestine which fill the lower part of the peritoneal cavity. Turn the great omentum upward and observe that its upper posterior border is attached to the **transverse colon,** a portion of the large intestine which crosses the peritoneal cavity from right to left.

Turn the transverse colon upward, together with the peritoneal fold which attaches it to the posterior wall of the peritoneal cavity, and identify the **duodenojejunal flexure.** At this point, which is slightly to the left of the midline, in the upper part of the umbilical region, the **duodenum** emerges from the posterior peritoneal wall to become continuous with the **jejunum,** the **second part of** the **small intestine.** The numerous coils of the jejunum and the **ileum** (the **third part of** the **small intestine**) fill the umbilical and hypogastric regions and also extend into the cavity of the pelvis minor. Draw them forward and observe that they are attached to the posterior wall by a broad, thick peritoneal fold, the **mesentery.**

In the right iliac region, the ileum ends by joining the **cecum,** the first part of the **large intestine.** Identify the **vermiform appendix.** This fingerlike process typically projects to the left from the lower end of the cecum, but it may turn upward behind the cecum or exhibit other variations in position. Running upward through the right iliac and lumbar regions, closely applied to the posterior wall, is the **ascending colon.** Under cover of the lower right border of the liver is the **right colic flexure,** at which the ascending colon becomes continuous with the **transverse colon.** At the **left colic flexure,** which is in the left hypochondriac region in relation to the lower part of the spleen, the transverse colon becomes continuous with the **descending colon.** The latter passes downward through the left lumbar region to become continuous in the left iliac region with the **sigmoid** or **pelvic colon,** which crosses the left side of the pelvic brim to enter the cavity of the pelvis minor.

Peritoneum

Now make a study of the peritoneum as a whole. The **peritoneum** may be subdivided, from its relation to other structures, as **visceral peritoneum,** i.e., peritoneum forming the **outer coat of** a visceral **organ; parietal peritoneum,** i.e., peritoneum forming the **walls of** the **peritoneal cavity;** and the peritoneum of the various peritoneal ligaments or mesenteries. These **ligaments** are double folds of peritoneum which help to hold the viscera in place and through which blood vessels and nerves reach the various intraperitoneal organs. They may represent the continuity of visceral with parietal perito-

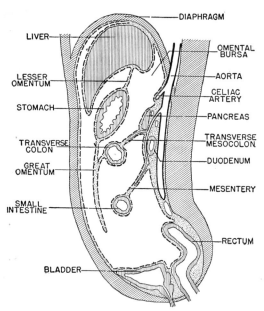

LIVER

LESSER
OMENTUM

STOMACH

TRANSVERSE
COLON

GREAT
OMENTUM

SMALL
INTESTINE

BLADDER

DIAPHRAGM

OMENTAL
BURSA

AORTA

CELIAC
ARTERY

PANCREAS

TRANSVERSE
MESOCOLON

DUODENUM

MESENTERY

RECTUM

FIG. 52. Diagrammatic midsagittal section through the abdominal cavity, showing the disposition of the peritoneum. In this, as in the four succeeding figures, the body wall is represented by diagonal shading and the organs by vertical shading. The peritoneum is represented by the broken line.

neum, or they may connect the visceral peritoneum of two or more organs. The parietal peritoneum is closely applied anteriorly and laterally to the inner surface of the abdominal wall, and superiorly to the inferior surface of the diaphragm. The posterior extent of the peritoneal cavity is not, however, so great as is that of the abdominal cavity, and numerous **structures** will be found at later stages of the dissection which are within the abdominal cavity but **behind** the **posterior parietal peri-**

toneum. Such structures are described as **retroperitoneal. Organs** which **project** freely **into** the **peritoneal cavity** and receive a coat of visceral peritoneum are described as **intraperitoneal.** However, such organs are not within the peritoneal cavity as the term intraperitoneal might suggest, since they are separated from the peritoneal cavity by their visceral covering of peritoneum. Inferiorly, the peritoneum descends below the pelvic brim, where its disposition will be observed when the pelvis is studied.

Observe the **falciform ligament of** the **liver.** This is a double fold of peritoneum which connects the **parietal peritoneum of** the **anterior abdominal wall** with the **visceral peritoneum** clothing the anterior surface **of** the **liver.** Its attachment to the anterior surface of the liver marks the junction of the right and left lobes of that organ. Inferiorly, it presents a free margin running downward and forward from the lower border of the liver toward the umbilicus. Within this free margin is contained the **ligamentum teres** of the liver, a cordlike structure representing the **obliterated umbilical vein** of the fetus.

Pass the hand upward over the right side of the liver and identify the **coronary ligament.** This is a broad **peritoneal fold** through which the peritoneum on the upper and posterior surfaces of the **liver** becomes continuous with the peritoneum on the under surface of the **diaphragm.** Its sharp, right free margin is known as the **right triangular ligament.** To the left of the attachment of the falciform ligament, connecting the diaphragmatic peritoneum with the peritoneum on the upper surface of the left lobe of the liver, is the narrow **left triangular ligament.**

Draw the left lobe of the liver forward and observe the **lesser omentum.** This is a flat peritoneal ligament which runs from the **lesser curvature of** the **stomach** and the upper border of the first part of the **duodenum** to the inferior surface of the **liver.** It is composed of **two layers of peritoneum,** anterior and posterior, which are closely applied to each other except near the right free margin, which runs from the duodenum to the lower part of the inferior surface of the liver. Around this margin the two layers are continuous with each other. Observe that near this **right free margin** the lesser omentum is **thick;** this is due to the presence within it of the **hepatic artery,** the **portal vein,** and the **bile duct.** At the lesser curvature, the peritoneum comprising the lesser omentum becomes continuous with the vis-

entery of the jejunum and ileum, and the sigmoid mesocolon. These should now be investigated (Figs. 52 to 56).

The **gastrophrenic ligament** is a short peritoneal fold running from the upper part of the greater curvature to the peritoneum covering the diaphragm. The **lienogastric ligament** is a double fold of peritoneum running from the left portion of the greater curvature to the hilus of the spleen. Running backward from the hilus of the spleen to join the parietal peritoneum on the posterior wall of the peritoneal cavity is the **lienorenal ligament,** so

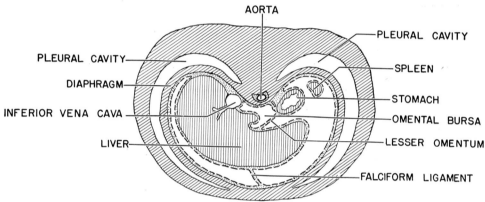

FIG. 53. Diagrammatic transverse section through the abdominal cavity at the level of the superior recess of the omental bursa. The peritoneum is represented by the broken line.

ceral peritoneum clothing the anterior and posterior surfaces of the stomach. At the liver, whose inferior surface it reaches along the line separating the right and left lobes, it becomes continuous with the visceral peritoneum on the inferior surface of the liver (Figs. 52 to 54).

The falciform ligament, the coronary and right and left triangular ligaments of the liver, and the lesser omentum are all derived from the **ventral mesentery of the embryonic gut.** The representatives in the adult of the **embryonic dorsal mesentery** are the gastrophrenic, lienorenal, and lienogastric ligaments, the great omentum, the transverse mesocolon, the mes-

called because it joins the posterior parietal peritoneum in front of the left kidney. The form, connections, and extent of the great omentum have been investigated.

The **transverse mesocolon** is a broad peritoneal ligament which runs upward and backward from the posterior surface of the transverse colon to the posterior wall of the peritoneal cavity. The **parietal peritoneum** on the posterior wall below the line of attachment of the transverse mesocolon is referred to as the **descending layer** of the **transverse mesocolon,** because it is continuous along this line of attachment with the posterior layer of the transverse mesocolon. Inferiorly, the descending layer of the transverse mesocolon becomes continuous with the anterior layer of the mesentery.

The **mesentery** is the **peritoneal ligament** which supports the **jejunum** and **ileum.** Posteriorly, its two layers become continuous with

attachment, giving the entire mesentery the form of a frill. Peritoneal fossae may be found near the duodenojejunal and the ileocecal junctions. These fossae may be the sites of intraperitoneal herniation.

The **ascending** and **descending colons** have

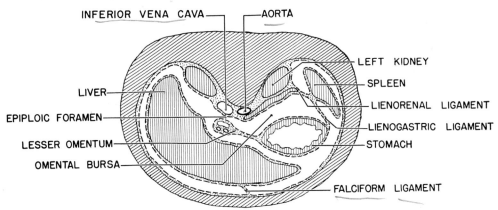

Fig. 54. Diagrammatic transverse section through the abdominal cavity at the level of the epiploic foramen. The peritoneum is represented by the broken line.

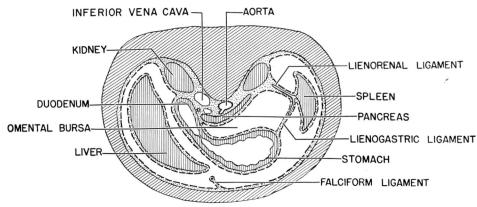

Fig. 55. Diagrammatic transverse section through the abdominal cavity slightly below the level of the epiploic foramen. The peritoneum is represented by the broken line.

the posterior parietal peritoneum along an oblique line running downward and to the right from the duodenojejunal flexure to the ileocecal junction; anteriorly, they become continuous with the visceral peritoneum clothing the jejunum and ileum. Its intestinal attachment is necessarily very much longer than its parietal

no mesenteries, being in contact posteriorly with the abdominal wall and covered by peritoneum only anteriorly and on their sides. The **cecum** is usually attached to the posterior wall by a short **mesocecum;** the **vermiform appendix** is usually also supported by a peritoneal fold, the **mesoappendix.** The **sigmoid colon** is suspended from the parietal peritoneum of the left iliac fossa by a peritoneal fold, the **sigmoid mesocolon,** which crosses the pelvic brim to enter the pelvis. The **phrenicocolic ligament** is a small, transverse, shelflike fold of peritoneum stretching from the lateral aspect of the upper part of the descending colon to the lower left portion of the diaphragm; the lower tip of the spleen usually rests upon its upper surface.

The portion of the peritoneal cavity which has so far been investigated is known as the

anteriorly by the posterior layer of the lesser omentum, inferiorly by the peritoneum on the first part of the duodenum, and posteriorly by parietal peritoneum which covers the inferior vena cava.

The omental bursa may now be opened from below by making an incision through the great omentum parallel to the greater curvature of the stomach and about ½ in. below it; this incision should not be carried far enough to the left and upward to sever the gastrosplenic liga-

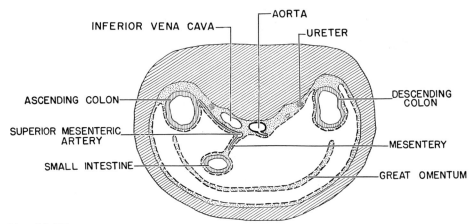

Fig. 56. Diagrammatic transverse section through the abdominal cavity near the middle of the umbilical and lumbar regions. The peritoneum is represented by the broken line.

greater peritoneal sac. There is another subdivision of the cavity, the **lesser sac,** or **omental bursa,** to which attention should now be turned. The omental bursa lies behind the lesser omentum, the stomach, and the upper anterior part of the great omentum. Its only **communication with** the **greater sac** is through an opening known as the **epiploic foramen,** which lies immediately behind the right free margin of the lesser omentum. If a finger is pushed upward and to the left along the inferior surface of the right lobe of the liver and behind the lesser omentum, it will pass through the epiploic foramen and enter the omental bursa. The epiploic foramen is bounded superiorly by peritoneum on the inferior surface of the liver,

ment. The boundaries of the omental bursa may then be explored through this opening.

The **pancreas** can usually be seen through the **ascending layer of** the **transverse mesocolon,** crossing the posterior abdominal wall just above the attachment of the transverse mesocolon.

Occasionally, the lower part of the omental bursa extends downward within the great omentum as far as its lower border. Usually, however, the anterior and posterior portions of the great omentum are firmly fused below, so that the cavity of the bursa rarely extends far below the lower border of the transverse colon (Fig. 52).

The highest portion of the **omental bursa** is

known as its **superior recess.** Observe that a small portion of the posterior surface of the right lobe of the liver projects into the superior recess. This is the **caudate lobe of the liver** and is the only part of the liver to be found in the wall of the omental bursa.

For further study of the stomach, it will be found helpful to remove the left lobe of the liver. The removal of the left lobe of the liver may be facilitated by making an incision

and greater curvatures and clean the vessels which supply the stomach with blood. The origins of these vessels will be seen somewhat later; they should now be cleaned only in relation to the stomach. In spare subjects they may sometimes be seen through the peritoneum without dissection (Fig. 57).

The **left gastric artery** reaches the upper end of the lesser curvature by passing through the left gastropancreatic fold. It runs downward

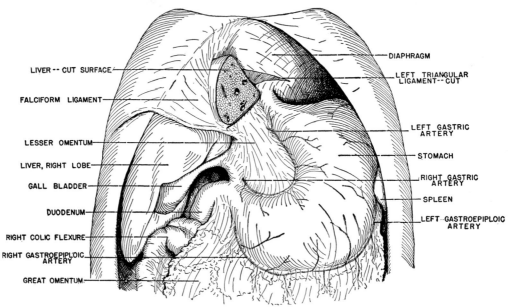

FIG. 57. The contents of the upper part of the abdominal cavity, seen from in front. The left lobe of the liver has been removed.

through the lower costal cartilages and into the peripheral part of the diaphragm on the left side and by retracting the costal cartilages laterally. Make an incision through the left lobe, starting anteriorly just to the left of the attachment of the falciform ligament and running straight backward to emerge just to the left of the attachment of the lesser omentum. To detach the left lobe from the diaphragm it will also be necessary to cut the left triangular ligament.

Cut through the peritoneum along the lesser

and to the right along the **lesser curvature** to anastomose with the **right gastric.** The **right gastroepiploic** should be found at the right end of the **greater curvature** and traced to the left, where it anastomoses with the **left gastroepiploic.** The left gastroepiploic reaches the left side of the greater curvature by passing forward within the lienogastric ligament and runs downward and to the right along the greater curvature. In the upper part of the greater curvature are the **short gastric arteries,** which also reach the stomach through the lienogastric ligament. All these vessels give branches to both surfaces of the stomach. A branch of the **left gastric passes** upward to the esophagus.

Remove the anterior layer of peritoneum from the right portion of the lesser omentum and expose and clean the structures which are contained within the **lesser omentum** in **front of** the **epiploic foramen.** The **hepatic artery** enters the lesser omentum through the right gastropancreatic fold and passes upward in the

the junction of **right** and **left hepatic ducts** from the two lobes of the liver. The common bile duct leaves the lesser omentum by descending behind the first part of the duodenum.

The **portal vein** is a wide channel which lies behind the hepatic artery and the bile duct. It enters the lesser omentum from behind the first part of the duodenum. In the omentum, it divides into **right** and **left branches,** which enter the **lobes of** the **liver.** Before its division,

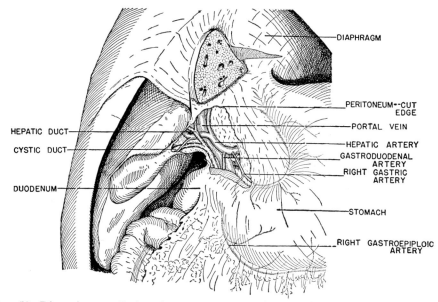

FIG. 58. Dissection to display the structures contained within the right margin of the lesser omentum.

omentum to end by dividing into **right** and **left hepatics,** which enter the right and left lobes of the liver. As it reaches the lesser omentum, the hepatic artery gives off the **right gastric,** whose entire course may now be seen, and the **gastroduodenal** artery, which passes downward behind the first part of the duodenum. The **common bile duct** is formed in the lesser omentum by the junction of the **cystic duct** and the **hepatic duct.** The **cystic duct** is the narrowed continuation of the **gall bladder.** It is accompanied by the **cystic artery,** a branch of the **right hepatic.** The **hepatic duct** is formed by

it receives the **coronary vein of** the **stomach,** which enters the omentum through the right gastropancreatic fold.

Cut the lesser omentum transversely and trace the **hepatic artery** back through the right gastropancreatic fold to its origin from the **celiac artery (trunk).** Clean the celiac trunk. This is a short, thick trunk which runs forward from the **abdominal aorta** just below the aortic hiatus of the diaphragm, behind the peritoneum on the posterior wall of the omental bursa, to break up into three branches, the **hepatic,** the **left gastric,** and the **splenic.** Cut through the

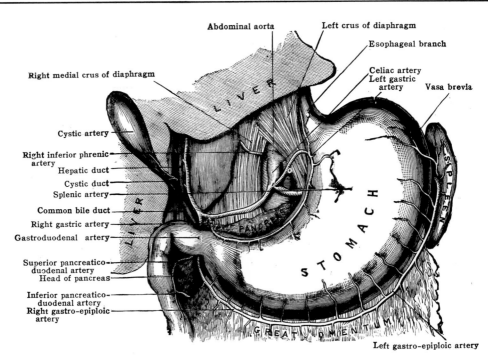

FIG. 59. The celiac artery and its branches. (*By permission from Schaeffer (ed.),* *"Morris' Human Anatomy,"* 11/e, *McGraw-Hill Book Company, Inc., Blakiston Division, New York,* 1953.)

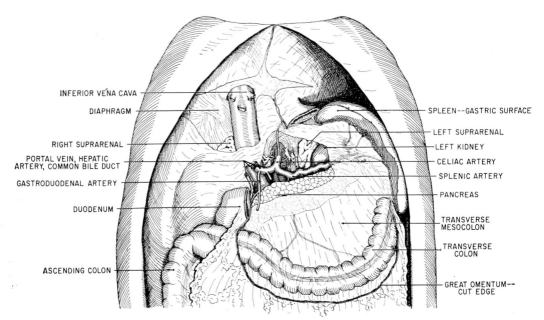

FIG. 60. The upper part of the abdominal cavity after removal of the stomach and liver, showing the stomach bed. A piece of parietal peritoneum has been removed from the posterior wall of the omental bursa.

peritoneum of the left gastropancreatic fold and trace the left gastric artery to the point at which it reaches the stomach. Clean the beginning of the splenic artery and observe that it runs to the left along the upper border of the pancreas, behind the peritoneum on the posterior wall of the omental bursa (Fig. 60).

Free and elevate the duodenum just beyond its junction with the pylorus. Turn the pyloric end of the stomach to the left and trace the **gastroduodenal artery** down behind the first part of the duodenum, where it ends by dividing into the **right gastroepiploic** and the **superior pancreaticoduodenal arteries.** The latter will be traced later down along the medial border of the duodenum. The right gastroepiploic should now be followed to the point at which it reaches the greater curvature.

Stomach

The **stomach** presents anterior and posterior surfaces which face respectively into the greater and lesser peritoneal sacs. Its borders are the curvatures already noted. The **esophagus** joins the stomach at the cardia, just below the diaphragm. The body of the stomach is divided into **cardiac** and **pyloric portions** by a notch in the lesser curvature, the **incisura angularis.** The pyloric portion is the narrower lower third, which joins the **duodenum.** The expanded upper end of the cardiac portion is known as the **fundus.**

Free and elevate the stomach. Then make an incision through the wall of the stomach along the greater curvature, extending the cut through the pyloric canal and into the superior part of the duodenum. Retract the cut edges of the stomach and duodenum and remove the food contents.

Observe that the **mucous membrane** is pitted by **minute depressions** which are more numerous toward the pylorus than at the fundus. Observe the **rugae.** These are projecting folds of the mucous membrane. In a distended stomach,

they are obliterated, but with contraction of the muscular wall of the stomach they appear, since the mucous membrane does not contract with the muscle.

The **pyloric canal** is the narrowed right end of the pylorus, leading to the **pyloric orifice,** the opening between the pylorus and the duodenum. Study the **pyloric sphincter.** This is a thick circular ring of smooth muscle by which the pyloric orifice is kept closed, except when food is passing from the stomach to the duodenum.

Study the **stomach bed,** the complex of structures upon which the posterior surface of the stomach rests. Observe that the lowest part of the stomach bed is formed by the **transverse colon.** Above this, the posterior surface of the stomach rests upon the **transverse mesocolon,** through which it is in relation with the coils of the **small intestine.** Above the parietal attachment of the transverse mesocolon, the stomach bed is formed to the right by the **parietal peritoneum** on the posterior wall of the omental bursa and to the left by the gastric surface of the **spleen.** The latter is, however, kept from direct contact with the posterior surface of the stomach by the lienogastric and lienorenal ligaments.

Remove the parietal peritoneum forming the upper right portion of the stomach bed and expose the retroperitoneal structures in relation to the posterior surface of the stomach. Crossing the posterior abdominal wall immediately above the attachment of the transverse mesocolon are the **body and tail of** the **pancreas.** Above the pancreas and immediately to the right of the spleen, a small portion of the anterior surface of the **left kidney** may be exposed; this is kept from contact with the posterior surface of the stomach only by the parietal peritoneum and some extraperitoneal areolar tissue. To the right of this area of kidney, the **left suprarenal gland** takes part in the formation of the stomach bed, and to the right of and above the suprarenal, the **left crus of** the **diaphragm** lies behind the highest part of the stomach.

Clean the **splenic artery.** It arises from the **celiac trunk** and crosses the posterior abdominal wall immediately above the pancreas, to which it gives numerous small branches. It passes between the two layers of the lienorenal ligament to reach the hilus of the spleen, where it terminates by dividing into three or four branches which enter the **spleen** and the **left gastroepiploic** and **short gastric arteries,** which pass forward through the lienogastric ligament to reach the stomach. The course of the splenic artery across the posterior abdominal wall is usually rather tortuous.

Spleen and Liver

Study the **spleen.** This organ is completely clothed with visceral peritoneum, except at its **hilus,** where it is joined by the lienorenal and lienogastric ligaments. Note that the tail of the pancreas extends as far as the hilus of the spleen. This is an important relationship and has to be considered in surgical removal of the spleen. It presents two primary surfaces. The **diaphragmatic surface** is smooth and convex and is in relation to the upper left portion of the diaphragm. The visceral surface is subdivided into three smaller surfaces, all of which converge toward the hilus. The largest and most anterior is the **gastric surface,** which is somewhat concave, and forms a portion of the stomach bed. The upper posterior portion is the **renal surface.** This is in relation to the upper left portion of the anterior surface of the left kidney, from which it is separated by peritoneum and extraperitoneal areolar tissue. The lowest portion is the **colic surface.** This is in contact with the left colic flexure and the phrenicocolic ligament. Starting at the hilus, bisect the spleen and note its internal structure.

The left lobe of the liver has already been removed. The right lobe should now be re-

moved for study of the surfaces of the liver. Cut through the falciform ligament from its free margin up to the point at which it joins the coronary and left triangular ligaments. Cut the right triangular ligament transversely and continue this incision to the left through the anterior layer of the coronary ligament to the point at which it joins the falciform ligament. As they pass to the left from the right triangular ligament, the anterior and posterior layers of the coronary ligament diverge, enclosing a broad area in the posterior surface of the right lobe of the liver, which is not covered with peritoneum. Free this area from the diaphragm and cut through the posterior layer of the coronary ligament. Sever the hepatic artery and the portal vein just below their division into right and left branches; cut the common bile duct at the same level. As another alternative, after cutting the coronary ligament and the hepatic veins, pull the liver downward and forward, leaving the hepatic artery, portal vein, and common bile duct intact. The liver can be rotated on the latter structures to study all its surfaces and replaced at any time for study of its relationships to the other viscera.

Immediately to the right of the caudate lobe, between it and the part of the posterior surface of the right lobe enclosed by the coronary ligament, the posterior surface of the liver partly encircles the **inferior vena cava.** All that remains to be done in removing the liver is to detach this portion of its posterior surface from the inferior vena cava. In doing this, it will be necessary to sever the **hepatic veins,** three or four short trunks which pass from the substance of the liver directly into the vena cava. After the right lobe has been removed, reattach the left lobe to it with pins and study the organ as a whole.

The superior, anterior, and right lateral surfaces of the **liver** are in contact with the **diaphragm** and present a rounded contour cor-

Liver - indespensable to life - largest organ -
3½ lbs. - R-hypochondriac region.

responding to the form of that structure. Near the median line, the inferior margin projects below the **costal arch,** bringing the lower part of the anterior surface into contact with the **anterior abdominal wall.**

The posterior surface of the liver is ordinarily described as including the bare area, the fossa for the vena cava, the caudate lobe, and a small upper right portion of the left lobe which is in contact with the esophagus. The **bare area** is the large triangular area of the right lobe, which is enclosed by the **coronary**

The **caudate lobe** lies between the fossa for the vena cava and the attachment of the lesser omentum. It is covered with visceral peritoneum, and, as already observed, it projects into the superior recess of the omental bursa.

The **inferior surface of** the **left lobe** is in contact with the lesser omentum and the upper part of the anterior surface of the **stomach.** The inferior surface of the right lobe exhibits numerous impressions corresponding to the structures with which it is in relation.

Closely applied to the inferior surface of

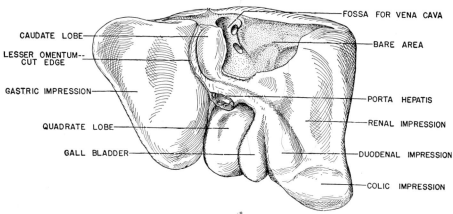

FIG. 61. The posterior and inferior surfaces of the liver.

and **right triangular ligaments.** It is in direct contact with the diaphragm, without the intervention of any peritoneum. Below and to the left this area is in contact with the **right suprarenal gland,** which here intervenes between the diaphragm and the liver. Dissect in the region from which the bare area was removed and expose the anterior surface of the right suprarenal (Fig. 60). Occasionally, the uppermost portion of the anterior surface of the right kidney is high enough also to come into relation with the bare area.

The **fossa for** the **vena cava** lies immediately to the left of the bare area. It sometimes almost entirely surrounds the vessel. Opening into it, the cut ends of the **hepatic veins** will be seen.

the **right lobe** is the **gall bladder.** The visceral peritoneum covering the inferior surface of the liver is reflected over the gall bladder, giving its free surface a serous coat of visceral peritoneum. Running to the left from the gall bladder into the lesser omentum is the **cystic duct.**

Observe the attachment of the lesser omentum. Toward its right margin it widens out to enclose the porta hepatis. The **porta hepatis** is the hilus of the liver, at which the **portal vein** and **hepatic artery** enter it and the **hepatic ducts** leave it.

In front of the porta hepatis and to the left of the gall bladder is a quadrangular portion of the inferior surface of the right lobe, the **quadrate lobe.** It is in contact with the pylorus and the beginning of the duodenum.

Immediately to the right of the constricted portion of the gall bladder is a variable **duodenal impression.** The part of the inferior surface which is most anterior and farthest to the right exhibits a **colic impression** where the liver is in contact with the right colic flexure. Above and behind the colic impression and occasionally extending on to the bare area is the broad **renal impression.** Here the right lobe of the liver is in relation to the anterior surface of the right kidney but separated from it by a layer of parietal peritoneum.

Open the **gall bladder** by a longitudinal incision running from the fundus to the neck and examine its interior. The interior of the gall bladder is stained dark green with **bile.** Observe that the lining membrane presents a ridged appearance and that toward the neck the ridges take on a spiral form. This is the **spiral valve** of the gall bladder, which is continued well into the **cystic duct.** Then dissect the gall bladder free from the surface of the liver and identify the **cystic artery.**

Detach the left lobe of the liver once more and study the cut surface of the organ. The larger cut vessels which will be seen are branches of the **portal vein** and tributaries of the **hepatic veins.** These two sets of veins can always be distinguished from each other by the fact that each branch of the **portal vein** is accompanied by a branch of the **hepatic artery** and a tributary of the **bile duct.** In addition, these three structures are enclosed in a fibrous sheath, constituting a **portal canal,** while the hepatic veins have very thin walls and appear to be in direct contact with the liver substance.

Large and Small Intestines

Turn the transverse colon and transverse mesocolon upward, draw the coils of jejunum and ileum downward and to the left so that the right surface of the mesentery faces an-

teriorly, and clean and study the superior mesenteric vessels. To do this, it will be necessary to remove a large, continuous piece of peritoneum constituting the posterior layer of the transverse mesocolon, the right layer of the mesentery, and the portion of the parietal peritoneum of the posterior abdominal wall which intervenes between these two mesenteries on the right side. The removal of this portion of the parietal peritoneum will expose the anterior aspect of the terminal part of the duodenum, and, enclosed within the bend of the duodenum, the lower part of the anterior surface of the head and neck of the pancreas (Fig. 62). Then make an incision through the parietal peritoneum just lateral to the ascending colon and a similar incision just lateral to the descending colon. By blunt dissection, free and elevate the ascending and descending colon and reflect them toward the midline of the body. This procedure, known as mobilization of the colon, simulates the primitive mesentery for the ascending and descending colon and exposes their blood supply. On the right side, the first part of the duodenum and part of the pancreas will be seen, while on the left side, the terminal part of the duodenum and the remainder of the pancreas will be exposed.

The **superior mesenteric artery** arises from the front of the **abdominal aorta** a short distance below the celiac artery. It enters the present area of dissection by passing downward behind the neck of the pancreas and in front of the lower part of the duodenum. The **superior mesenteric vein** lies to the right of the artery and often overlaps it anteriorly. The tributaries of the vein, which correspond to the branches of the artery, may be removed in cleaning the arteries, but the trunk of the vein should be retained.

In front of the lower part of the duodenum, the superior mesenteric artery reaches the root of the mesentery. It then runs downward and to the right across the posterior abdominal wall along the root of the mesentery. Its terminal portion enters the mesentery to reach the lower part of the ileum.

The first branch of the superior mesenteric, the **inferior pancreaticoduodenal,** is at present the ascending branch anastomoses with the right branch of the **middle colic.** Arising usually somewhat below the right colic, but sometimes by a common stem with it, is the **ileocolic branch.** This runs downward and to the right across the posterior abdominal wall, to give

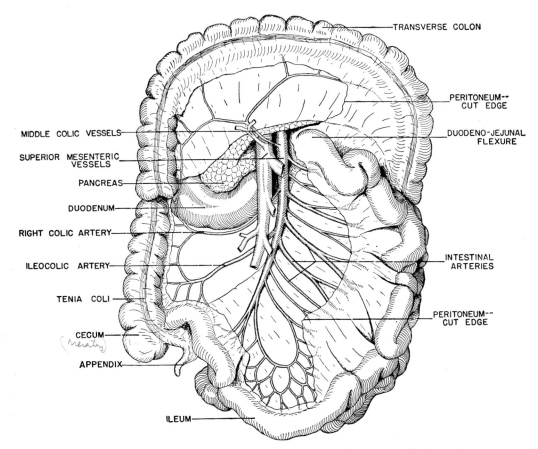

FIG. 62. Dissection to display the superior mesenteric artery and its branches.

hidden by the pancreas. Just below the pancreas the superior mesenteric gives rise to the **middle colic artery.** This vessel enters the transverse mesocolon, where it divides into **right** and **left branches** which supply the **transverse colon.** Somewhat lower is the **right colic artery,** which crosses the right side of the posterior abdominal wall behind the parietal peritoneum and divides into **ascending** and **descending branches** which supply the **ascending colon;** branches to the **cecum, appendix,** and terminal part of the **ileum.** Its terminal branches anastomose with each other and with the descending branch of the right colic.

In its passage along the root of the mesentery, the **superior mesenteric artery** gives rise to a series of from 12 to 16 **intestinal arteries** which run forward through the mesentery to supply the **jejunum** and ileum. Each intestinal artery divides into two branches, which unite with similar branches from adjacent arteries to form a series of **arterial loops** or **arcades** in the mesentery. From these arcades other branches arise, which also unite to form smaller arches as they approach the intestine. Observe the manner in which these arterial arcades change from the upper to the lower end of the mesentery. In the **upper part of** the **mesentery** there is usually only **one set of arterial arches,** giving branches directly to the gut, while toward the **lower end of** the **ileum** there may be as many as **four or five sets of arches.** Observe also that the amount of **fat** contained **within** the **mesentery** around the arterial arches **increases from above downward;** if the mesentery is held up to light, large translucent areas may be seen within the arterial arches of its upper portion, while in the lower portion the translucent areas are much smaller, due to the larger amount of fat present.

Study the jejunum and ileum. Together they measure on the average about 22 ft in length. The division between jejunum and ileum is an arbitrary one, the **jejunum** being the **upper two-fifths** and the **ileum** the **lower three-fifths.** It is based on the fact that there is a gradual change in the character of the intestinal wall from the duodenojejunal flexure to the ileocolic junction, so that the lower end of the ileum exhibits some very different characteristics from the upper end of the jejunum.

Section the jejunum about 1 in. below the duodenojejunal flexure; section the ileum about 1 in. from its junction with the cecum; cut through the mesentery along the entire length of its intestinal attachment; and remove the jejunum and ileum. Open the gut by longitudinal incisions in the wall at intervals along its length and compare the characteristics of its lining in different regions.

Observe that the **circular folds of** the **mucous membrane** are largest and closest together in the upper part of the jejunum and almost entirely lacking in the lower part of the ileum.

The wall of the jejunum is in general somewhat thicker than that of the ileum. Attempt to find some **aggregate lymph nodules.** These are collections of **solitary lymph nodules** occurring in oval patches which may be as much as 5 or 6 cm in length. They are **largest** and **most numerous in** the **lower** part of the **ileum.** In old age they seem frequently to disappear entirely.

Observe the external characteristics of the **large intestine.** A surgeon, working in a circumscribed area in the peritoneal cavity, cannot depend on diameter as a criterion if he is in doubt as to whether he is dealing with a bit of small or large intestine. There are, however, two features which are purely characteristic of the large gut. These are the teniae coli and the epiploic appendages.

The **teniae coli** are **three longitudinal bands** which traverse the length of the large intestine. They are caused by part of the longitudinal muscle of the large intestine being aggregated into these three bands. Between the teniae, the wall of the large intestine is thrown into three longitudinal series of **sacculations.** All three **teniae begin at** the **base of** the **vermiform process.**

The **epiploic appendages** are small outpocketings, filled with **fat,** of the **peritoneum** covering the large intestine. They are found throughout its length.

The **cecum** is usually entirely covered with peritoneum, though in some cases the upper part of its posterior surface is not covered and is in direct contact with the abdominal wall. Open the cecum by an anterior longitudinal incision and observe the **ileocecal orifice.** This orifice, at which the ileum joins the cecum, has the form of an anteroposterior slit in the medial wall of the cecum. It is bounded by a superior and an inferior lip, which constitute the **valve of** the **colon** and represent a partial protrusion of the ileum into the colon. Below the ileocecal orifice, identify the **orifice of** the **vermiform appendix,** which may be freely

Treitz

open, or may be guarded by a fold of mucous membrane, the **valve of** the **vermiform process.**

The ascending colon is not covered posteriorly by peritoneum but is in direct contact with the extraperitoneal tissue of this portion of the abdominal wall. Observe, however, that the transverse mesocolon does not extend so far to the right as it does to the left. Consequently, the **first part of** the **transverse colon,** just to the left of the right colic flexure, has **no mesentery,** and its posterior surface comes into direct contact with the anterior surfaces of the **right kidney** and the descending portion of the **duodenum** as it crosses them.

Duodenum and Pancreas

The **duodenum** is the **first part of** the **small intestine.** It is about 10 in. in length and its course has the form of a C-shaped curve whose concavity encircles the **head of** the **pancreas.** It is described as consisting of superior, descending, and inferior portions. Except for the superior portion, which begins at the pylorus and is partly covered on its posterior surface by peritoneum, the duodenum is firmly fixed to the posterior abdominal wall and is covered only anteriorly by peritoneum. Its descending portion, where it is crossed anteriorly by the transverse colon, has no peritoneal covering whatever.

The **superior part** runs upward and to the right from the pylorus for about 2 in. The peritoneum on its upper border forms the lower boundary of the epiploic foramen. Below the right lobe of the liver, it turns downward to join the **descending part.** The descending portion runs downward for about 3 or 4 in., lying behind the peritoneum and in front of the medial portion of the anterior surface of the right kidney, the right renal vessels, and the right border of the inferior vena cava. It then bends to the left as the **inferior (horizontal) part** which crosses the median plane, running to the left and upward, to bend forward and

join the jejunum at the **duodenojejunal flexure,** as already noted. In addition to the peritoneum, a band of retroperitoneal fibrous and muscle tissue (**Treitz's ligament**) extends from the left crus of the diaphragm to the duodenojejunal flexure to help support it in place. Observe that it is crossed anteriorly, near the median plane, by the **superior mesenteric vessels,** and usually also, slightly more to the left, by the root of the mesentery. Posteriorly, it is in relation to the inferior vena cava and the aorta.

The **pancreas** is an elongated gland consisting of head, neck, body, and tail. The **head** is the flattened portion which fills the concavity of the duodenal curve. Anteriorly, it is covered by peritoneum and crossed by the parietal attachment of the right end of the transverse mesocolon. Posteriorly, it rests against the inferior vena cava. Observe that its lower portion, the **uncinate process,** projects to the left behind the **superior mesenteric vein.** The **neck** is a short constricted portion, running upward and to the left from the upper part of the head to join the body. It rests posteriorly against the beginning of the portal vein.

The **body of** the **pancreas** runs to the left and somewhat upward across the posterior abdominal wall. The line of attachment of the transverse mesocolon usually follows the border separating anterior and inferior surfaces, so that the former faces into the omental bursa and comes into relation, through the peritoneum covering it, with the posterior surface of the stomach. The inferior surface of the pancreas faces downward into the greater sac. The posterior surface has no relation to peritoneum and crosses the aorta and the upper part of the superior mesenteric artery; it is in relation also to the anterior surface of the left kidney. The **tail of** the **pancreas** is the narrowed left extremity of the body. It usually extends forward through the lienorenal ligament to come into contact with the **hilus of** the **spleen.**

Detach the tail, body, and neck of the pancreas from the posterior abdominal wall and turn them forward to expose the structures behind them. Observe that the splenic vein runs to the right behind the upper border of the pancreas. The **splenic vein** is formed at the hilus of the spleen by the junction of the **short gastric** and **left gastroepiploic veins** and several **veins from** the **spleen.** It traverses the lienorenal ligament and passes to the right across the posterior abdominal wall. Behind the neck of the pancreas, it joins the **superior mesenteric vein** to form the **portal vein,** which then passes upward behind the first part of the duodenum and into the lesser omentum. Clean the terminal portion of the inferior mesenteric vein, which ascends behind the pancreas to join the splenic vein. Occasionally, it lies farther to the right, opening into the superior mesenteric vein near the termination of the latter. The **left renal vein** may usually also be seen behind the body of the pancreas, crossing from the left kidney to the inferior vena cava in front of the aorta and behind the superior mesenteric artery (Fig. 64).

Clean the **pancreaticoduodenal arteries.** The origin of the **superior pancreaticoduodenal** behind the superior part of the duodenum as a branch of the **gastroduodenal** has already been seen. Trace it downward along the medial border of the descending part, where it will be found to give branches to the duodenum and the head of the pancreas. The **inferior pancreaticoduodenal artery** arises from the **superior mesenteric** near the lower border of the pancreas. It runs downward and to the right between the inferior part of the duodenum and the head of the pancreas, giving branches to both, and ends by anastomosing with the superior pancreaticoduodenal. The inferior pancreaticoduodenal occasionally arises as a branch of the first intestinal branch of the superior mesenteric.

The **common bile duct** has already been seen to be formed within the right margin of the lesser omentum by the junction of the **cystic** and **hepatic ducts** and to descend behind the first part of the duodenum. Trace it now downward between the descending part of the duodenum and the head of the pancreas to the point at which it enters the wall of the duodenum.

Dissect in the substance of the pancreas and clean and study its ducts. The **pancreatic ducts** lie nearer to the posterior than the anterior surface of the gland and, consequently, can be more readily exposed from behind. The ducts are small, thin-walled, and usually white or grey in color. The **main duct begins in** the **tail** of the pancreas and passes to the right through the body, receiving small ducts from the numerous lobules along its course. It then passes downward and to the right through the neck and head and accompanies the **common bile duct** in the medial wall of the descending part of the duodenum. The **accessory duct** is smaller; it **begins in** the lower part of the **head** and runs upward through the substance of the pancreas to open into the descending part of the duodenum above the main duct. The two ducts often communicate within the substance of the pancreas.

Open the **duodenum** and study its interior. Observe that the **circular folds of** the **mucosa** are large and numerous. Find the **duodenal papilla.** This is a small elevation at about the middle of the medial wall of the descending portion of the duodenum, at the summit of which is the common orifice of the **main pancreatic** and **common bile ducts.** Just above this narrow common opening, the lumen may be dilated forming the hepatopancreatic ampulla (of Vater). The papilla is usually at the upper end of a longitudinal fold of the mucosa, the **plica longitudinalis.**

Clean and study the inferior mesenteric vessels (Fig. 64). The **inferior mesenteric artery** is much smaller than the superior mesenteric. It arises from the front of the lower part of the **abdominal aorta** and runs downward and to the

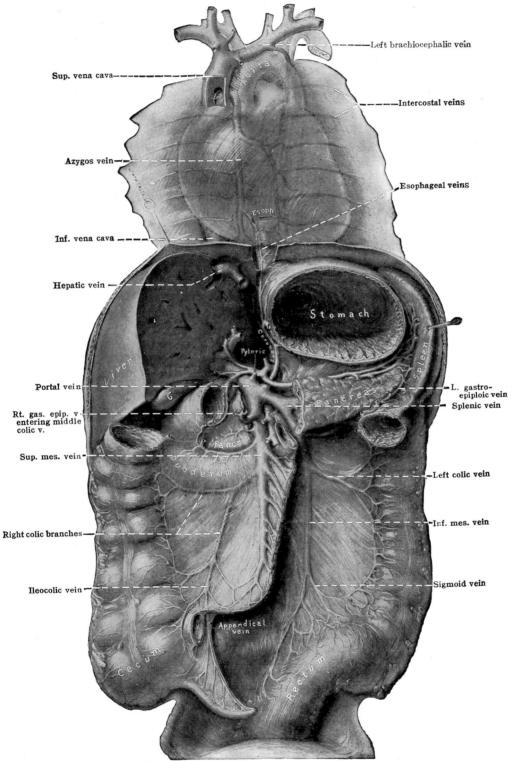

FIG. 63. The portal vein and its major tributaries. (*By Brödel.*)

left behind the peritoneum on the posterior abdominal wall. Its first branch is the **left colic artery.** This vessel runs to the left behind the peritoneum and divides into **ascending** and **descending branches,** which supply the **descending colon;** the ascending branch anastomoses with the left branch of the middle colic artery.

The tributaries of the **inferior mesenteric vein** correspond to the branches of the artery. The trunk of the vein does not, however, accompany the artery but ascends behind the peritoneum on the left side of the posterior abdominal wall to pass behind the pancreas and join the splenic vein.

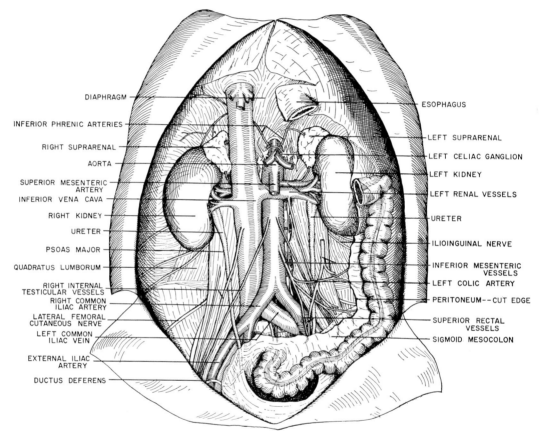

FIG. 64. Dissection of the retroperitoneal structures on the posterior abdominal wall.

Below the left colic, several **sigmoid branches** arise from the **inferior mesenteric.** These pass forward in the sigmoid mesocolon to supply the **sigmoid colon.** They form anastomosing loops with one another, with the descending branch of the left colic, and with the superior hemorrhoidal artery. The **superior hemorrhoidal (rectal)** is the direct continuation of the **inferior mesenteric,** which crosses the pelvic brim to enter the pelvis minor.

Free, elevate, and retract cephalad the spleen, pancreas, and duodenum in order to study the subjacent structures. Later replace these viscera to study their relationships to the adjacent organs.

Suprarenals and Kidneys

The **suprarenal glands** are of irregular shape and are flattened anteroposteriorly. The **left**

Single { hypogastric ganglia
Inf. mes. "
Sup. "
Celiac "

Paired phrenic g.
" Suprarenal g.
uterine

suprarenal is in relation anteriorly with the posterior surface of the stomach through the parietal peritoneum of the stomach bed; the lower part of its anterior surface often lies behind the pancreas. The anterior surface of the **right suprarenal** is overlapped on the left by the inferior vena cava but is elsewhere in contact with the liver.

The lower lateral portion of the posterior surface of each **suprarenal** is in contact with the upper medial part of the anterior surface of the corresponding **kidney;** above the kidney, each suprarenal rests posteriorly against the **diaphragm.** Make a transverse incision through the middle of the suprarenal glands. Note the outer **cortical** and inner **medullary parts** of these glands.

The height to which the kidneys rise in the abdominal cavity is somewhat variable, a circumstance which can be readily understood from a knowledge of the embryology of these organs. In most cases, however, the lower pole of each kidney lies well above the iliac crest. Observe that the upper medial portion of the anterior surface of each kidney is in direct contact with the posterior surface of the suprarenal.

The anterior surface of the **right kidney** is in direct contact near its medial border with the descending portion of the **duodenum.** To the right of this, it presents a broad area which is in relation through the parietal peritoneum with the inferior surface of the **liver.** Below the liver, this surface is in contact, without the intervention of any peritoneum, with the right **colic flexure.** The lowest and most medial portion of the anterior surface of the right kidney comes into relation, through the peritoneum, with the coils of the **small intestine.** The **left kidney** is crossed anteriorly by the **pancreas.** Above the pancreas, it is in relation with the renal surface of the **spleen** and the posterior surface of the **stomach,** from both of which it is separated by parietal peritoneum. Below the pancreas it is in relation to the right

with coils of **small intestine** and to the left with the left **colic flexure.**

The relations of the posterior surfaces of the kidneys can be better appreciated when the posterior abdominal wall has been studied.

The **hilus of** each **kidney** is an oval area at the middle of its medial border, where the renal artery enters it and the renal vein and the ureter leave it. The **renal arteries** are branches of the abdominal aorta; the **renal veins** drain into the inferior vena cava. Near the hilus, the vein is usually the most anterior and the ureter the most posterior of the three structures, but this relation is not constant. Observe that the left renal vein crosses anterior to the aorta and the right renal artery posterior to the vena cava. It is not uncommon to find more than one artery passing from the aorta to the kidney on one or both sides. As it emerges from the hilus, the **ureter** is wide. Its diameter contracts, and it passes downward and medially across the posterior abdominal wall toward the pelvic brim.

Without severing the renal vessels or the ureter, make a longitudinal section through the kidney from the lateral border to the hilus and study the cut surfaces. Observe that the **kidney** substance exhibits a differentiation into two parts, cortex and medulla. The **cortex** is the lighter-colored peripheral portion. The inner, **medullary portion** is made up of a variable number of **renal pyramids,** which converge toward the center of the kidney and end there as rounded projections, the **renal papillae.** The uriniferous tubules empty into the calyces at the apices of the papillae. The potential central cavity of the kidney is the **renal sinus,** but this cavity contains fat, the renal vessels, and the dilated upper part of the ureter, the **renal pelvis.** The peripheral part of the renal pelvis is in the form of funnel-shaped sacs, the **calyces,** which surround the ends of the papillae.

Clean and study the **celiac plexus.** This is a nerve plexus of the autonomic system which

Renal fascia - fascia of Gerota

receives fibers from the **vagi** and from the **sympathetic trunks;** the latter reach it through the greater and lesser splanchnic nerves. It consists of the two **celiac ganglia** and their **branches** of communication. Each celiac ganglion is, in reality, a group of several closely connected ganglia (Fig. 64). The **left celiac ganglion** lies on the left crus of the diaphragm between the aorta and the left suprarenal gland. Cut carefully into the substance of the diaphragm to expose the **left greater splanchnic nerve,** which pierces the diaphragm to end in the ganglion.

The **right celiac ganglion** occupies a similar position on the right side but is for the most part covered anteriorly by the inferior vena cava. The right and left ganglia are connected by branches which pass transversely, above and below the celiac trunk. The **branches of** distribution of the **celiac plexus** are the various **sympathetic plexuses** which accompany the **abdominal aorta** and its branches.

Abdominal Aorta and Inferior Vena Cava

Clean and study the **abdominal aorta** and the **inferior vena cava.** In cleaning the aorta, observe the **aortic plexus.** This is a **sympathetic nerve plexus** which is connected above with the celiac plexus and also receives branches from the lumbar portion of the sympathetic trunk. From it arise subordinate plexuses which accompany the branches of the aorta to the viscera. Observe the **hypogastric plexus** which leaves the aorta at the level of the origin of the common iliac arteries and courses over the sacral promontory into the pelvis.

The **abdominal aorta** begins at the **aortic hiatus of** the **diaphragm** as a continuation of the descending portion of the **thoracic aorta.** It descends in front of the bodies of the first four lumbar vertebrae to end, usually, in front of the **fourth lumbar** by dividing into the **right** and **left common iliac arteries.** Anteriorly and to the left, it is in relation to the parietal peritoneum of the posterior abdominal wall, except

where other structures intervene between the aorta and the peritoneum. These structures are the pancreas, the inferior part of the duodenum, the splenic vein, the left renal vein, and portions of some of its own branches. To the right, it is in relation with the inferior vena cava, with the exception that its most superior portion is separated from the vena cava by the right crus of the diaphragm.

The **unpaired branches** which arise from the anterior aspect of the aorta have already been studied. The **paired branches** should now be investigated (Fig. 64).

The **inferior phrenic arteries** arise from the aorta between the two crura of the diaphragm. They pass upward and laterally across the inferior surface of the **diaphragm.** Observe that the right artery passes behind the inferior vena cava and the left behind the esophagus. One or both of the inferior phrenics may be found to arise from the celiac; the left inferior phrenic occasionally arises from the left gastric. The inferior phrenic usually gives a **superior suprarenal branch** to the suprarenal gland.

The **middle suprarenal arteries** are small vessels, not always present, which arise from the lateral aspects of the **aorta** at about the same level as the origin of the superior mesenteric. They cross the crura of the diaphragm to reach the suprarenal glands.

The **renal arteries** have already been observed as large lateral branches of the aorta which supply the kidneys. Before it reaches the hilus of the kidney, each renal artery usually gives an **inferior suprarenal branch** to the suprarenal gland. The right renal artery crosses behind the inferior vena cava.

The **internal spermatic (testicular) arteries** arise from the front of the **aorta** somewhat below the origin of the superior mesenteric. They pass downward and laterally across the posterior abdominal wall to reach the deep inguinal ring, from which point their further course has already been seen. In its passage across the posterior abdominal wall, the testicular artery crosses in front of the ureter. The **ovarian arteries** are the homologues in the female of the testiculars in the male. Superiorly, their course is similar; inferiorly, however, they do not diverge so far laterally but cross in front of the common iliac arteries to enter the pelvis minor.

The **common iliac arteries** are short, thick trunks which run downward and laterally from the termination of the **aorta** to end opposite the lumbosacral articulation by dividing into the **external iliac** and the **hypogastric (internal iliac) arteries.** They have no other branches. Observe that the left common iliac artery is crossed anteriorly by the superior rectal vessels and also that each common iliac is crossed anteriorly by the ureter and, in the female, by the ovarian vessels.

In addition to the branches described above, there arise from the **posterior aspect of** the **abdominal aorta** four pairs of **lumbar arteries** and a single middle sacral artery. The lumbar arteries may be studied to better advantage somewhat later; the **middle sacral** may be found now, emerging from behind the left common iliac vein and running downward in front of the body of the fifth lumbar vertebra into the pelvis.

The **inferior vena cava** is formed, to the right of the body of the **fifth lumbar vertebra** and behind the right common iliac artery, by the junction of the **right** and **left common iliac veins.** The common iliac veins are at their origin somewhat medial and posterior to the terminations of the common iliac arteries. Ob-serve that the left common iliac vein is considerably longer than the right. It runs upward, medial to the left common iliac artery, to join the right vein behind the right common iliac artery, receiving in its course the middle sacral vein.

From its origin, the **vena cava** ascends on the posterior abdominal wall to an orifice in the **tendinous portion of** the **diaphragm.** It lies in front of the right sides of the bodies of the lumbar vertebrae and the medial border of the right psoas major muscle. Its upper portion rests posteriorly against the diaphragm. Here it is elsewhere in contact with the liver, as previously observed. Below the liver, it is in relation anteriorly and to the right with the parietal peritoneum, except where it is covered by the pancreas and duodenum. The largest tributaries of the inferior vena cava, above the common iliac veins, are the **renal veins.** Observe that while the vena cava receives directly the **right suprarenal** and **right testicular (or ovarian) veins,** the **left suprarenal** and **left testicular veins** join the **left renal vein.** The vena cava also receives the **inferior phrenic veins** and three or four **hepatic veins.**

Draw the vena cava forward and, dissecting carefully behind it, attempt to determine how many of the **lumbar veins** join it. There are four pairs of lumbar veins, corresponding to the lumbar arteries, but they do not always all join the vena cava. The upper ones usually drain into the right and left ascending lumbar veins, which pass through the diaphragm as the azygos and hemiazygos veins, respectively.

Diaphragm and Posterior Abdominal Wall··

Study the **diaphragm.** This is the great dome-like sheet of muscular and fibrous tissue which **separates** the **thoracic** and **abdominal cavities.** It consists of a **peripheral muscular portion** and a **central tendinous portion.** The muscle fibers which constitute the peripheral portion are described as taking origin at their peripheral attachments and as being inserted into the central tendon. Starting anteriorly, the diaphragm originates by two small slips from the back of the **xiphoid process;** then on each side by a series of six slips from the inner surfaces of the **cartilages of** the **lower** six **ribs,** which interdigitate with the slips of origin of the transversus abdominis; between the cartilage of the twelfth rib and the vertebral column, the diaphragm takes origin from the **lateral** and **medial lumbocostal arches.** Its most posterior portion arises from the lumbar vertebrae by means of the **right** and **left crura.**

The **posterior abdominal wall,** below the diaphragm and lateral to the vertebral column, is formed by the **psoas major** and **quadratus lumborum muscles.** The **lumbocostal arches** are thickenings in the fascia covering the anterior surfaces of these muscles. They cannot always be demonstrated as distinct structures, but the origin of the diaphragm from the quadratus and psoas fascia is constant. The **medial lumbocostal arch** typically crosses the **psoas major** from the body to the transverse process of the second lumbar vertebra; the **lateral arch** crosses the **quadratus** from the same transverse process to the twelfth rib (Fig. 65).

The **crura** are the thickest and most fleshy portions of the diaphragm. The **right crus** is larger and descends lower than the left; it arises from the bodies of the first three lumbar vertebrae. The **left crus** arises from only the first two lumbar vertebrae. The lowest portions of both crura are tendinous. As they ascend,

the crura approach each other, and their fibers cross and mingle with each other in front of the aorta. Observe that the **aortic hiatus** is thus not an actual opening in the diaphragm but a passage behind it. The **aorta** is protected from constriction when the diaphragm contracts by a fibrous arch which connects the medial borders of the two crura in front of the aorta and forms the actual border of the aortic hiatus.

Clean and study the psoas and quadratus muscles. In cleaning the psoas, watch for the **genitofemoral nerve,** which emerges through its substance and runs downward and laterally on the anterior surface of the muscle. In cleaning the quadratus, preserve the **subcostal, iliohypogastric,** and **ilioinguinal nerves,** all of which will be found emerging from behind the lateral border of the psoas and crossing the anterior surface of the quadratus.

First observe whether or not the **psoas minor** is present. This small muscle arises from the sides of the **bodies of** the **twelfth thoracic** and **first lumbar vertebrae.** Its fleshy body narrows to a flat tendon which passes down on the anterior surface of the psoas major to be inserted on the **pecten of** the **pubis.** It is very often lacking on one or both sides.

The **psoas major** arises by a series of fleshy bundles from the **intervertebral discs** of all the lumbar vertebrae and from a series of **fibrous arches** which bridge across the sides of the bodies of the lumbar vertebrae between the discs. Observe that the lumbar arteries pass around the sides of the bodies of the upper four lumbar vertebrae behind these fibrous arches. The psoas major also has a deep origin from the **transverse processes of** the **lumbar vertebrae.** The muscle fibers form a fusiform belly, which crosses the ilium above the brim of the pelvis, where it lies lateral to the external iliac artery. It leaves the abdomen by passing behind the inguinal ligament into the thigh, where it is inserted on the **lesser trochanter of the femur.**

The **quadratus lumborum** is a flat muscle lying lateral to the upper part of the psoas major between the twelfth rib and the iliac crest. It arises from the posterior part of the

articulation as one of the terminal branches of the **common iliac** and runs forward on the pelvic brim, at the medial border of the psoas major, to pass behind the medial part of the **inguinal ligament.** Beyond this point, it is continued into the thigh as the **femoral artery.** It is crossed superiorly near the inguinal liga-

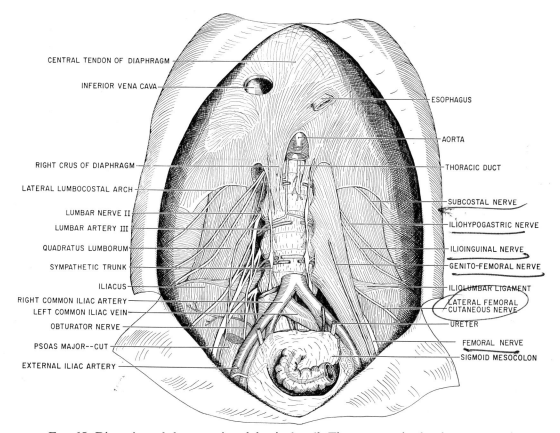

CENTRAL TENDON OF DIAPHRAGM
INFERIOR VENA CAVA
ESOPHAGUS
AORTA
RIGHT CRUS OF DIAPHRAGM
THORACIC DUCT
LATERAL LUMBOCOSTAL ARCH
SUBCOSTAL NERVE
LUMBAR NERVE II
ILIOHYPOGASTRIC NERVE
LUMBAR ARTERY III
ILIOINGUINAL NERVE
QUADRATUS LUMBORUM
GENITO-FEMORAL NERVE
SYMPATHETIC TRUNK
ILIOLUMBAR LIGAMENT
ILIACUS
LATERAL FEMORAL CUTANEOUS NERVE
RIGHT COMMON ILIAC ARTERY
LEFT COMMON ILIAC VEIN
URETER
OBTURATOR NERVE
FEMORAL NERVE
PSOAS MAJOR--CUT
SIGMOID MESOCOLON
EXTERNAL ILIAC ARTERY

FIG. 65. Dissection of the posterior abdominal wall. The psoas major has been removed on the right side to display the lumbar plexus.

internal lip of the **iliac crest,** from the **iliolumbar ligament,** the **transverse processes of** the lower three or four **lumbar vertebrae,** and the deep surface of the **anterior lamella of** the **lumbodorsal fascia.** Some fibers pass upward to be inserted on the lower border of the **twelfth rib** and the **transverse processes** of the upper two or three **lumbar vertebrae.**

Clean the external iliac vessels. The **external iliac artery** arises opposite the lumbosacral

ment by the ductus deferens (or the round ligament of the uterus). Just before it passes behind the inguinal ligament, it gives rise to its only branches, the **inferior epigastric** and deep circumflex iliac arteries. The full course of the inferior epigastric has already been traced. The **deep circumflex iliac** artery arises from the lateral side of the external iliac and runs laterally and upward along the line of junction of the iliac fascia with the inguinal ligament.

At the anterior superior iliac spine, it pierces the transversus muscle to run posteriorly along the iliac crest between the transversus and the internal oblique, where it has already been exposed. The **external iliac vein** begins behind the inguinal ligament as a continuation of the **femoral vein.** From this point to its termination in the common iliac it lies just medial to the artery.

Below the iliac crest the posterolateral portion of the abdominal wall is formed by the **iliacus muscle.** This is a broad flat muscle which fills the **iliac fossa,** from the bony surface of which it takes origin. Its fibers pass downward and medially behind the inguinal ligament to **join** the **tendon** of insertion **of** the **psoas major.** The iliacus is covered internally by a fairly dense fascial layer, the **iliac fascia,** which joins the inguinal ligament anteriorly. In removing this fascia to expose the muscle, do not injure the **lateral femoral cutaneous nerve.** This nerve will be found emerging from behind the psoas and running laterally across the iliacus. It enters the thigh by passing behind the inguinal ligament just medial to the anterior superior spine of the ilium. Passing behind the inguinal ligament immediately lateral to the psoas, in the groove between the psoas and iliacus will be found the **femoral nerve.** This large nerve emerges from behind the psoas and passes into the thigh behind the inguinal ligament (Fig. 65).

Clean and study the lumbar portions of the **sympathetic trunks.** Each sympathetic trunk enters the abdomen by passing through or behind the corresponding **crus of** the **diaphragm.** It then runs downward on the anterior surfaces of the lumbar vertebrae just medial to the psoas major. Each trunk usually exhibits **four lumbar ganglia,** which send **rami communicantes** to the first four **lumbar nerves.** From each trunk, branches pass forward to the **aortic plexus.** Inferiorly, the sympathetic trunks pass downward over the sacral promontory into the pelvis. Observe that the right trunk lies behind the inferior vena cava and the left one is crossed anteriorly by the left common iliac vessels.

Draw the aorta forward and display the four pairs of **lumbar arteries** arising from its posterior aspect. These pass backward and laterally around the bodies of the first four lumbar vertebrae, dorsal to the sympathetic trunks, and behind the psoas, which they supply. In their further course, they are usually behind the quadratus lumborum.

Dissecting in the areolar tissue behind the aorta, attempt to display the **cisterna chyli.** This is the lower expanded portion of the **thoracic duct.** It lies in front of the body of the second lumbar vertebra and receives the lymphatic vessels from all parts of the body below the diaphragm. From the cisterna, the thoracic duct ascends through the aortic hiatus into the posterior mediastinum of the thorax.

Portions of the **ilioinguinal, iliohypogastric, lateral femoral cutaneous, genitofemoral,** and **femoral nerves** have already been displayed in relation to the muscles of the posterior abdominal wall. These nerves are all derived from the **lumbar plexus.** The distribution of the iliohypogastric and ilioinguinal nerves was followed in the dissection of the anterior abdominal wall. If the **genitofemoral nerve** is now traced downward on the psoas, it will be found to terminate by dividing into two branches, the external spermatic (genital) and the lumboinguinal (femoral). The **genital nerve** has already been traced into the deep inguinal ring as the nerve of supply of the **cremaster muscle.** The **femoral branch** crosses the iliacus to pass behind the inguinal ligament into the thigh.

The **lumbar plexus** lies deeply within the substance of the **psoas major muscle.** For its display, it will be necessary to cut away the psoas major carefully. Start the dissection by following the genitofemoral nerve upward and posteriorly into the psoas muscle. Then remove the longitudinal strands of this muscle piecemeal to expose the lumbar plexus. When the plexus is exposed, it will be seen to be derived from the **anterior primary divisions** of the first four **lumbar nerves.** The branches which arise from the plexus are the iliohypogastric, ilioinguinal, femoral, genitofemoral, lateral femoral cutaneous, and obturator nerves. Some portion of each of these nerves, with the exception of the obturator, has already been seen. The **obturator nerve** arises within the psoas by three roots, which are derived from the anterior primary divisions of the second, third, and fourth lumbar nerves. It emerges from the medial border of the psoas and enters the pelvis minor by passing downward behind the common iliac vessels (Fig. 65).

The **femoral nerve** is the largest branch of the lumbar plexus. It also is derived from the second, third, and fourth lumbar nerves. It emerges from the lateral border of the psoas, from which point its further abdominal course has already been seen; it gives **twigs** of supply **to** the **iliacus muscle.**

The **genitofemoral nerve** has two roots, which are derived from the first and second lumbar nerves. The **iliohypogastric** and **ilioinguinal nerves** are both derived from the first lumbar nerve, though they often also receive a communication from the last thoracic. Observe that, as they emerge from the lateral border of the psoas to cross the quadratus lumborum, these two nerves are in relation with the posterior surface of the kidney. The **lateral femoral cutaneous nerve** is derived from the second and third lumbars; it is sometimes represented by two smaller nerves, which cross the iliacus at some distance from each other.

In addition to these branches, the **four roots of** the **lumbar plexus** give **twigs** of supply directly **to** the **psoas** and **quadratus muscles.** From the fourth and fifth lumbar nerves a large branch (**lumbosacral trunk**) descends to join the sacral plexus. A small branch known as the **accessory obturator nerve** is sometimes found to arise from the third and fourth lumbar nerves; it descends along the medial border of the psoas and enters the thigh by crossing the pecten of the pubis.

Perineum ·

The **perineum** is a diamond-shaped area at the lower end of the trunk, between the thighs. It corresponds to the **inferior pelvic aperture,** and, as a distinct region of the body, it is separated from the pelvic portion of the abdominal cavity by the **pelvic diaphragm.** In the erect posture, the surface area of the perineum is reduced to a narrow groove running forward from the **coccyx to** the **pubis, between** the **thighs.** For its dissection, it is therefore necessary to tie the body in the lithotomy posi-

tion, with the thighs widely spread and the inferior pelvic aperture facing upward. Throughout the dissection, it should be borne in mind that with the body in this position structures which are anatomically superior or inferior will appear to the dissector in exactly the reverse positions.

A knowledge of the pelvic skeleton is essential for a proper dissection of the perineum. Before starting the dissection, study an articulated bony pelvis, preferably one with the ligaments still in place. Observe that the most **anterior point of** the **perineum** is represented in the skeleton by the lower end of the **pubic symphysis;** this bony surface is covered by the **arcuate ligament** of the pelvis. **Posteriorly,** the perineum is limited by the **coccyx.** Its widest lateral extent is about midway between the symphysis and the coccyx and is limited on each side by the **tuberosity of** the **ischium.** Its **anterolateral boundary** is formed on each side by the **inferior rami of** the **pubis and** the **ischium. Posterolaterally,** the perineum is bounded by the **sacrotuberous ligament** which

a **posterior, anal triangle.** At the **anal orifice,** which appears in the anal triangle, the skin of the perineum becomes continuous with the mucous membrane of the anal canal.

Male Perineum

Note the location of the anal orifice. Then make two incisions through the skin of the perineum: (1) a median longitudinal incision running from the upper posterior part of the skin of the scrotum backward to a point about 1 in. above the tip of the coccyx (this incision must encircle the anal orifice); (2) a trans-

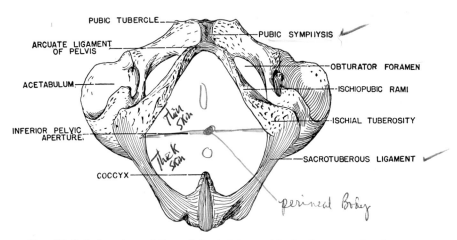

Fig. 66. Inferior view of the pelvic skeleton, with the ligaments in place.

stretches from the lower end of the sacrum and the coccyx to the ischial tuberosity. As the dissection proceeds, it will be found that this ligament is covered externally by the lower part of the **gluteus maximus muscle,** so that the lower border of this muscle may be regarded as forming on each side the posterolateral boundary of the perineum. The ischiopubic rami, the ischial tuberosity, and the coccyx may be palpated from the surface and should be identified before the skin is reflected.

The perineum is arbitrarily subdivided by an imaginary transverse line running between the anterior portions of the two ischial tuberosities into an **anterior, urogenital triangle** and

verse incision running from a point about 1 in. lateral to the ischial tuberosity on one side across in front of the anus to a similar point on the other side. By this means four triangular flaps of skin will be marked out. The two anterior flaps should be reflected forward and laterally, the two posterior flaps backward and laterally.

Skin the remaining part of the scrotum and dissect the terminal course of the posterior scrotal vessels and nerves. Then divide the scrotum in the midline and reflect the testes and their coverings laterally to each side. Now trace the nerves posteriorly into the superficial fascia of the urogenital triangle.

The reflection of skin will expose the **superficial fascia** of the perineum. In the **anal triangle,** this layer differs from the same layer in other parts of the body only in its **extreme thickness.** In the **urogenital triangle,** it is thinner. The superficial fascia over the urogenital triangle of the perineum, just like that over the lower abdominal wall, was assumed to be, and can be artificially dissected into, an outer fatty and an inner membranous layer. However, sections of this tissue from normal cadavers and from patients in whom this tissue was infiltrated with extravasates showed that the subcutaneous tissue here, as in the other parts of the body, consists of only one layer.* This one layer is made up of alveoli of fat embedded in strands or sheets of collagenous and elastic fibers. These fibers attach to the periosteum or deep fascia in certain areas of the body, but there is no definite subdivision of this tissue into an outer fatty and an inner membranous layer.

The **inner membranous layer (Colles' fascia)** was thought to be attached posteriorly to the urogenital diaphragm and laterally to the ischiopubic rami and anteriorly to be continuous with the dartos around the scrotum and penis and with the membranous layer (**Scarpa's fascia**) over the ventral abdominal wall. The potential space formerly described as existing between **Colles' fascia** and the **inferior layer of** the **urogenital diaphragm** was known as the **superficial perineal pouch.** This old concept of a subdivision of the superficial fascia into two definite layers is revised in the chapters on the male and female perineum.

Cut down through the superficial fascia along the midline of the urogenital triangle and reflect it to each side. This must be done with care to avoid injury to the **superficial perineal nerves.** As the layer is reflected, it will be found to be continuous laterally over the ischiopubic

* Based on the studies of Tobin and Benjamin (*Surg. Gynec. & Obst.,* **88:** 545, 1949).

rami with the same layer of fascia on the medial aspect of the thigh and posteriorly with the superficial fascia of the anal triangle.

The deeper fibers of the **superficial fascia** attach **laterally** to the margins of the **ischiopubic rami. Posteriorly,** this **fascia** extends **into** the **anal triangle** but also **attaches to** the **posterior** free **margin of** the **urogenital diaphragm. Anteriorly,** however, it is continuous through the **dartos tunic** of the scrotum and, around the sides of the penis and scrotum, with the **superficial fascia** on the lower part of the **anterior abdominal wall.**

Identify the **central point of** the **perineum.** This is a tendinous septum in the midline of the body a short distance in front of the anus. Then clean the **external sphincter ani muscle.** This is a thick ring of muscle fibers, running backward from the **central point to** the tip of the **coccyx** and encircling the anus. As it is cleaned, small branches of the **inferior hemorrhoidal nerve and artery** will be found emerging from the fat on each side to enter the muscle (Fig. 67).

The **perineal nerve** divides into superficial and deep branches. The **superficial branches** are two or three **posterior scrotal nerves.** These are **cutaneous nerves** to the skin of the urogenital triangle and the posterior part of the scrotum.

The **deep branches supply** the **muscles,** which should now be cleaned. Observe that these nerves are all accompanied by branches of the perineal artery.

The **superficial transverse perineal muscle** is a small paired muscle, variable in size and degree of development and, consequently, often difficult to demonstrate. It arises from the inner surface of the anterior part of the **ischial tuberosity** and is inserted at the **central point of** the **perineum,** where it blends somewhat with the external sphincter ani and the bulbocavernosus.

The ischiocavernosus and bulbocavernosus

are thin sheets of muscle which cover the external surfaces of the structures forming the **root of** the **penis.** These structures are the **bulb of** the **urethra** and the two **crura** of the **penis.**

The bulbocavernosus and all ischiocavernosus muscles are embedded in a layer of fascia —the **deep** (Buck's) **fascia of** the **penis.** This

The **bulb of** the **urethra** lies in the median plane. It is attached above to the undersurface of the inferior fascial layer of the urogenital diaphragm. Anteriorly, it narrows to become continuous with the **corpus cavernosum urethrae.** Each **crus penis** is attached to the corresponding ischiopubic rami and the inferior surface of the lateral parts of the urogenital

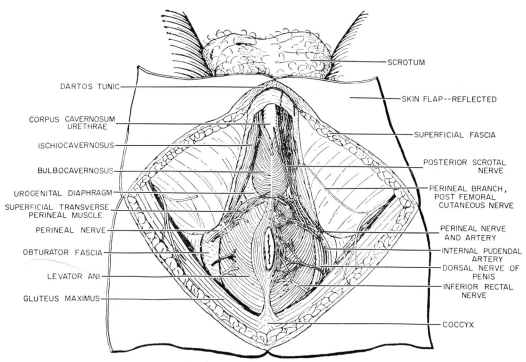

DARTOS TUNIC

CORPUS CAVERNOSUM URETHRAE

ISCHIOCAVERNOSUS

BULBOCAVERNOSUS

UROGENITAL DIAPHRAGM

SUPERFICIAL TRANSVERSE PERINEAL MUSCLE

PERINEAL NERVE

OBTURATOR FASCIA

LEVATOR ANI

GLUTEUS MAXIMUS

SCROTUM

SKIN FLAP--REFLECTED

SUPERFICIAL FASCIA

POSTERIOR SCROTAL NERVE

PERINEAL BRANCH, POST FEMORAL CUTANEOUS NERVE

PERINEAL NERVE AND ARTERY

INTERNAL PUDENDAL ARTERY

DORSAL NERVE OF PENIS

INFERIOR RECTAL NERVE

COCCYX

FIG. 67. Superficial dissection of the male perineum. Alcock's canal has been opened on the left side. Most of the terminal branches of the inferior rectal and perineal nerves and vessels have been removed on the right side.

fascia is thin over these muscles but is thick over the shaft of the penis where it is in the form of a figure eight. The **two crura** and the **deep vessels and nerves** are enclosed in the **upper compartment,** whereas the **corpus cavernosum urethrae** is in the **lower compartment.** This fascia attaches to the suspensory ligament of the penis. The part enclosing the corpus cavernosum urethrae helps to limit the spread of urine extravasated through a perforation in the ventral wall of the penile urethra.

diaphragm. They run forward and medially and unite in front of the lower part of the pubic symphysis to form the **corpus cavernosum penis.** Each is covered by an ischiocavernosus muscle.

The **bulbocavernosus** arises from the **central point of** the **perineum** and from a **median raphe** running forward on the undersurface of the bulb. From this origin, its fibers diverge to surround the bulb and be inserted into the fascia of the **urogenital diaphragm** and the **dor-**

sal surface of the **corpus cavernosum urethrae.** Some of its most anterior fibers reach the dorsum of the corpus cavernosum penis. Each **ischiocavernosus** arises from the inner aspect of the **ramus of** the **ischium** and is inserted into the lateral aspect of the **anterior part of** the **crus.** Make an incision through the bulbocavernosus muscle along the midventral line of the corpus cavernosum urethrae and reflect the two

end. At this point, the **urethra pierces** the **urogenital diaphragm to enter** the **bulb.** Attempt to display the small **artery to** the **bulb,** which pierces the diaphragm on each side of the urethral orifice to enter the bulb. Draw the bulb forward to expose the lower surface of the urogenital diaphragm. Find the **dorsal nerve of** the **penis** and the **internal pudendal artery,** which here pierce the inferior fascial layer of

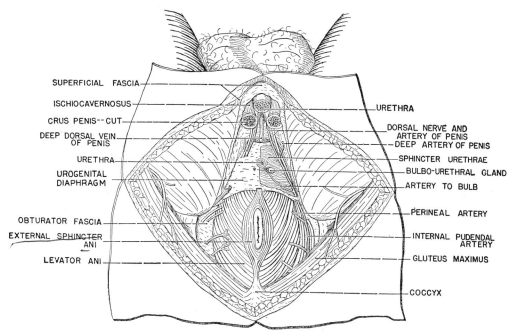

FIG. 68. Deep dissection of the male perineum. The crura penis and the bulb of the urethra have been removed. The inferior fascia of the urogenital diaphragm has been removed on the left side to expose the structures of the deep pouch.

parts of the muscle laterally. The ischiocavernosus muscle should also be reflected from the ventral surface of each crus.

Free and elevate the crura from the ischiopubic rami and complete the separation of the three components of the penis. Then dissect between the bulb and the crus and expose the lower surface of the **urogenital diaphragm.** Attempt to separate the bulb from the diaphragm and observe that it is firmly attached superiorly to the diaphragm at a point in the midline about ½ in. in front of its posterior

the urogenital diaphragm under cover of the crura. Just as it emerges from the urogenital diaphragm, the **internal pudendal artery** terminates by dividing into the **deep artery of** the **penis,** which enters the crus, and the **dorsal artery of** the **penis,** which accompanies the dorsal nerve forward onto the dorsum of the penis (Fig. 68).

The inferior surface of the urogenital diaphragm is now exposed. Clean its sharp anterior border, the **transverse ligament of** the **pelvis.** Observe that this lies just behind the arcuate ligament, which covers the lower border of the pubic symphysis, and that the **deep dorsal vein of** the **penis** enters the pelvic cavity by passing through the narrow interval between the transverse and arcuate ligaments.

The dissection of the anal triangle consists principally in the display of the boundaries and contents of the two **ischiorectal fossae.** Each ischiorectal fossa is a potential space lying lateral to the lower end of the **anal canal.** The superomedial boundary of each is formed by the inferior surface of the **pelvic diaphragm,** which separates the fossa from the pelvic cavity. The lateral wall of each ischiorectal fossa is formed by a layer of fascia known as the **obturator fascia,** which clothes the inner surface of the obturator internus muscle; this muscle intervenes between the obturator fascia and the inner surface of the ischium. Posteriorly, the ischiorectal fossa is bounded by the **sacrotuberous ligament** and the lower border of the **gluteus maximus muscle.** The ischiorectal fossa is filled by an **ischiorectal fat pad** within which the **inferior rectal nerves and vessels** ramify. The highest part, or roof, of the ischiorectal fossa is formed by the line along which the pelvic diaphragm joins the obturator fascia.

Insert the blade of a scalpel into the fat pad of the ischiorectal fossa about 1 in. lateral to the anal orifice. The blade should enter the fat pad in a lateral direction, at about a 30° angle from the transverse plane of the perineum, and penetrate the fat pad to a depth of 2 in. Then insert a finger into the opening made by the scalpel and palpate the boundaries of the ischiorectal fossa. Flex the finger and palpate the structures crossing from the lateral to the medial part of the fossa. These are the inferior rectal vessels and nerves.

First clean the lower border of the gluteus maximus muscle between the coccyx and the ischial tuberosity. Then proceed to the removal of the ischiorectal plug of fat to display the walls of the fossa and the inferior rectal nerves and vessels. This dissection is generally considered difficult only because it is tedious. The fat must be carefully removed, and the vessels and nerves preserved. The **pelvic diaphragm,** which forms the medial wall of the fossa, consists of the **levator ani** and **coccygeus muscles** and **their fascial coverings.** These muscles are often very thin, and care is necessary to avoid breaking through them into the pelvic cavity.

When the dissection is complete, it will be seen that the **inferior rectal vessels** and **nerves** emerge from the obturator fascia to run medially through the ischiorectal fossa and ramify about the lower end of the **anal canal.** Emerging from the obturator fascia at the anterior end of the lateral wall of the ischiorectal fossa, the **perineal nerve** and **artery** may be identified. These structures pierce the obturator fascia, run forward for a short distance in the anterolateral angle of the ischiorectal fossa, and enter the superficial fascia of the perineum (Fig. 67).

The arteries and nerves thus exposed in the ischiorectal fossa are derived from the **pudendal nerve** and the **internal pudendal artery.** Before emerging into the fossa, they are lodged in a **canal in** the **obturator fascia** known as **Alcock's canal.** Alcock's canal runs forward in the lateral wall of the ischiorectal fossa from the **lesser sciatic foramen to** the **posterior edge of** the **urogenital diaphragm.** Open this canal on one side and display the structures it contains.

The **pudendal nerve** is derived from the **sacral plexus.** It usually divides into its two terminal branches, the perineal nerve and the dorsal nerve of the penis, before entering the perineum. Consequently, these two nerves will be found separately in the canal. The **perineal nerve** usually lies below the internal pudendal artery and leaves the canal in company with the perineal branch of the artery. The **dorsal nerve of** the **penis** lies above the artery. This nerve and the internal pudendal artery leave the anterior end of the canal by entering between the two fascial layers of the urogenital diaphragm. The **inferior rectal nerve** may enter the posterior end of Alcock's canal separately or may arise within it as a branch of the perineal nerve.

Now reflect the inferior layer of fascia of the urogenital diaphragm to open the **deep pouch of** the **perineum.** This is the space enclosed between the two fascial layers of the urogenital diaphragm itself and contains the structures described below.

The **sphincter urethrae** is a thin muscle which stretches across between the ischiopubic rami of the two sides and encircles the membranous urethra. It is continuous posteriorly with the **deep transverse perineal muscle,** which also stretches across between the ischiopubic rami.

The **second** or **membranous portion of** the male **urethra** is short and traverses the urogenital diaphragm from above downward. It is continuous with the **third** or **cavernous portion of** the **urethra.** The **bulbourethral glands** are embedded in the deep transverse perineal muscle a short distance behind the urethra. Their fine ducts pierce the inferior fascia of the diaphragm to enter the **bulb** and join the third part of the **urethra.**

The dorsal nerve of the penis and the internal pudendal artery were previously seen to enter the urogenital diaphragm at the anterior end of Alcock's canal. They may now be traced forward along the lateral margin of the deep pouch to the point at which they were found to leave it by piercing the inferior fascia. Observe that while in the deep pouch the **internal pudendal artery** gives rise to the **artery to** the **bulb,** which pierces the inferior fascia independently to enter the bulb, as already noted.

Female Perineum

The **urogenital triangle of** the **female** perineum includes the **urethral orifice** and the **ex-** ternal genital organs, which should be studied before any dissection is done.

The **mons pubis** is an elevation of the skin in front of the pubic symphysis which is caused by the presence of a thick layer of adipose tissue. Extending downward and backward from the mons pubis on each side are the **labia majora,** folds of skin and fascia, which diminish in size posteriorly and meet a short distance in front of the anus. Between the two labia majora is the **urogenital fissure,** which contains the **urethral** and **vaginal orifices.** Overlapped by the labia majora are two much thinner integumental folds, the **labia minora,** which lie on each side of the vaginal orifice. Anteriorly, they converge and each divides into two folds. The lower fold from each **labium minus** is attached to the undersurface of the **clitoris** to form the **frenulum clitoridis.** The upper fold from each labium minus unites with the fold from the other side above the clitoris to form the **preputium clitoridis.** Between the frenulum and the preputium, the **glans clitoridis** will be seen. The region between the labia minora and behind the clitoris is known as the **vestibule.** The **vaginal orifice** will be seen opening into the posterior part of the vestibule. It may or may not be partly guarded by a fold of the mucous membrane, the **hymen.** The **urethral orifice** is a small slitlike opening in the wall of the vestibule slightly anterior to the vaginal orifice. On each side of the vaginal orifice, the minute opening of the **duct of** the **greater vestibular gland** may be seen.

Make two incisions through the skin: (1) a median longitudinal incision from the mons pubis backward to a point about 1 in. above the tip of the coccyx; this incision must bifurcate to encircle the labia minora and again to encircle the anus; (2) a transverse incision passing in front of the anus from a point about 1 in. lateral to the ischial tuberosity on one side to a similar point on the other side. Four flaps of skin will thus be marked out; the two anterior ones should be reflected forward and laterally and the two posterior ones backward and laterally.

The **superficial fascia** of the female urogenital triangle is the same as that of the male.

Dissect the course of the **perineal nerve** and **artery** in the superficial fascia of the urogenital triangle. Observe that they give, as in the male, deep and superficial branches. The **deep branches** of the perineal nerve supply the

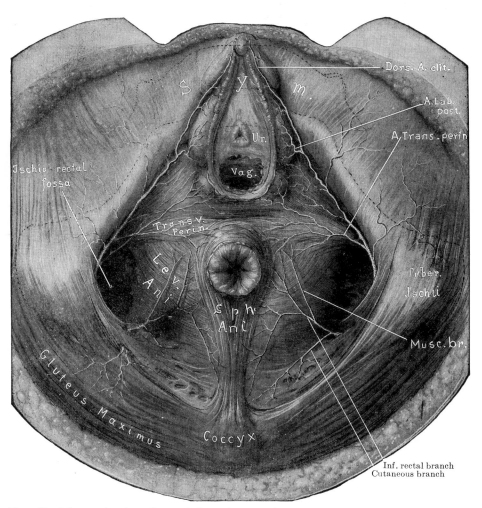

Fig. 69. The perineal and rectal branches of the internal pudendal arteries in the female. (*By Brödel.*)

The fascia is, however, divided into **two parts by** the presence of the **urogenital fissure.** Its lateral and posterior attachments are the same as in the male, and it should be cleaned as in the male. Observe that in the labia majora and the mons pubis this superficial fatty layer is very thick.

superficial muscles; the superficial branches are known as the **posterior labial nerves** and supply the **skin of** the **labia.**

The **superficial transverse perineal muscle** is similar to the same muscle in the male but is usually poorly developed. The **ischiocavernosus** is also present but is much smaller than the same muscle in the male. It arises from the **ramus of the ischium** near the tuberosity and covers the **crus clitoridis,** upon which it is inserted. The **bulbocavernosus** is divided into two halves which lie one on each side of the **vestibule,** closely applied to the external surface of the two halves of the **bulb of the vestibule.** Posteriorly, the muscle arises from the **central point of the perineum;** anteriorly, its two halves

toridis, the small rounded elevation which was already seen at the anterior end of the urogenital fissure between the preputium and the frenulum clitoridis.

Carefully reflect the bulbocavernosus muscle to expose the **bulb of the vestibule.** It consists of two oblong halves, composed principally of **erectile tissue,** situated on each side of the vestibule. Remove the bulb from the inferior

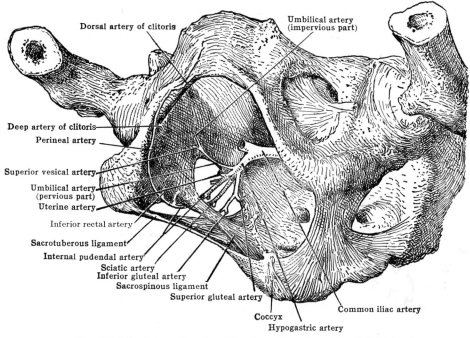

Fig. 70. The internal pudendal artery (female). (*By Brödel.*)

converge to be attached to the **sides of the clitoris.**

Examine the clitoris. The **body of the clitoris,** which corresponds to the corpus cavernosum penis, is formed in front of the lower border of the pubic symphysis by the junction of the two crura. The **crura,** which diverge widely from each other posteriorly along the medial borders of the pubic arch, correspond to the crura of the penis and, like them, each is covered by the **ischiocavernosus muscle.** From the symphysis, the body of the clitoris projects downward for a short distance to terminate at the **glans cli-**

surface of the urogenital diaphragm to expose the inferior fascial layer of the diaphragm. As the bulb is being removed, watch for the **artery** which pierces the inferior fascia **to** enter the **bulb** and the greater vestibular glands. Each **greater vestibular gland** lies under cover of the posterior end of the corresponding half of the bulb of the vestibule. From it a long duct passes into the wall of the vestibule to open lateral to the vaginal orifice.

Remove the crus clitoridis from its attachment to the ischiopubic rami. As the crus is reflected, secure the **dorsal nerve of the clitoris** and the **internal pudendal artery,** which emerge through the inferior fascia of the urogenital diaphragm under cover of the crus. Observe that the internal pudendal artery here divides into its terminal branches, the **deep and dorsal arteries of** the **clitoris.** The former immediately enters the crus; the latter proceeds anteriorly with the dorsal nerve to reach the dorsum (anterior surface) of the body of the clitoris.

The dissection of the anal triangle in the female is precisely the same as in the male, and the same structures will be exposed as in the male, with the exception that the place of the **dorsal nerve of** the **penis** is taken by the **dorsal nerve of** the **clitoris,** which is considerably smaller than the corresponding nerve in the male.

The **urogenital diaphragm** has the same fascial and muscular layers in the female as in the male and the same lateral attachments; its free anterior margin forms, as in the male, the **tranverse ligament of** the **pelvis.** It is, however, not so complete a partition as in the male, since it is pierced by the **vaginal canal** as well as the **urethra.** The dorsal nerve of the clitoris and the internal pudendal artery traverse the lateral margin of the urogenital diaphragm from its posterior border, which corresponds to the anterior end of Alcock's canal, to the point at which they have been seen to pierce the inferior layer of fascia. While it is within the diaphragm, the **internal pudendal artery** gives rise to the **artery to** the **bulb.**

Pelvis Minor ·

The cavity of the **pelvis minor** is the **lowest** and most posterior **portion** of the general **abdominal cavity.** It communicates freely with the abdomen proper at the **pelvic brim.** The **pelvic cavity** is bounded anteriorly and laterally by the internal surfaces of the **coxal (hip) bones,** covered by the **obturator internus muscles** and the **obturator fascia,** and posteriorly by the anterior surface of the **sacrum,** which is also covered internally by **fascia.** Inferiorly, the pelvic cavity is separated from the perineum by the **pelvic diaphragm.** The pelvic diaphragm is composed of two paired muscles, the **levator ani** and the **coccygeus,** covered on both their superior and their inferior surfaces by a layer of fascia. The fascia covering the inferior surface of the pelvic diaphragm is usually thin and has already been seen in the dissection of the perineum, where it forms the medial wall of the ischiorectal fossa. The superior fascial layer

of the pelvic diaphragm is known as the **visceral layer of** the **endopelvic fascia;** it not only covers the superior surfaces of the muscles of the pelvic diaphragm but also splits to form fascial sheaths in which the pelvic viscera are more or less completely enclosed. The fascia covering the internal surfaces of the obturator internus muscle (obturator fascia) and its extension across the front of the sacrum are known as the **parietal pelvic fascia.** The parietal fascia, from which in large part the muscles and fascia of the pelvic diaphragm arise, not only forms the lateral wall of the cavity of the pelvis minor, but extends into the perineum as well, where it has been seen to form the lateral wall of the ischiorectal fossa.

The **peritoneum** extends below the pelvic brim, but does not reach so far as the pelvic diaphragm. Consequently, a considerable portion of the pelvic cavity is extraperitoneal. The principal contents of the pelvic portion of the peritoneal cavity are coils of the **small intestine,** which have already been removed, and the **sigmoid colon.** In the female, however, the **uterus** is clothed with peritoneum and projects upward and forward into the pelvic peritoneal cavity.

The dissection of the pelvis can be most satisfactorily done in four stages: first, the observation and study of the disposition of the the peritoneum within the pelvis minor should be left undisturbed for the present. Next, identify the various **structures** which enter or leave the pelvis by **crossing** the **pelvic brim** external to the peritoneum.

Running upward toward the umbilicus from behind the pubic symphysis will be found the **urachus** or **middle (median) umbilical ligament.** Somewhat lateral to this on each side, also running toward the umbilicus, is the **lateral**

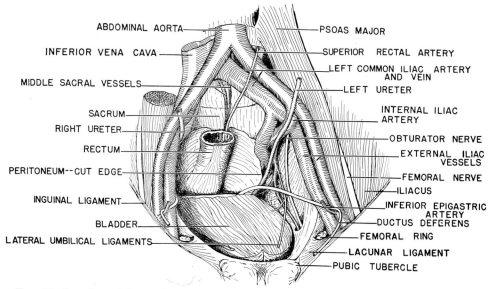

FIG. 71. Interior of the male pelvis, seen from above and slightly to the right. Most of the pelvic peritoneum has been removed.

pelvic peritoneum; second, the removal of the peritoneum and study of the structures occupying the extraperitoneal space; third, the study of the visceral pelvic fascia and the pelvic viscera which it encloses, during which the pelvis will be split into two halves; and, finally, the study of the muscles of the pelvic diaphragm and the pelvic wall.

The male and female pelvis should be compared at each stage of the dissection.

Male Pelvis Minor

Any peritoneum which still remains in place above the pelvic brim should be removed, but **(medial) umbilical ligament,** a cordlike structure representing the umbilical artery of the fetus. Still more laterally, the **ductus deferens** descends into the pelvis, having first crossed the external iliac artery and vein shortly before their passage behind the inguinal ligament. The **ureter** crosses the pelvic brim on each side at about the point where the common iliac arteries terminate. Here also the large **internal iliac artery and vein** descend into the pelvis. Running downward in front of the sacrum, the **middle sacral vessels** should be identified, and slightly to the left of these vessels the superior rectal vessels cross in front of the left common iliac vessels to run downward into the pelvis minor. An obturator artery will occasionally be found running downward across the brim of the pelvis slightly anterior to the ductus deferens. In such cases, it is a branch of the inferior epigastric or of the external iliac artery. In most cases, however, the **obturator artery** does not cross the brim of the pelvis but arises within the cavity of the pelvis minor as a branch of the hypogastric.

Next, study the disposition of the **peritoneum** within the pelvis. Anteriorly, it covers the **superior surface of** the **bladder.** If this viscus is empty and its walls contracted, as is frequently the case in cadavers, its outline is not readily apparent through the peritoneum. From the superior surface of the bladder, the peritoneum is reflected upward on each side onto the **lateral wall of** the **pelvis.** This portion of the peritoneum is sometimes called the lateral **false ligament of** the **bladder.** At the posterior border of the bladder, the peritoneum is reflected downward for a short distance over the **posterior surface of** the **bladder** and then upward onto the **front of** the **rectum.** It should be observed that here the rectum is covered only anteriorly by peritoneum. Slightly higher, it is covered anteriorly and on the sides and, still higher, where it is joined by the sigmoid colon, it is entirely covered by peritoneum. The **sigmoid colon** ends in front of the third sacral vertebra; it is completely covered with peritoneum and attached to the posterior left wall of the pelvis by the lower end of the **sigmoid mesocolon.**

The pelvic portion of the peritoneal cavity is divided into **three pairs of** more or less clearly defined **fossae by peritoneal folds and ridges.** The **sacrogenital folds** are horizontal folds of the peritoneum running from the posterior surface of the bladder in a curve backward and laterally toward the sacrum. If the rectum and bladder are both contracted, these folds are usually clearly visible, with a

sharp free margin, within which, near the bladder, the seminal vesicles can be felt. If one or both of these viscera are distended, the folds may be partly or wholly obliterated. Between this fold and the rectum on either side is the **pararectal fossa** of the peritoneal cavity. The two pararectal fossae communicate freely with each other in front of the rectum and behind the bladder. The two pararectal fossae and their communication together form the **rectovesical peritoneal pouch.**

The **ureter,** as it passes downward and medially external to the pelvic peritoneum, generally causes a distinct peritoneal ridge, which is parallel and anterior to the sacrogenital fold. The peritoneum between the sacrogenital fold and the ureteral ridge forms on each side of the floor of the middle or **genital peritoneal fossa** of the pelvis. The peritoneum on the side wall of the pelvis anterior to the ureteral ridge and lateral to the upper surface of the bladder (i.e., the lateral false ligament of the bladder) forms the floor of the **paravesical peritoneal fossa.** The **ductus deferens** can usually be seen through the peritoneum, crossing first the paravesical and then the genital fossa; when it reaches the sacrogenital fold, it turns abruptly downward behind the bladder.

Remove the peritoneum from the pelvic cavity, except for that part of the peritoneum covering the superior surface of the bladder and that over the anterior surface of the rectum and the intervening rectovesical pouch. The peritoneum detached from the rest of the pelvic wall is cut away and discarded.

The satisfactory dissection of the pelvic contents depends to a large extent on the realization that there is a considerable amount of **fatty areolar tissue between** the **peritoneum** and the **fascia lining** the **pelvic wall** and enclosing the pelvic viscera. This tissue is to be removed as the structures embedded in it are cleaned.

Clean first the **ductus deferens.** It lies on the

side wall of the pelvis immediately external to the peritoneum, crossing in turn the superior vesicle artery, the obturator nerve and vessels, and the ureter. Here it turns downward behind the bladder and enters the visceral pelvic fascia; its further course will be followed later.

Follow the **lateral (medial) umbilical ligament** backward across the pelvic wall and observe that it springs from the **internal iliac artery,** of which it was, in fact, the original direct continuation. Two or three small vessels will be found to arise from it and pass to the bladder. These are the **superior vesical arteries.** Distal to the origin of the last of these the lateral umbilical ligament is a solid cord. Proximal to that point it is a patent vessel of small caliber.

The **obturator nerve** has already been seen to arise from the lumbar plexus above the pelvic brim, which it crosses external to the common iliac vessels. It will be found emerging from the medial side of the psoas major muscle behind the internal iliac artery and running forward across the pelvic wall to enter the **obturator canal.** Entering the obturator canal just below the nerve is the **obturator artery** and below it, the **obturator vein.** The parietal pelvic fascia is prolonged into the thigh through the obturator canal to form a sheath from the obturator nerve and vessels. Trace the obturator artery back to the **internal iliac,** of which it is usually a branch. It may arise from the internal iliac by a common stem with the umbilical or with some other branch or branches of the internal iliac.

Clean the pelvic portion of the **ureter.** It runs downward and forward in front of the internal iliac artery to the posterolateral angle of the bladder. Here, just below the point at which it is crossed anteriorly by the ductus deferens, it also enters the visceral pelvic fascia.

Attention should next be directed to the **bladder.** The bladder presents a superior surface which is completely covered with peritoneum, a posterior surface covered only on its upper part, and two inferolateral surfaces which are devoid of peritoneum and in relation to the pelvic wall and pelvic diaphragm. The **urachus or middle umbilical ligament** runs upward from the apex of the bladder, at which the superior and the two inferolateral surfaces meet. If the apex is pulled upward and backward, the inferolateral surfaces may easily be detached from the pelvic wall, exposing a space known as the **cave of Retzius,** which intervenes **between** the **pelvic wall and** the **inferolateral surfaces of** the **bladder.** This is a potential rather than an actual space, since it is narrow and filled with fatty areolar tissue. Its importance lies in the fact that an effusion of fluid into it, as from a rupture of the bladder, may readily spread laterally as far as the internal iliac arteries and upward into the extraperitoneal space at the sides of the pelvic and abdominal cavities.

As the bladder is turned upward and backward, it will be seen that while its inferolateral surfaces can be readily detached from the pelvic wall, its neck is firmly attached to the pelvic floor. The **neck of** the **bladder** is the region to which the two inferolateral surfaces and the posterior surface converge. It lies immediately above the **prostate gland,** which is enclosed in a heavy sheath of the visceral fascia. When the fatty areolar tissue has all been removed from the cave of Retzius, two white fascial bands will be seen running forward from the neck of the bladder to be attached to the inner surface of the body of the pubis on each side of the pubic symphysis. These are the **anterior true ligaments of** the **bladder** or **puboprostatic** (pubovesical) **ligaments** and represent thickenings of the visceral layer of the endopelvic fascia.

Now attempt to define the line along which the pelvic diaphragm springs from the pelvic wall. Push the peritoneum of the pararectal fossa over, open the cave of Retzius widely by displacing the bladder, and remove all the fatty areolar tissue which may remain. The object of this dissection is to clean the upper surface of the lateral part of the pelvic diaphragm and the parietal fascia.

With the aid of reference to a bony pelvis, locate by touch the pelvic surface of the **spine of the ischium.** If the fascia has been carefully cleaned, a **tendinous fascial band** will be seen running from the **spine** in a curve upward and forward to the **lower border of the obturator canal.** Anterior to the obturator canal, the same band turns downward and forward across the internal surface of the pubic bone as far as the anterior end of the anterior true ligament of the bladder. This band is the **arcus tendineus,** or tendinous arch, and marks the line along which the pelvic diaphragm springs from the pelvic wall. From the ischial spine to the obturator canal, the **pelvic diaphragm** (i.e., the levator ani muscle and the visceral pelvic fascia which covers it superiorly) arises from the **obturator fascia;** anterior to the obturator canal, the diaphragm arises directly from the **internal surface of the pubic bone.**

The obturator fascia, which forms the lateral boundary of the pelvic cavity, is the same layer which extends down into the perineum to form the lateral wall of the ischiorectal fossa. It will now be apparent that the **obturator fascia** is seen within the pelvis minor only posterior to the obturator canal. Here the fibers of the **obturator internus muscle** can usually be seen through the fascia, or a portion of the fascia may be removed to expose them. It will also be apparent that the **pelvic diaphragm** does not stretch horizontally across the pelvis but runs downward as well as medially from each side, so that the diaphragm as a whole has roughly the **shape of an inverted dome.** This should explain the apparent contradiction that the inferior surface of the pelvic diaphragm forms the medial wall of the ischiorectal fossa. If one hand is now introduced

through the perineum into the ischiorectal fossa and the other hand into the pelvis from above, the entire thickness of the pelvic diaphragm may be felt between the two hands.

The **visceral fascia** forming the uppermost layer of this lateral portion of the pelvic diaphragm is a single layer in direct relation to the upper surface of the levator ani muscle, which can usually be seen through it. As it approaches the midline anterior to the rectum, the visceral fascia is prolonged upward over the posterior surface of the prostate gland and still higher encloses the seminal vesicles, which lie behind the posterior surface of the bladder. This portion of the visceral fascia is known as the **rectovesical** (rectogenital) **fascia.** Still more anteriorly, the visceral fascia is prolonged upward over the anterior surface of the prostate and the inferolateral surfaces of the bladder and is known as **vesical fascia.**

The pelvis is now to be split into two parts for the further study of the viscera. The pelvic viscera and skeleton will be separated into equal halves.

Insert a probe, a director, or a catheter into the urethra and with a sharp knife bisect the corpus cavernosum urethrae by cutting down to the instrument inserted into the urethra from both the dorsal and ventral surfaces of the corpus cavernosum urethrae.

Cut through the midline of the pubic symphysis and extend the cut posteriorly through the pelvic viscera (bladder, prostate, and rectum) to the sacrum. Sever one common iliac vessel at the level of the fourth lumbar vertebra. Then divide the ureter near the renal pelvis and tie it to the testicular vessels, which should also be severed near their origins. Reflect the aorta and vena cava to one side and make a saw cut through the coccyx, sacrum, and lumbar vertebrae. Make a clean transverse cut through the soft tissues above the iliac crest to the intervertebral disc between the third and fourth lumbar vertebrae. This procedure should be done on either the right or left side and that lower quadrant of the body removed. The ureter and the testicular vessels should be cut only on that side of the body from which the lower quadrant is to be removed. Review the course of the lower spinal nerves (cauda equina) within the dura and the spinal canal. Locate and dissect the dorsal root ganglia on the lower lumbar and sacral nerves.

devoid of peritoneum, since it lies below the lowest part of the rectovesical peritoneal pouch. The lowest part of the rectum turns downward and backward, almost at right angles from the upper part, then runs downward and forward, passing through the **pelvic diaphragm** to reach the **anus**. This is the **anal canal** (or anal part). Trace the **superior rectal artery** downward along the posterior surface of the rectum. It

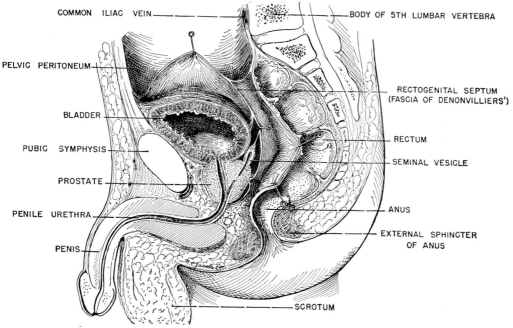

COMMON ILIAC VEIN

BODY OF 5TH LUMBAR VERTEBRA

PELVIC PERITONEUM

RECTOGENITAL SEPTUM
(FASCIA OF DENONVILLIERS')

BLADDER

RECTUM

PUBIC SYMPHYSIS

SEMINAL VESICLE

PROSTATE

PENILE URETHRA

ANUS

PENIS

EXTERNAL SPHINCTER
OF ANUS

SCROTUM

FIG. 72. Sagittal section through the male pelvis. The ischiorectal fossa has not been dissected. The rectum and its intrinsic fascia are retracted dorsally. The peritoneum over the superior surface of the bladder is retracted cephalad.

Dissect the **peritoneum** from the superior surface of the bladder and from the anterior surface of the rectum. Retract the peritoneum upward and note the **fascial septum** (rectogenital septum or **fascia of Denonvilliers**), which extends from the pelvic peritoneum downward to the pelvic floor between the seminal vesicles and prostate anteriorly and the rectum posteriorly (Fig. 72).

Clean the **rectum** and observe that there is a considerable portion of it which is entirely

divides into two main branches, one passing to each side of the rectum to anastomose with the right and left **middle rectal arteries.** These are branches of the internal iliac. The course of the superior rectal artery should be sought where it reaches the upper part of the anal canal.

Clean the **prostate.** It rests upon the upper surface of the middle of the urogenital diaphragm. The two levator ani muscles do not meet in the midline anteriorly, and the **gap in** the **pelvic diaphragm** thus left between their free margins is closed below by the **urogenital diaphragm**. The **prostate** is enclosed in a strong **sheath** derived from the visceral fascia. Posteriorly, this fascia cannot easily be separated from the gland. Anteriorly and at the sides, the **pudendal plexus of veins** will be found to intervene between the gland and its fascial covering. The **dorsal vein of** the **penis** enters beneath the pubic symphysis and above the anterior border of the urogenital diaphragm to join this plexus. Above the prostate clean each **seminal vesicle.** Each also is enclosed in a tough fascial sheath which must be removed to expose the contour of the vesicle. It rests against the posterior surface of the bladder. Along its medial border will be found the terminal part of the **ductus deferens** also enclosed in the fascia.

For a detailed study of the structure and relations of the bladder, prostate, and seminal vesicles, these organs should be retracted medially from the pelvic wall and the pelvic blood vessels should be studied. In this study, particular attention should be paid to the **internal iliac artery** and its branches. The veins of the pelvis are numerous, often plexiform in character, and drain into the internal iliac vein. If they obscure the dissection, they should be cut away and discarded.

The **internal iliac artery** has already been seen to arise from the **common iliac** and run down into the pelvis, crossing the pelvic brim opposite the sacroiliac articulation, where it lies medial to the external iliac vein and usually anterior to the internal iliac vein. The internal iliac artery gives rise to visceral and parietal branches. The **visceral branches** are the umbilical, inferior vesical, and middle rectal; the **parietal branches** are the iliolumbar, lateral sacral, obturator, internal pudendal, and superior and inferior gluteal. These branches are constant in their occurrence, but the manner in which they arise from the main

trunk is subject to great variation. The **umbilical artery,** which has already been seen, may be regarded as the direct continuation of the main trunk. The **superior gluteal, inferior gluteal,** and internal pudendal arteries always arise in that order from above downward, but any two or all three may arise by a common stem; the inferior gluteal and internal pudendal very frequently do so. All other branches may arise directly from the internal iliac or indirectly by any combination of common stems. The iliolumbar and lateral sacral very often arise in common with the superior gluteal. Identify the various branches and trace them so far as their course lies within the pelvis.

The **iliolumbar artery** runs upward and laterally to cross the pelvic brim external to the common iliac artery and vein, where it divides into iliac and lumbar branches. The **iliac branch** runs laterally behind the psoas major to enter the deep surface of the **iliacus;** the **lumbar branch** runs upward behind the **psoas,** supplying it and the **quadratus lumborum.**

The **lateral sacral** runs downward and medially over the anterior surface of the sacrum. There are frequently two lateral sacrals. The **superior gluteal** leaves the pelvis through the **upper part of** the **greater sciatic foramen.** The **inferior gluteal** and **internal pudendal** have a longer course in the pelvis, which they leave through the **lower part of** the **greater sciatic foramen** just above the spine of the ischium. The obturator has already been traced.

The **inferior vesical** and **middle rectal vessels,** which often arise in common, run medially through the fatty areolar tissue above the pelvic diaphragm. The former supplies the lower part of the **bladder** and the **prostate;** the latter reaches the side wall of the **rectum,** along which it sends branches to anastomose with the superior and inferior rectals.

Clean the **posterior surface of** the **bladder** and observe its relations. It lies above the

prostate and is in direct contact with the anterior surfaces of the **seminal vesicles,** which separate its lower part from the rectum. The terminal portions of the **deferent ducts** cross the posterior surface of the bladder along the medial borders of the seminal vesicles. The uppermost portion of the posterior surface is covered by peritoneum and forms the anterior boundary of the rectovesical pouch. The ureter joins the upper lateral angle of the bladder, where the posterior, superior, and inferolateral surfaces converge.

The **mucous membrane** lining the **bladder** is thrown into **irregular folds** over most of its surface when the bladder is empty. In the area known as the **trigone of** the **bladder** (trigonum vesicae), however, it is always **smooth.** This is a triangular area corresponding to the lower portion of the posterior surface. It is bounded below by the internal **urethral orifice,** which is at the neck of the bladder and leads downward into the first or prostatic portion of the urethra, and above on each side by the **ureteral orifice,** which is slitlike in appearance. Observe the **plica ureterica,** a curved transverse ridge extending between the two ureteral orifices. Pass a probe through one of these orifices into the ureter and observe that the ureter runs for some distance within the wall of the bladder before opening into its interior.

Return to the posterior aspect of the bladder and attempt to demonstrate by dissection that each **seminal vesicle** is in reality a single long tube which is folded backward and forward on itself so that it presents a lobulated appearance. At its lower medial angle, immediately above the prostate, this tube narrows to form the **excretory duct of** the **seminal vesical.**

The **ductus deferens,** as it runs downward and medially along the medial border of the seminal vesicle, widens to form the **ampulla of** the **ductus deferens.** This terminates below by joining the excretory duct of the seminal vesicle to form the **ejaculatory duct.** The two

ejaculatory ducts pass through the substance of the prostate gland to join the **prostatic portion of** the **urethra.**

The **prostate gland** occupies the interval between the anterior portions of the two levator ani muscles. Superiorly, it rests against the bladder and inferiorly against the upper surface of the urogenital diaphragm. It is traversed by the **first portion of** the **urethra.** If the entire course of the prostatic urethra was not exposed by the midline cut used to bisect the pelvic viscera, dissect off that part of the prostrate which still covers the prostatic urethra.

Observe the **urethral crest.** This is a median longitudinal ridge on the posterior wall of the prostatic urethra. It is most prominent at about its middle, where it enlarges to form the **seminal hillock** (colliculus seminalis). At the summit of the hillock is the orifice of a **small blind pouch,** the **prostatic utricle,** which runs backward for a varying distance into the substance of the prostate. Just below and to each side of the orifice of the **prostatic utricle** are the small terminal **orifices of** the **ejaculatory ducts.** The ducts of the prostate gland itself open by a number of minute orifices on each side of the urethral crest; these may often be made apparent by squeezing the prostate.

The second or **membranous portion of** the **urethra** traverses the **urogenital diaphragm.** It is short and narrower than the prostatic portion, and its wall presents no features of particular interest.

The third or **cavernous portion of** the **urethra** is much the longest of the three, traversing the whole length of the **corpus cavernosum urethrae** to terminate at the glans penis. The **bulbourethral glands** open into the cavernous portion about $\frac{1}{2}$ in. from its beginning. Its terminal dilated portion is known as the **fossa navicularis.**

Reflect the pelvic viscera medialward and clean the muscles of the pelvic diaphragm by removing the visceral fascia. Note branches of the second, third, and fourth sacral nerves to the pelvic viscera. The **levator ani** is a broad sheet of muscle whose line of origin is the same as that along which the visceral fascia arises. Anterior to the obturator canal, it springs directly from the **internal surface of** the **pubic bone;** posterior to the obturator canal, it springs from the internal surface of the **obturator fascia** along a curved line extending downward and backward to the **spine of** the **ischium.** Anteriorly, the muscle presents a free margin which passes backward and medially around the side of the prostate to join, behind the prostate and in front of the rectum, the **muscle of** the **opposite side.** More posteriorly, the levator ani is inserted into the side of the **rectum** and, still more posteriorly, it passes behind the rectum to join the muscle of the opposite side. The most posterior fibers are inserted upon the **coccyx.** Its nerve of supply, which is derived from the **fourth sacral,** should be sought running forward on its superior surface.

The **coccygeus** arises from the **spine of** the **ischium** and spreads out as it passes medially to be inserted on the **coccyx** and lower part of the **sacrum.** It is often more tendinous than muscular.

Observe that a portion of the **parietal pelvic fascia** covers the front of the sacrum above the coccygeus muscle. This is continuous on each side with the obturator fascia. The sacral nerves and the piriformis muscle lie external to it. The internal iliac artery and the beginning of its branches lie, as has been seen, internal to the parietal fascia. The parietal branches of the internal iliac pierce the parietal fascia as they leave the pelvis.

Female Pelvis Minor

Leaving the peritoneum within the pelvic cavity intact, remove all the peritoneum above the brim of the pelvis, identifying at the same time the various **structures** which **cross** the

brim external to the peritoneum. These are the **urachus** or **median umbilical ligament,** the **lateral (medial) umbilical ligament** (umbilical artery), the **round ligament of** the **uterus,** the **ureter,** and also the **middle sacral, superior rectal, hypogastric,** and **ovarian blood· vessels.** The urachus, the medial umbilical ligament, the ureter, and the middle sacral, superior rectal, and internal iliac vessels are the same as in the male. The ovarian vessels cross the pelvic brim a short distance anterior to the ureter. The **round ligament** occupies a position similar to that of the **ductus deferens** in the male, having first crossed the external iliac vessels near the inguinal ligament.

Now study the disposition of the **peritoneum** within the pelvic cavity. As in the male, the peritoneum covers the **superior surface of** the **bladder,** from which it is reflected upward onto the pelvic wall on each side as the **lateral false ligament of** the **bladder,** which forms the floor of a peritoneal fossa known as the **paravesical fossa.** This fossa is bounded posteriorly on each side, as in the male, by a peritoneal ridge caused by the ureter, but in the female it is subdivided into a large anterior and a small posterior portion by the **broad ligament of** the **uterus,** which should now be studied.

Diseased conditions of the female reproductive organs are very common in cadavers, and it is important to know in this dissection whether or not one is dealing with a perfectly normal case. The following description applies to a normal, healthy, and moderately young individual and may not in all cases suit the subject under observation (Fig. 73).

At the posterior border of the bladder, the peritoneum is reflected downward for a very short distance onto the posterior surface of the **bladder and then up onto** the front of the **uterus,** thus forming the floor of a shallow peritoneal fossa, the **vesicouterine pouch.** The uterus is almost entirely clothed with peritoneum. Normally it is bent so that its anterior surface faces not only forward but downward and overhangs the bladder. The **broad ligament** is a double fold of peritoneum which stretches on each side from the lateral border of the **uterus to the side wall of** the **pelvis.** Superiorly, it presents a free border in which the **uterine tube** is contained; at this border, the two layers of peritoneum which compose the **broad ligament** are continuous with each other. At its

toneal fold, the **mesovarium,** which supports the ovary. The **ovary** is a small oval body completely enclosed in peritoneum. The portion of the broad ligament above the mesovarium is known as the **mesosalpinx;** the portion below it is the **mesometrium.** As they run downward and medially below the pelvic brim to reach the ovary, the ovarian vessels cause a peritoneal ridge in relation to the posterior

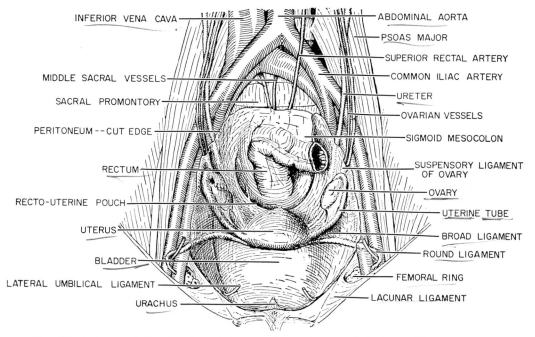

INFERIOR VENA CAVA — ABDOMINAL AORTA
— PSOAS MAJOR
MIDDLE SACRAL VESSELS — SUPERIOR RECTAL ARTERY
— COMMON ILIAC ARTERY
SACRAL PROMONTORY — URETER
— OVARIAN VESSELS
PERITONEUM - - CUT EDGE — SIGMOID MESOCOLON
RECTUM — SUSPENSORY LIGAMENT OF OVARY
RECTO-UTERINE POUCH — OVARY
UTERUS — UTERINE TUBE
— BROAD LIGAMENT
BLADDER — ROUND LIGAMENT
— FEMORAL RING
LATERAL UMBILICAL LIGAMENT — LACUNAR LIGAMENT
URACHUS

FIG. 73. Interior of the female pelvis, seen from above and in front. The peritoneum has been removed above the pelvic brim but remains in place within the pelvis minor.

medial border, the broad ligament joins the lateral border of the uterus, and here its two layers of peritoneum are continuous with the peritoneum covering the anterior and posterior surfaces of the uterus. Along its lateral and inferior borders, the anterior and posterior peritoneal layers of the broad ligament are reflected anteriorly and posteriorly to become continuous with the peritoneum lining the pelvic wall and pelvic floor.

Projecting posteriorly from the lateral part of the broad ligament is a short double peri-

surface of the lateral part of the broad ligament, known as the **suspensory ligament of** the **ovary.** Projecting from the anterior surface of the broad ligament another peritoneal fold will be seen; in this the **round ligament** is enclosed.

The female pelvic peritoneal cavity also presents, as does the male, middle, or genital, and pararectal peritoneal fossae. The **middle fossa** is bounded anteriorly on each side by the ureteral ridge and posteriorly by the recto-uterine fold. The **rectouterine** folds are similar to the sacrogenital folds of the male. They pass backward and laterally from the lower part of the posterior surface of the uterus toward the sacrum and may be wholly or partially obliterated by distention of the bladder or rectum. The two **pararectal fossae** communicate freely with each other in front of the rectum and behind the uterus, the whole forming the **rectouterine peritoneal pouch.** The lowest portion of the anterior wall of the rectouterine pouch is formed by the peritoneum not on the uterus but on the **vagina,** since the peritoneum is carried downward below the lower border of the uterus onto the uppermost portion of the posterior surface of the vagina before being reflected backward and upward onto the front of the rectum.

At the upper lateral end of the broad ligament, the **uterine tube** usually turns downward and backward so that its **fimbriated end** comes into close relation with the **ovary.** The open end of this tube is the only place at which the peritoneum is normally pierced. At the edges of this opening, the peritoneum becomes continuous with the mucous membrane lining the tube. Insert the point of the scissors into this opening and open the **tube** along its whole length, on the left side of the pelvis. Observe that it joins the **upper lateral angle of** the **uterus.** Cut through the peritoneum on the front of the broad ligament on the same side to expose the **round ligament.** This is a fibrous cord containing smooth muscle tissue, which is attached to the uterus just below its junction with the uterine tube. Cut through the posterior layer of the broad ligament along the left lateral margin of the uterus and expose the **uterine artery.** It runs up along the lateral border of the uterus, to which it sends branches, between the two layers of the broad ligament and is accompanied by a plexus of veins. Branches of it may be followed laterally through the broad ligament, toward the ovary, where they anastomose with the ovarian artery.

Now clean the **structures** which occupy the **extraperitoneal space** by removing the fatty areolar tissue in which they are embedded. The structures to be cleaned are the **ureter,** the **umbilical artery** (lateral umbilical ligament), and the **obturator vessels** and **nerve.** These structures are substantially the same as in the male. Observe, however, that the ureter crosses below the inferior border of the broad ligament to reach the upper lateral angle of the bladder. The **uterine artery** has already been seen running upward along the lateral border of the uterus; now follow it backward and laterally from the lower part of this border through the extraperitoneal space to the **internal iliac artery,** of which it is a branch. Study the **cave of Retzius,** which is the same as in the male.

The **bladder** presents the same surfaces as in the male; a superior surface, which, as has been seen, is covered with peritoneum and is in relation to the anterior surface of the uterus and coils of the small intestine; two inferolateral surfaces, which, as in the male, are in relation to the pelvic diaphragm and form the inner boundaries of the cave of Retzius on each side; and a posterior surface, which rests against the anterior wall of the vagina, except in its most superior part, where it is separated by peritoneum from the lowest part of the anterior surface of the uterus.

Remove all the fatty areolar tissue from the case of Retzius and the extraperitoneal space above it and clean the upper surface of the pelvic diaphragm and the pelvic wall. The superior surface of the **pelvic diaphragm** is formed by the visceral layer of the **pelvic fascia,** which covers the upper surface of the **levator ani muscle.** It springs, as in the male, from the side wall of the pelvis, along a fascial band known as the **arcus tendineus,** which runs from the ischial spine to the lower border of the obturator canal, and then downward and medially across the **internal surface of** the **pubis** toward the symphysis. Posterior to the obturator canal, the diaphragm arises from the **parietal fascia** covering the internal surface of the obturator internus muscle; anterior to the canal, it arises directly from the bone.

This lateral portion of the **visceral fascia** is a single layer, in direct relation to the upper surface of the levator ani muscle, which may be seen through it; it is known as the **rectal fascia.** Posteriorly, the rectal fascia is continued across the midline behind the rectum, still as a single

The pelvis is now to be split into two parts. The procedure for dividing the pelvis is the same as in the male.

Clean the **rectum.** It will now be apparent that there is a considerable portion of the rectum which is entirely devoid of peritoneum. The rectum is the same as in the male, except for the anterior relations of its lower portion, which is in direct contact with the **posterior wall of** the **vagina.**

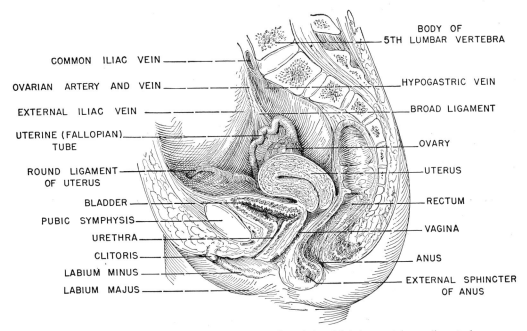

COMMON ILIAC VEIN

OVARIAN ARTERY AND VEIN

EXTERNAL ILIAC VEIN

UTERINE (FALLOPIAN) TUBE

ROUND LIGAMENT OF UTERUS

BLADDER

PUBIC SYMPHYSIS

URETHRA

CLITORIS

LABIUM MINUS

LABIUM MAJUS

BODY OF 5TH LUMBAR VERTEBRA

HYPOGASTRIC VEIN

BROAD LIGAMENT

OVARY

UTERUS

RECTUM

VAGINA

ANUS

EXTERNAL SPHINCTER OF ANUS

FIG. 74. Midsagittal section through a female pelvis which has not been dissected.

layer, to become continuous with the same layer on the other side. Anterior to the rectum, as it approaches the midline, the visceral fascia is prolonged upward to form a **fascial covering for** the **vagina** and still higher onto the wall of the **uterus.** More anteriorly, it is prolonged upward onto the sides of the **bladder.** Running forward from the neck of the bladder to the internal surface of the pubis slightly lateral to the midline, it presents a thickening, the **anterior pubovesical ligament,** or anterior true ligament of the bladder.

By carefully removing the posterior layer of the **broad ligament,** attempt to demonstrate the **epoophoron** and the proper ligament of the ovary. The former is a vestigial structure representing a part of the **mesonephros** of the embryo, which lies between the two layers of the peritoneum of the mesosalpinx. The **ovarian ligament** is a band of smooth muscle and fibrous tissue which runs from the medial end of the **ovary to** the lateral border of the **uterus,** also lying between the two layers of peritoneum.

Now clean and study the **internal iliac artery**

and its branches. To do this, most of the peritoneum and the extraperitoneal areolar tissue must be removed. The arteries are the same in the female as in the male, with the addition of the **uterine branch,** whose course has already been seen.

The interior of the **female bladder** does not differ from that of the male. The **female urethra** is a short canal with a fibrous and muscular wall which lies immediately anterior to the vagina and ends below in the vestibule. It corresponds to the portion of the prostatic urethra in the male which lies above the opening of the prostatic utricle.

Draw the bladder forward and separate its posterior surface from the anterior surface of the vagina, to which it is loosely attached. At the same time, separate the posterior surface of the urethra from the vagina. Study the wall and interior of the **vagina.** It is a wide canal whose anterior and posterior surfaces are usually in contact. Observe the **rugae vaginales,** transverse ridges found on both walls. Observe

that the uterus projects downward into the upper part of the vagina, into which it opens by a small circular or oval aperture, **the external uterine orifice.** The portions of the vaginal canal which extend upward, anterior and posterior to this lower portion of the uterus, are known as the **anterior** and **posterior fornices of** the vagina.

Observe that there is a constriction of the lumen of the uterus about ½ in. above the external orifice. This is the **internal orifice of** the **uterus** and marks the junction of the **body** or upper portion **of the uterus with** the **cervix** or lower portion. The lining of the canal of the cervix is usually thrown into folds, while the lumen of the body has a smooth lining.

Retract the vagina and uterus medialward. Clean and study the **muscles of** the **pelvic diaphragm.** These do not differ from the same muscles in the male. The **gap** left **between** the two **levator ani muscles** anteriorly, which is filled in the male by the prostate, is filled in the female by the **vagina and urethra.**

Superior Extremity ·

Surface Anatomy

Certain body landmarks should be identified before the skin is reflected from the superior extremity. The **humerus** is for the most part thickly covered by muscle, being subcutaneous only at its distal end, where the **lateral** and **medial epicondyles** form the subcutaneous bony prominences at each side of the elbow. The broad bony prominence at the back of the elbow is made by the **olecranon process of** the **ulna.** Continuing distad into the forearm from the olecranon is the dorsal border of the **ulna,** which is subcutaneous throughout its length

and ends on the dorsomedial aspect of the wrist in the **styloid process of** the **ulna.** The **radius** is more deeply placed, but its distal portion can usually be felt rather easily through the thin muscles and tendons which cover it. The bony projection at the lateral side of the wrist is the **styloid process of** the **radius.**

When the axilla was dissected, an incision was made in the skin, crossing the anterior aspect of the arm transversely a little below the shoulder. This incision should now be extended to encircle the arm at this level. Then make a median longitudinal incision through the skin on the front of the arm and the forearm, extending from the upper transverse incision distad to the front of the wrist. Make two transverse incisions, one across the front of the wrist from the medial to the lateral border and another in front of the elbow from the medial to the lateral epicondyle. This will mark out four skin flaps on the front of the arm and forearm. These should be reflected medially and laterally. Starting at the upper transverse incision on the back of the arm, reflect the skin downward off the back of the arm and forearm. The skin of the entire arm and forearm will then have been reflected in a single piece, which will remain attached only at the back of the wrist, where it is still continuous with the skin on the back of the hand.

The skin should now be reflected from the hand by the following incisions: (1) a median longitudinal incision through the skin of the palm from the middle of the transverse incision already made across the wrist to the tip of the middle finger; (2) a transverse incision across the palm at the proximal ends of the fingers; (3) an oblique incision from the middle of the front of the wrist to the tip of the thumb; (4) longitudinal incisions, from incision 2, distally along the middle of the volar surfaces of the index, ring, and little fingers to their tips. Starting with these incisions, reflect the skin, first from the volar and then the dorsal surfaces of the hand and fingers, and remove it completely from the extremity.

Cutaneous Veins and Nerves

The **superficial veins** of the upper extremity are numerous and variable. They often may be seen to better advantage in the living arm than in the cadaver. The two largest and most constant are the **cephalic vein** and the **basilic vein.** These veins begin at the lateral (radial) and medial (ulnar) ends, respectively, of a **venous arch** on the **dorsum of** the **hand.** The **cephalic vein** should be found at the **lateral side of** the wrist and traced upward through the superficial fascia along the **lateral side of** the volar aspect of the **forearm.** Passing in front of the lateral side of the elbow, it ascends on the **lateral aspect of** the **arm.** The last part of its course is in the groove between the pectoralis major and deltoid muscles, and its termination in the **axillary vein** behind the clavicle. The **basilic vein** ascends along the **ulnar border of** the **forearm,** crosses in front of the medial side of the elbow to reach the **medial aspect of** the **arm,** and, at about the middle of the arm, pierces the deep fascia to join the **deep veins** which accompany the brachial artery. The **median cubital vein** is a large connecting channel usually present in front of the elbow. It runs upward and medially from the **cephalic to** the **basilic vein.**

Clean and study the **cutaneous nerves** of the arm, forearm, and hand. These should be identified at the points at which they pierce the deep fascia and their distributions traced. The main trunks and branches lie in relation to the deep surface of the superficial fascia, which should be removed from the arm and forearm as the nerves are cleaned. Clean first the nerves on the anterior aspect of the extremity.

The origins of the medial brachial and medial antibrachial cutaneous nerves from the medial cord of the brachial plexus have already been seen. The **medial brachial cutaneous** nerve pierces the deep fascia at about the middle of the medial aspect of the arm, usually just medial to the terminal part of the basilic vein. It descends on the medial side of the arm and just above the elbow turns posteriorly to supply the skin over the olecranon. The **medial antibrachial nerve** pierces the deep fascia slightly lower in the arm and usually lies just lateral to the basilic vein. It divides into an **anterior and** a **posterior branch.** Both of these descend into the forearm and supply the skin on the anteromedial and posteromedial aspects of the forearm as far down as the wrist.

The **lateral antibrachial cutaneous nerve** is a direct continuation of the **musculocutaneous nerve.** It will be found piercing the deep fascia on the anterolateral aspect of the arm a short distance above the elbow, usually close to the cephalic vein. It is distributed to the skin on the lateral and anterolateral aspects of the forearm as far as the base of the thumb.

Turn to the back of the arm and identify the posterior and lateral brachial cutaneous nerves. The **posterior brachial cutaneous nerve** is a branch of the **radial nerve;** it pierces the deep fascia on the posteromedial aspect of the arm near the border of the deltoid muscle and is distributed to the skin on the back of the arm below the deltoid. The **lateral brachial cutaneous nerve** is a branch of the **axillary nerve;** it pierces the deep fascia at about the middle of the posterior border of the deltoid and runs upward and laterally to supply the skin covering the lower half of that muscle.

The **dorsal antibrachial cutaneous nerve** is a branch of the **radial nerve;** its two terminal branches usually pierce the deep fascia on the dorsolateral aspect of the arm separately. The **superior branch** is relatively small; it appears about 2 in. above the lateral epicondyle and is distributed to the lower half of the lateral and anterolateral aspects of the arm. The **inferior branch** is large; it emerges slightly below the superior branch, descends behind the lateral epicondyle, and supplies the skin on the back of the forearm as far as the wrist.

Clean the **cutaneous nerves** on the **dorsum of** the **hand.** The **superficial radial nerve** emerges from under cover of the lateral border of the brachioradialis and winds dorsally around the lateral side of the distal part of the forearm just proximal to the wrist. Reaching the lateral side of the dorsum of the wrist, it divides into branches which supply the skin on the lateral half of the dorsum of the hand, the dorsal surfaces of the thumb, index, and middle fingers, and, usually, the lateral side of the

dorsum of the ring finger. The **posterior cutaneous branch of** the **ulnar nerve** will be found winding dorsally around the medial border of the wrist to be distributed to the skin on the medial half of the dorsum of the hand, the dorsum of the little finger, and the medial side of the dorsum of the ring finger. The cutaneous nerves on the palmar surface of the hand and fingers can be dissected and studied to better advantage after a deeper dissection of this region is done subsequently.

Deltoid Region

Clean the deltoid. The **deltoid** is the large, thick, triangular muscle which forms the fleshy prominence of the shoulder. It arises by fleshy fibers from the anterior border and upper surface of the lateral third of the **clavicle** and the lateral border and upper surface of the **acromion** and by an aponeurosis from the **spine of** the **scapula.** Its fibers converge laterally and inferiorly to join a strong tendon which is inserted into the **deltoid tuberosity of** the **humerus** between the biceps and the lateral head of the triceps.

Cut the deltoid away from its origin and reflect it downward and laterally toward its insertion. As this is done, care must be taken to avoid injury to the **axillary nerve** and the **posterior humeral circumflex artery,** which ramify on its deep surface.

Now turn to the axilla. Review the **brachial plexus** and the **axillary artery** and their branches, and remove any traces of axillary fat which may remain. Identify the muscles by which the vertebral border of the scapula attaches to the axial skeleton. Identify the insertion of the **pectoralis minor** on the upper surface and medial border of the **coracoid process of** the **scapula.** Clean the **common tendon of origin of** the **coracobrachialis and** the **short head of** the **biceps brachii** from the tip of the coracoid process and follow these muscles into the arm. Observe that they separate from each other below the coracoid process, the coracobrachialis lying medial to the biceps, and that the long head of the biceps, here narrow and tendinous, emerges from under cover of the anterior border of the deltoid to join the short head on its lateral side. The proximal portions of these muscles rest deeply against the anterior aspect of the humerus and are embraced anteriorly by the tendon of insertion of the pectoralis major and posteriorly by the tendons of

Observe that the musculocutaneous nerve enters the medial border of the muscle and passes obliquely downward through its substance to emerge under cover of the biceps. The coracobrachialis is supplied by a branch of the **musculocutaneous nerve,** which usually arises proximal to the point of entry of the main trunk into the muscle.

Clean the **biceps brachii.** The origin of its **short head** has already been seen. The **long**

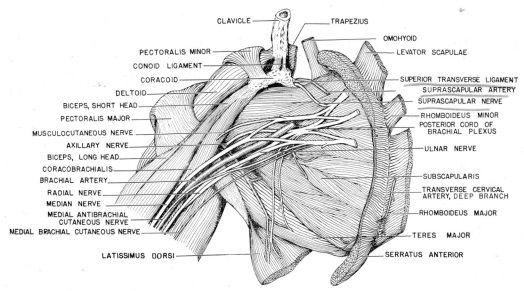

FIG. 75. Anterior aspect of the shoulder region after removal of the extremity from the trunk.

the latissimus dorsi and the teres major (Fig. 75).

Flexor Region of Arm

The coracobrachialis should now be cleaned to its insertion. Be careful, however, not to injure the brachial artery or the median nerve, which cross its surface. The **coracobrachialis** is a bandlike muscle whose fibers extend almost straight downward from their origin to be inserted into the **medial surface of** the **humerus** above the middle of the shaft. It is partially overlapped on its lateral side by the biceps.

head arises within the capsule of the shoulder joint from the **upper border of** the **glenoid fossa of the scapula.** Its tendon may be seen now emerging from the capsule and descending in the intertubercular sulcus to join the short head. The fusiform belly of the biceps narrows below to a strong tendon which enters the cubital fossa, where its insertion on the **tuberosity of** the **radius** may be seen more satisfactorily later. As the distal part of the biceps is being cleaned, clean also the **lacertus fibrosus (aponeurosis of biceps).** This is a thickened fibrous band which passes medially and distally, from the distal part of the medial border of the biceps, to join the deep fascia on the proximal part of the medial side of the forearm. Draw the biceps forward and secure the nerves of supply which it receives from the **musculo-cutaneous nerve.**

The entire course of the **musculocutaneous nerve** may now be followed. It arises in the axilla as a branch of the **lateral cord of** the **brachial plexus.** It passes downward and laterally to enter the **coracobrachialis,** which it supplies. Emerging from the coracobrachialis, it lies behind the biceps and descends between the **biceps** and the **brachialis,** both of which muscles it supplies. A short distance above the elbow, it emerges from behind the lateral border of the biceps and pierces the deep fascia as the **lateral antibrachial cutaneous nerve,** whose further course has been traced. The brachialis is the thick fleshy muscle which lies behind the biceps in the lower part of the arm. Its attachments may be seen more satisfactorily later in the dissection. It should be noted now, however, that it is a large muscle and forms one of the main constituents of the anterior compartment of the arm.

The **arm,** below the level of the insertions of the deltoid and the coracobrachialis, is divided into **two compartments,** an **anterior and** a **posterior,** which are separated from each other by the humerus and the lateral and medial intermuscular septa. The **lateral and medial intermuscular septa** are strong aponeurotic fascial bands which stretch laterally and medially from the lateral and medial supracondylar ridges of the humerus to the deep surface of the deep fascia covering the lateral and medial surfaces, respectively, of the arm. They end inferiorly at the epicondyles and superiorly by blending with the fascia covering the deltoid and the coracobrachialis, respectively. The **anterior compartment** contains the brachialis and the lower part of the biceps and origins of the brachioradialis and extensor carpi radialis longus muscles and

is traversed by the brachial artery and the median and musculocutaneous nerves. The **posterior compartment** contains the lower part of the triceps; through it pass the radial and ulnar nerves and the profunda brachii artery, which will be dissected later.

Clean the **brachial artery.** This vessel begins at the lower border of the teres major as a continuation of the **axillary** and descends on the anteromedial aspect of the arm to terminate in front of the elbow by dividing into the **radial and ulnar arteries.** It is superficial throughout its course, with the exception that it is crossed superficially at about the middle of the arm by the median nerve and it may be somewhat overlapped anteriorly by the biceps. Near its termination, it is crossed by the lacertus fibrosus. The medial antibrachial cutaneous nerve also usually crosses its proximal portion superficially. Deeply, it rests successively from above downward on the triceps, the coracobrachialis, and the brachialis muscles. In the proximal part of its course the ulnar nerve lies on its medial side but soon passes posteriorly, away from the artery. The median nerve may also be cleaned at this time. It lies at first lateral to the artery but crosses it at about the middle of the arm and, from that point to the termination of the artery, lies on its medial side. The **median nerve** has **no branches in the arm,** though it is not uncommon to find a twig of communication between it and the musculocutaneous nerve (Fig. 76).

In addition to numerous muscular branches, the **brachial artery** gives rise to the profunda brachii and the superior and inferior ulnar collateral arteries. The **profunda brachii** is a large branch which arises from the medial side of the brachial near the beginning of the latter. Running distad and posteriorly, it passes between the medial and long heads of the triceps, in company with the **radial nerve,** to reach the back of the arm, where its further course will be seen later. The **superior ulnar collateral**

usually arises at about the level of the insertion of the coracobrachialis. It runs downward and posteriorly and pierces the upper part of the medial intermuscular septum to join the ulnar

2 in. above its bifurcation and runs medially across the brachialis to divide into an anterior and a posterior branch. The **posterior branch** pierces the medial intermuscular septum to

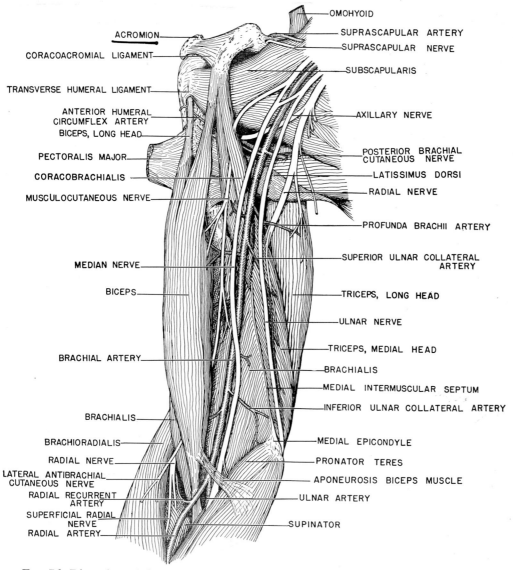

OMOHYOID
SUPRASCAPULAR ARTERY
SUPRASCAPULAR NERVE
SUBSCAPULARIS
AXILLARY NERVE
POSTERIOR BRACHIAL CUTANEOUS NERVE
LATISSIMUS DORSI
RADIAL NERVE
PROFUNDA BRACHII ARTERY
SUPERIOR ULNAR COLLATERAL ARTERY
TRICEPS, LONG HEAD
ULNAR NERVE
TRICEPS, MEDIAL HEAD
BRACHIALIS
MEDIAL INTERMUSCULAR SEPTUM
INFERIOR ULNAR COLLATERAL ARTERY
MEDIAL EPICONDYLE
PRONATOR TERES
APONEUROSIS BICEPS MUSCLE
ULNAR ARTERY
SUPINATOR

ACROMION
CORACOACROMIAL LIGAMENT
TRANSVERSE HUMERAL LIGAMENT
ANTERIOR HUMERAL CIRCUMFLEX ARTERY
BICEPS, LONG HEAD
PECTORALIS MAJOR
CORACOBRACHIALIS
MUSCULOCUTANEOUS NERVE
MEDIAN NERVE
BICEPS
BRACHIAL ARTERY
BRACHIALIS
BRACHIORADIALIS
RADIAL NERVE
LATERAL ANTIBRACHIAL CUTANEOUS NERVE
RADIAL RECURRENT ARTERY
SUPERFICIAL RADIAL NERVE
RADIAL ARTERY

FIG. 76. Dissection of the anteromedial aspect of the arm. The biceps has been slightly displaced anterolaterally.

nerve, which it accompanies distad on the outer surface of the medial head of the triceps and behind the medial epicondyle. The **inferior ulnar collateral** arises from the brachial about

reach the back of the medial epicondyle; the **anterior branch** descends in front of the medial epicondyle, where its termination is at present hidden by the muscles which arise there.

Cubital Fossa

Now define the boundaries of the cubital fossa and clean its contents. The **cubital fossa** is the triangular space at the front of the elbow. The **base** of the triangle is formed by an imag-

tad, is the point where these two muscles meet. The **pronator teres** is the most lateral of the superficial group of muscles of the forearm which take origin by a common tendon from the **medial epicondyle of** the **humerus.** From

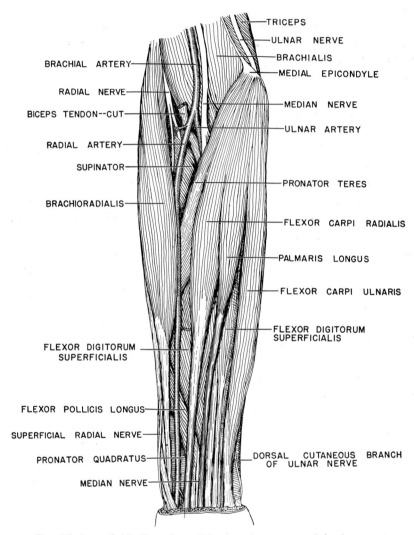

FIG. 77. Superficial dissection of the anterior aspect of the forearm.

inary transverse **line** drawn **between** the **two epicondyles.** Its **medial boundary** is formed by the lateral border of the **pronator teres;** its **lateral boundary** by the medial border of the **brachioradialis.** Its **apex,** which is directed dis-

this origin, its fibers pass distad and laterally across the front of the forearm to be inserted on the middle third of the **lateral surface of** the **radius;** its insertion is covered by the brachioradialis. The brachioradialis is ordinarily grouped with the extensor muscles which spread over the back of the forearm and hand. It acts, however, principally as a flexor of the elbow and does not reach the hand at all. It may, therefore, be cleaned well and studied now (Figs. 76 and 77).

The **brachioradialis** arises from the upper two-thirds of the lateral **supracondylar ridge of** the **humerus** and from the anterior surface of the **lateral intermuscular septum.** Its upper portion lies, therefore, in the anterior compartment of the arm, where it overlaps the lateral part of the brachialis. It extends distad along the lateral side of the anterior surface of the forearm and gives rise to a strong flat tendon which is inserted into the base of the **styloid process of** the **radius.** The most proximal portion of another muscle will also be seen in the anterior compartment. This is the **extensor carpi radialis longus,** which arises from the **lateral supracondylar ridge** immediately distal to the origin of the brachioradialis.

The **floor of** the **cubital fossa** is formed proximad by the lower part of the **brachialis** and distad by the **supinator.** Its **roof** is formed by **skin** and **fascia** and is crossed by the **biceps aponeurosis.**

Clean first the radial and ulnar arteries. The **radial artery** passes distad and somewhat laterally from its origin, crossing in front of the tendon of the biceps, to leave the cubital fossa at its apex, where it lies in front of the pronator teres and is somewhat overlapped anteriorly by the brachioradialis. Near its origin it gives rise to the **radial recurrent artery.** This vessel runs laterally on the supinator and then turns proximad to ascend in front of the lateral epicondyle between the brachialis and the brachioradialis (Fig. 76).

The **ulnar artery** runs distad and medially to leave the cubital fossa by passing deep to the pronator teres. In the fossa it gives rise to the anterior and posterior ulnar recurrent arteries, which may rise separately or by a common

stem. The **anterior ulnar recurrent** ascends between the pronator teres and the brachialis to anastomose with the anterior branch of the inferior ulnar collateral. The **posterior ulnar recurrent** passes medially, deep to the pronator teres. The further courses and anastomoses of the recurrent arteries can be seen to better advantage during the dissection of the joints.

Clean the **deep head of** the **pronator teres.** This is a very small slip, sometimes entirely lacking, which arises from the medial border of the **coronoid process of** the **ulna** and joins the large superficial head. If it is present, it will be found to intervene **between** the **ulnar artery** and the **median nerve.** The median nerve passes distal through the cubital fossa, lying medial to the brachial artery, and medial and anterior to the ulnar artery. It leaves the fossa by passing between the two heads of the pronator teres. In the fossa, it gives a twig of supply to the pronator teres.

Clean the **insertion of** the **biceps.** This is on the **tuberosity of** the **radius** and is overlapped by the pronator teres. Spread the proximal parts of the brachioradialis and the extensor carpi radialis longus laterally away from the brachialis to expose the terminal part of the radial nerve. The **radial nerve** enters the anterior compartment of the arm by piercing the lateral intermuscular septum close to the lateral supracondylar ridge of the humerus. It is accompanied by a branch of the **profunda brachii artery,** which here anastomoses with the radial recurrent. After giving branches to the brachioradialis and the extensor carpi radialis longus and one or two small twigs to the brachialis, the nerve ends by dividing into the superficial and deep radial nerves. The **superficial radial nerve** is a cutaneous branch; it passes distal in the forearm under cover of the brachioradialis (Fig. 76). Some distance above the wrist, it emerges from behind the lateral border of that muscle and winds dorsally around the lateral side of the wrist to reach the dorsum of the hand. The **deep radial nerve** passes from view at present by entering the substance of the supinator.

Displace the brachioradialis and the pronator teres as far to the lateral and medial sides as can conveniently be done and clean and study the **brachialis.** This muscle arises from the entire **anterior surface** of the **distal half of** the **humerus,** from the entire anterior surface of the **medial intermuscular septum,** and from the anterior surface of the **lateral intermuscular septum** proximal to the origin of the brachioradialis. Its distal portion lies in front of the capsule of the elbow joint, to which it is closely bound, and narrows to a strong tendon which is inserted on the **tuberosity of** the **ulna.** Its nerve supply is derived chiefly from the **musculocutaneous nerve,** but it receives additional small twigs from the **radial.**

Flexor Region of Forearm and Hand

Turn to the anterior aspect of the forearm. The **anterior and medial portions of** the **forearm** are occupied by the **muscles** which **flex** the **wrist and fingers** and **pronate** the **hand.** These muscles are arranged in **three layers,** the most superficial of which should now be cleaned. The muscles of the **superficial layer** arise by a common tendon from the **medial epicondyle of** the **humerus** and from the **deep fascia** which invests their proximal portions. They spread distad and laterally over the anterior aspect of the forearm, becoming distinct from one another 2 or 3 in. distal to the medial epicondyle.

The **pronator teres** near its insertion is crossed by the radial artery and overlapped by the brachioradialis. The **flexor carpi radialis** narrows to a rounded tendon which descends along the medial side of the radial artery and enters the palm superficially, where its insertion on the **base of** the **second** and **third metacarpals** may better be seen later.

The **flexor carpi ulnaris** arises by the common tendon from the **medial epicondyle** but

has a second head of origin from the medial border of the **olecranon** and from an aponeurosis attached to the proximal two-thirds of the dorsal border of the **ulna.** It is inserted into the **pisiform bone.** Observe that the **ulnar nerve** passes behind the medial epicondyle and enters the forearm by passing deep to a fibrous arch which unites the two heads of origin of the flexor carpi ulnaris.

The tendon of the **palmaris longus** crosses the middle of the front of the wrist, lying, in the distal part of the forearm, immediately in **front of** the **median nerve,** and is inserted into the **palmar aponeurosis.** In about 12 per cent of cases this muscle is absent; in such cases the median nerve is superficial just above the wrist.

Clean the **palmar aponeurosis.** This is a dense thickening of the **deep fascia of** the **palm,** which radiates from the tendon of the palmaris longus toward the bases of the fingers, where it divides into four slips which join the **fibrous sheaths** by which the **flexor tendons** are held in place against the palmar surfaces of the phalanges.

Reflect the palmar aponeurosis, together with the attached tendon of insertion of the palmaris longus and the palmaris brevis, cephalad from the palm. This must be carefully done to avoid injury to the **superficial palmar arterial arch** and the terminal part of the **median nerve,** which lie immediately subjacent to the aponeurosis in the palm of the hand. As it is reflected, the palmar aponeurosis should be cut away at the bases of the fingers, where its four divergent slips join the fibrous sheaths of the flexor tendons (Fig. 78).

Divide the pronator teres about 1 in. medial to its insertion; free and elevate the tendons of the flexor carpi radialis, the palmaris longus, and the flexor carpi ulnaris. As this is done, secure and clean the nerves which enter their deep surfaces. The **pronator teres** is supplied by a branch of the **median nerve** which arises

STUdy intervactions ↓

in the cubital fossa. The **flexor carpi radialis** and the **palmaris longus** are supplied by branches arising from the **median nerve** under cover of the pronator teres. The **flexor carpi**

muscle, the **flexor digitorum sublimis (superficialis)**. It arises in part from the **medial epicondyle** of the **humerus,** in common with the more superficial muscles; it has, however, a

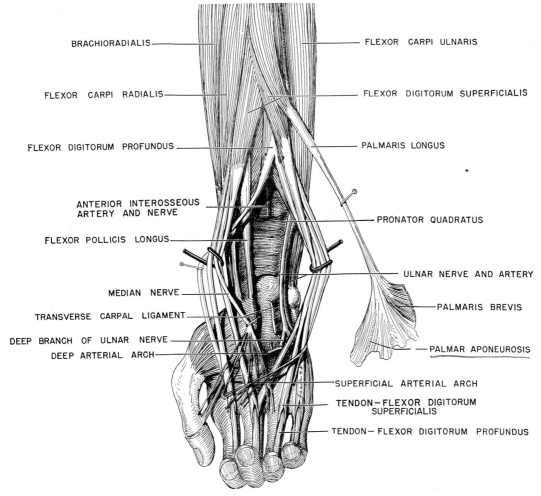

BRACHIORADIALIS

FLEXOR CARPI RADIALIS

FLEXOR DIGITORUM PROFUNDUS

ANTERIOR INTEROSSEOUS ARTERY AND NERVE

FLEXOR POLLICIS LONGUS

MEDIAN NERVE

TRANSVERSE CARPAL LIGAMENT

DEEP BRANCH OF ULNAR NERVE

DEEP ARTERIAL ARCH

FLEXOR CARPI ULNARIS

FLEXOR DIGITORUM SUPERFICIALIS

PALMARIS LONGUS

PRONATOR QUADRATUS

ULNAR NERVE AND ARTERY

PALMARIS BREVIS

PALMAR APONEUROSIS

SUPERFICIAL ARTERIAL ARCH

TENDON—FLEXOR DIGITORUM SUPERFICIALIS

TENDON—FLEXOR DIGITORUM PROFUNDUS

FIG. 78. Deep dissection of the flexor region of the forearm and hand. The palmar aponeurosis, with the embedded palmaris brevis, is reflected medially and upward with the tendon of the palmaris longus. The transverse carpal ligament is cut. The median nerve and the tendons of the flexor digitorum superficialis and profundus, with their mucous sheaths, are elevated and retracted to each side. The courses of the flexor tendons on the fingers are freed and elevated from their osteofibrotic canals.

ulnaris is supplied by two or three twigs from the **ulnar nerve** in the upper part of the forearm.

The **second layer** of the anterior aspect of the forearm is represented by a single large

more extensive origin from the medial borders of the **ulnar tuberosity** and the **coronoid process of** the **ulna,** from the **oblique line on** the anterior surface of the **radius,** and from a **fibrous arch** which bridges across the gap **be-**

tween its **ulnar and radial origins.** Observe that the median nerve and the ulnar artery pass into the forearm behind this fibrous arch. As the wrist is approached, the muscle divides into **four tendons, of which those for the middle and ring fingers** are **superficial** and those for the **index and little fingers** lie **behind them.** All four tendons pass behind the transverse carpal ligament, where they are enclosed in a single mucous sheath which is common to them and to the four tendons of the flexor digitorum profundus, to enter the palm of the hand.

It is advisable at this stage of the dissection to clean the palmar carpal and transverse carpal ligaments. The **transverse carpal ligament** (**flexor retinaculum**) is a strong, dense, fibrous band, which stretches across the carpus, and, together with the palmar surfaces of the carpal bones, completes an osteofibrous tunnel through which the flexor tendons of the digits and the trunk of the median nerve enter the palm. It is attached laterally to the **navicular** and **greater multangular bones** and medially to the **pisiform** and the **hook of** the **hamate.** The tendon of the flexor carpi radialis pierces the lateral end of the transverse carpal ligament as it crosses the wrist. The ulnar nerve and artery cross the medial end of the ligament superficially to enter the palm. They are held in place against the transverse carpal ligament by the **palmar carpal ligament (palmar retinaculum).** The latter is a thinner fibrous band which is attached medially to the **pisiform bone** and the **hook of** the **hamate** and laterally to the anterior surface of the **transverse carpal ligament.**

The **deepest layer** of the anterior muscles of the forearm includes the **flexor pollicis longus,** the **flexor digitorum profundus,** and the **pronator quadratus.** Before studying these muscles in detail, however, it is best to study the course in the forearm of the radial and ulnar arteries and the median and ulnar nerves. The **radial artery** is **superficial** throughout its course **in** the

forearm, with the exception that distal to the apex of the cubital fossa, it is overlapped for a variable distance on its lateral side by the brachioradialis. Deeply, it rests successively against the tendon of the biceps, the supinator, the insertion of the pronator teres, the radial head of the flexor digitorum superficialis, the flexor pollicis longus, the pronator quadratus, and the anterior surface of the radius. Just proximal to the wrist, it turns laterally and dorsally toward the back of the wrist, where its further course will be traced later.

In addition to the radial recurrent artery, the **radial artery** gives rise in the forearm to numerous small muscular branches and to an anterior radial carpal and a superficial palmar branch. The **palmar radial carpal** is a small branch which passes medially across the distal end of the radius, deep to the flexor tendons, to anastomose with the **palmar carpal branch of** the **ulnar artery.** The **superficial palmar branch** arises just as the radial turns dorsally at the wrist and runs forward over or through the short muscles of the ball of the thumb to take part in the formation of the **superficial palmar arch.**

Detach the radial head of origin of the flexor digitorum superficialis from the radius and displace the muscle medially. Then clean the ulnar artery. The **ulnar artery** in the **proximal half of** the **forearm** is **covered by** the four muscles of the **superficial layer and** by the **flexor digitorum superficialis.** It is also crossed, under cover of the pronator teres, by the median nerve, which here passes from its medial to its lateral side. In the **distal half of** the **forearm,** the **ulnar artery** is more **superficial,** being merely overlapped by the tendon of the flexor carpi ulnaris. Deeply, it rests first upon the brachialis and then, for the remainder of its course through the forearm, upon the flexor digitorum profundus; at the wrist, it crosses the medial end of the transverse carpal ligament superficially to enter the palm.

The origin of the **ulnar recurrent arteries** has already been seen. The further course of the **posterior ulnar recurrent** may now be traced. It ascends between the flexors digitorum superficialis and profundus to pass behind the medial epicondyle and anastomose with the **superior ulnar collateral** and the posterior branch of the **inferior ulnar collateral.**

The **common interosseous artery** arises from the **ulnar** near the point where that vessel is crossed by the median nerve. It passes backward and distal between the adjacent borders of the flexor pollicis longus and the flexor digitorum profundus and shortly divides into the posterior and the anterior interosseous arteries. The **dorsal interosseous** passes straight backward, between the proximal ends of the radius and ulna, and above the proximal border of the interosseous membrane to reach the dorsal aspect of the forearm. The **anterior interosseous** passes distal in front of the interosseous membrane, where it is covered by the overlapping borders of the flexor pollicis longus and the flexor digitorum profundus. Near its origin, however, it gives rise to a branch known as the **median artery,** which accompanies the **median nerve.** While usually small and unimportant, the median artery is occasionally considerably enlarged and may accompany the nerve into the hand and take part in the formation of the superficial palmar arch.

In its course through the forearm, the **ulnar artery** gives rise to numerous **muscular branches.** Near the proximal border of the transverse carpal ligament, it gives rise to a **dorsal ulnar carpal branch** which winds medially and dorsally to reach the dorsal surface of the carpus. The **palmar ulnar carpal** branch arises at about the same level and passes laterally deep to the flexor tendons to anastomose with the **palmar radial carpal.**

The **ulnar nerve** enters the forearm by passing **between** the two **heads of** the **flexor carpi ulnaris.** In its whole course through the fore-arm, it is covered only by that muscle. Proximad, the ulnar nerve is separated from the ulnar artery by the flexor digitorum superficialis, but distad it closely accompanies the artery, lying on the medial side of the latter. In the proximal part of the forearm, the ulnar nerve gives branches which supply the **flexor carpi ulnaris** and the **medial portion of** the **flexor digitorum profundus;** in the distal part of the forearm, it gives rise to the **posterior cutaneous branch** whose distribution to the skin on the **dorsum of** the **hand** has already been traced and to a small **palmar cutaneous branch,** which passes in front of the ulnar artery to reach the skin on the medial half of the **palm.** Near the distal border of the transverse carpal ligament, the ulnar nerve terminates by dividing into a **deep** and a **superficial branch.**

The **median nerve** runs almost vertically through the forearm, to pass behind the transverse carpal ligament, in company with the flexor tendons, into the hand. In the upper two-thirds of the forearm, it lies between the flexors digitorum superficialis and profundus; in the distal third, it is covered superficially only by the tendon of the palmaris longus. In the cubital fossa, or just distal to it under cover of the pronator teres, it gives rise to branches which supply the **pronator teres,** the **flexor carpi radialis,** the **palmaris longus,** and the **flexor digitorum superficialis.** Slightly more distad, it gives rise to a branch known as the **anterior interosseous nerve;** this nerve accompanies the anterior interosseous artery along the anterior surface of the interosseous membrane and is distributed to the **flexor pollicis longus,** the lateral part of the **flexor digitorum profundus,** and the **pronator quadratus.** Immediately above the transverse carpal ligament, the median nerve gives a small **palmar cutaneous branch,** which crosses the ligament superficially to supply the skin of the lateral half of the palm.

The transverse carpal ligament should be divided by a longitudinal incision. All of the long flexor tendons to the fingers, together with their synovial sheaths, should be elevated to facilitate the dissection of the deeper structures in both the distal forearm and in the hand. The fibrous sheaths over the flexor tendons of the fingers may be opened at this time to facilitate the elevation of the flexor tendons and straightening of the fingers (Fig. 78).

Now clean the **deep (anterior) muscles.** The **flexor digitorum profundus** has a wide, fleshy origin from the **proximal two-thirds** of the anterior and the medial surfaces of the **ulna** and the adjacent part of the **interosseous membrane;** it also derives some fibers from the deep surface of the aponeurosis of the flexor carpi ulnaris on the dorsal border of the ulna. The muscle gives rise to **four tendons** which pass into the hand side by side, deep to the transverse carpal ligament and the tendons of the flexor digitorum superficialis. The **flexor pollicis longus** arises from the **middle half** of the anterior surface of the **radius** and from the adjacent portion of the **interosseous membrane;** the origin of this muscle is limited proximolaterally by the line of origin of the radial head of the flexor digitorum superficialis. Its tendon passes deep to the transverse carpal ligament, where it lies lateral to the first tendon of the flexor digitorum profundus.

Spread the flexors digitorum profundus and pollicis longus apart to expose the pronator quadratus and the anterior interosseous artery and nerve. The **pronator quadratus** is a flat, quadrangular muscle which arises from the medial side of the **distal fourth of** the anterior surface of the **ulna.** Its fibers pass transversely to be inserted on the anterior surface of the **radius.**

The **anterior interosseous artery** descends in front of the interosseous membrane, supplying branches to the deep flexors. It ends at the proximal border of the pronator quadratus by dividing into posterior and anterior terminal branches. The larger **posterior branch** pierces

the interosseous membrane to reach the back of the forearm. The **anterior branch** descends deep to the pronator quadratus to anastomose with the **anterior carpal branches** of the **radial** and **ulnar arteries.** The **anterior interosseous nerve** accompanies the artery. It is distributed to the three **deep muscles** and also sends a twig which accompanies the anterior branch of the artery to the wrist joint.

Clean and study the superficial palmar arch and the superficial branch of the ulnar nerve (Fig. 79). The **superficial palmar arch** is formed principally by the continuation of the **ulnar artery** into the palm but is usually completed on its lateral side by the **superficial palmar branch of** the **radial artery.** As it reaches the distal border of the transverse carpal ligament, the ulnar artery gives off a **deep branch,** which accompanies the deep branch of the ulnar nerve deeply into the palm by passing between the short muscles of the little finger. The superficial arch crosses the palm at about the level of the middle of the metacarpal bones. The superficial palmar branch of the radial artery may cross the base of the thenar eminence superficially to join the arch or may pass deep to the abductor pollicis brevis. The branches of the superficial palmar arch are somewhat variable but usually include a **proper palmar digital artery** for the medial side of the little finger and three **common palmar digital arteries.** The latter pass distad superficial to the three medial interosseous spaces; at the bases of the interdigital clefts, each divides into two proper digital arteries, which supply the medial side of the index finger, both sides of the middle and ring fingers, and the lateral side of the little finger.

The superficial branch of the **ulnar nerve** terminates in the palm by dividing into three **palmar digital branches,** which are distributed to the skin of both sides of the little finger and the medial side of the ring finger.

Attempt to demonstrate the **two synovial**

sheaths which envelop the flexor tendons as they pass behind the transverse carpal ligament. One (the **radial bursa**) encloses the **tendon of** the **flexor pollicis longus** and extends from near the proximal border of the transverse carpal ligament almost to the insertion of the tendon. The second (the **ulnar bursa**) close the **tendons of** the **index, middle,** and **ring fingers** within their fibrous sheaths. These extend, in each case, from the level of the metacarpophalangeal point to the base of the terminal phalanx.

The **fibrous sheaths** of the flexor tendons may also be investigated at this time. These are

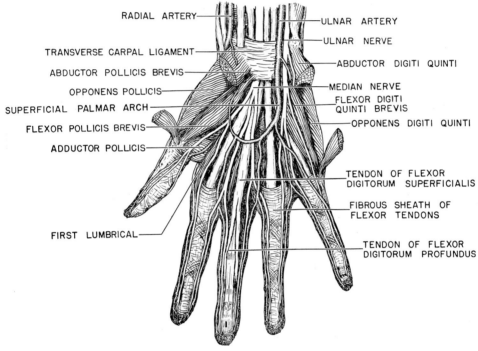

RADIAL ARTERY

TRANSVERSE CARPAL LIGAMENT

ABDUCTOR POLLICIS BREVIS

OPPONENS POLLICIS

SUPERFICIAL PALMAR ARCH

FLEXOR POLLICIS BREVIS

ADDUCTOR POLLICIS

FIRST LUMBRICAL

ULNAR ARTERY

ULNAR NERVE

ABDUCTOR DIGITI QUINTI

MEDIAN NERVE

FLEXOR DIGITI QUINTI BREVIS

OPPONENS DIGITI QUINTI

TENDON OF FLEXOR DIGITORUM SUPERFICIALIS

FIBROUS SHEATH OF FLEXOR TENDONS

TENDON OF FLEXOR DIGITORUM PROFUNDUS

FIG. 79. Superficial dissection of the palm after removal of the palmar aponeurosis. The fibrous sheath has been removed from the middle finger to expose the insertions of the flexor tendons. The normal relations of the transverse carpal ligament to the flexor tendons, the vessels, and nerves are shown.

encloses the **four tendons of** the **flexor digitorum superficialis** and the **four tendons of** the **flexor digitorum profundus**. It begins about 1 in. proximad to the proximal border of the transverse carpal ligament and extends distad for about 1 in. beyond the distal border of the ligament. Its most **medial portion,** however, is prolonged distad to enclose the two **flexor tendons for** the **little finger,** within their fibrous sheath, as far as the base of the terminal phalanx. **Three** individual **synovial sheaths** en-

bands of fibrous tissue which are attached to the margins of the phalanges and bridge across the palmar aspects of the latter, thus forming in each finger an **osteofibrous canal** through which the flexor tendons pass to their insertions. Their strongest portions, known as the **digital vaginal ligaments,** lie opposite the bodies of the first and second phalanges of each finger (Fig. 79).

Trace the distribution of the **median nerve** in the palm. As it emerges from under cover of the transverse carpal ligament, the median nerve terminates by dividing into three **common palmar digital nerves.** The first of these, passing distad and laterally, supplies the short abductor, the short flexor, and the opponens of the thumb, the first lumbrical muscle, and then it divides into three **proper palmar digital nerves,** which supply the skin on both sides of the thumb and the lateral side of the index finger. The second and third common palmar digital branches each divide into two proper palmar digitals, which supply the medial side of the index finger, both sides of the middle finger, and the lateral side of the ring finger. The second common palmar digital usually also gives a twig to the second lumbrical.

Now study the **long flexor tendons** in the palm. Observe that, as they emerge from under cover of the transverse carpal ligament, the tendons of the long flexors diverge toward the bases of the fingers, the tendon of the **flexor superficialis** lying in each case **superficial to** that of the **flexor profundus.** Open the fibrous sheath in all of the fingers by a longitudinal incision to study the manner of insertion of the two tendons. This procedure will also aid in straightening out the fingers, which are usually fixed in the flexed position, to facilitate the deeper dissection of the hand. Observe that in front of the body of the first phalanx the **tendon of** the **flexor superficialis is pierced by the tendon** of the **flexor profundus.** The **superficialis tendon** is then inserted on the **base of** the **second phalanx,** while the **tendon of** the **profundus** passes distad to be inserted on the **base of** the **terminal phalanx** (Figs. 78 and 79).

Elevate the tendons of the flexor digitorum sublimis. Then clean the **lumbrical muscles.** These are four small muscles which arise in the distal part of the palm from the **tendons of** the **flexor digitorum profundus.** The **first** arises from the lateral border of the tendon for the index finger and the **second** from the lateral

border of the tendon for the middle finger; the **third** and **fourth** originate, each from the adjacent sides of the tendons between which they lie. Each passes distad around the lateral side of the base of a finger and ends in a slender tendon which is inserted into the corresponding **extensor tendon** on the dorsum of that finger.

With the elevation of the flexor tendons and lumbrical muscles, note a potential space which is located between these tendons and muscles and the deeper palmar interosseous muscles and the metacarpal bones. This space is divided by a fibrous septum along the shaft of the middle metacarpal bone into two compartments. A medial compartment (the **midpalmar space)** is beneath the tendons to the ring, middle, and little fingers and their accompanying lumbrical muscles. A lateral compartment (the **thenar space)** is found between the deep surface of the tendon to the index finger, with its accompanying lumbrical muscle, and the superficial surface of the adductor pollicis muscle.

Clean the **short muscles of** the **little finger** which together form the **hypothenar eminence** on the medial side of the palm. The **abductor digiti quinti (minimi)** is the most medial; it arises from the **pisiform bone** and is inserted into the medial side of the **base of the first phalanx** of the little finger. The **flexor digiti quinti (minimi) brevis** arises from the **hook of** the **hamate** and the medial end of the **transverse carpal ligament** and is inserted **with** the **abductor.** The opponens digiti quinti (minimi) is covered superficially by the short flexor, with which it is often partially blended. The **opponens** arises from the **hook of** the **hamate** and the adjacent border of the **transverse carpal ligament** and is inserted into the whole length of the medial palmar surface of the **fifth metacarpal.** All three of these muscles are supplied by twigs from the **deep branch of** the **ulnar nerve.** Observe that the deep branches of the ulnar nerve and artery pass between the origins of the abductor and the flexor brevis as they sink into the palm.

Clean the **short muscles of** the **thumb** which form the **thenar eminence,** or ball of the thumb. Of these, the **abductor pollicis brevis** is the most superficial. It arises from the **greater multangular (trapezium) bone** and the lateral end of the **transverse carpal ligament** and is inserted into the lateral side of the base of the **first phalanx** of the thumb. When it has been cleaned, it should be detached from its origin and reflected toward its insertion to expose the deeper muscles. The **opponens pollicis** is a thick, fleshy muscle which arises from the **trapezium** bone and the adjacent part of the **transverse carpal ligament** and is inserted into the lateral side of the entire palmar surface of the **metacarpal** of the thumb. The **flexor pollicis brevis** is divided into a deep and a superficial portion by the tendon of the flexor pollicis longus. The **superficial portion** lies along the medial side of the opponens pollicis and covers the tendon of the flexor longus. It arises from the **trapezium** and the **transverse carpal ligament** and is inserted into the base of the **first phalanx,** just medial to the insertion of the abductor brevis. Divide the superficial head of the short flexor close to its origin and turn it laterally to its insertion. Trace the tendon of the **long flexor** to its insertion at the base of the **terminal phalanx** of the thumb. The small **deep head of** the **flexor pollicis brevis** may now be seen; it arises from the **trapezoid** bone and runs laterally and distad deep to the tendon of the flexor longus to be inserted **with** the **superficial head.**

The **adductor pollicis** arises by two heads, which may be clearly distinguished from each other by the fact that the deep palmar arch passes medially into the palm between them. The **oblique head** arises from the **capitate** and the bases of the **second** and **third metacarpals;** the **transverse head** arises from the palmar

aspect of the shaft of the **third metacarpal.** The two heads converge toward a tendon which is inserted into the medial side of the base of the **first phalanx** of the thumb.

To render the deep palmar arch accessible for study, retract the tendons of the flexor digitorum superficialis, flexor digitorum profundus, and flexor pollicis longus upward (Fig. 78). The lateral end of the deep palmar arch is covered by the oblique head of the adductor pollicis. This, as well as the deep head of the short flexor, should, therefore, be divided close to its origin and turned laterally. The **deep palmar arch** begins at the base of the first interosseous space, where the radial artery enters the palm. The arch is formed principally by the palmar continuation of the **radial artery** but is completed medially by the **deep branch of** the **ulnar artery,** which enters the palm under cover of the flexor digiti quinti brevis. If the latter muscle is now detached from its origin and reflected, the full course of the deep palmar arch will be exposed. It crosses the palm at the level of the bases of the metacarpal bones, resting deeply against the proximal portions of the interosseous muscles. Its two largest branches arise from its lateral end, at the base of the first interosseous space. The **princeps pollicis** passes along the metacarpal of the thumb, under cover of the oblique head of the adductor, and at the base of the first phalanx divides into two branches which are distributed to the two sides of the volar aspect of the thumb. The **lateral palmar artery of** the **index finger** passes distad, under cover of the transverse head of the adductor, to reach the lateral side of the index finger. In addition to these branches, the deep palmar arch gives rise to three **palmar metacarpal branches,** which descend in the three medial interosseous spaces to anastomose with the palmar digital branches of the superficial arch.

The **deep branch of** the **ulnar nerve** accompanies the medial part of the deep palmar arch.

It is distributed to the three **short muscles of the little finger, the third** and **fourth lumbricals, the adductor pollicis,** and all of the **interosseous muscles.**

The **interossei** are small muscles which occupy the interosseous spaces. They are arranged in two groups, consisting of **three palmar** and **four dorsal interossei.** Detach the transverse head of the adductor pollicis from its origin and reflect it laterally. Then clean and study the interossei. The **first palmar interosseous** muscle arises from the medial palmar surface of the second metacarpal and is inserted into the medial side of the base of the first phalanx of the index finger. The **second** and **third palmar interossei** arise from the lateral palmar surfaces of the fourth and fifth metacarpals, respectively, and are inserted into the lateral sides of the bases of the first phalanges of the ring and little fingers. The **dorsal interossei** lie on a slightly deeper plane; one dorsal interosseous muscle is found in each space, each arising from the adjacent sides of two metacarpals. The **first** and **second** are inserted into the lateral sides of the bases of the first phalanges of the index and middle fingers, respectively. The **third** and **fourth** are inserted into the medial sides of the bases of the first phalanges of the middle and ring fingers. In addition to these insertions, the tendons of the interossei are also attached to the long extensor tendons of the fingers.

Extensor Region of Arm

Turn to the back of the arm and clean the **triceps brachii.** The lower part of this muscle occupies the entire posterior compartment of the arm. It arises by three heads which are all inserted by a common tendon on the olecranon of the ulna. The origin of the **long head** is from the **axillary border of** the **scapula.** The medial and lateral heads arise from the posterior aspect of the humerus; the origins of these two heads

are separated by the spiral sulcus for the radial nerve. The **lateral head** arises from the superior lateral portion of the posterior surface of the **humerus.** The origin of the medial head is lower and much more extensive and is partly covered by both the long and the lateral heads. The **medial head** arises from the entire posterior surface of the **humerus** below and medial to the radial groove, from the entire posterior surface of the **medial intermuscular septum,** and from the lower part of the posterior surface of the **lateral intermuscular septum.** The **common tendon** of insertion of the triceps forms a strong aponeurotic band on the posterior surface of the distal part of the muscle; it is inserted into the proximal surface of the **olecranon.** Observe that the **ulnar nerve** lies on the external surface of the **medial head,** close to the medial intermuscular septum as it descends through the arm to pass behind the medial epicondyle. It is joined at about the middle of the arm by the **superior ulnar collateral artery,** which here pierces the medial intermuscular septum. Separate the three heads of the triceps as completely as possible to expose the **radial groove.** Clean the radial nerve and the profunda brachii artery.

The **radial nerve** arises in the axilla from the **posterior cord of** the **brachial plexus.** It crosses the subscapularis, the teres major, the tendon of the latissimus dorsi, and the long head of the triceps and then enters the **radial groove** on the back of the humerus by passing between the long and medial heads of the triceps. Three branches arise from the radial nerve before it enters the radial groove. The first of these is the **posterior brachial cutaneous nerve,** whose distribution to the skin on the back of the arm has already been traced. The second supplies the **long head of** the **triceps.** The third is distributed to the **medial head;** it is sometimes known as the **ulnar collateral nerve** from the fact that it descends on the external surface

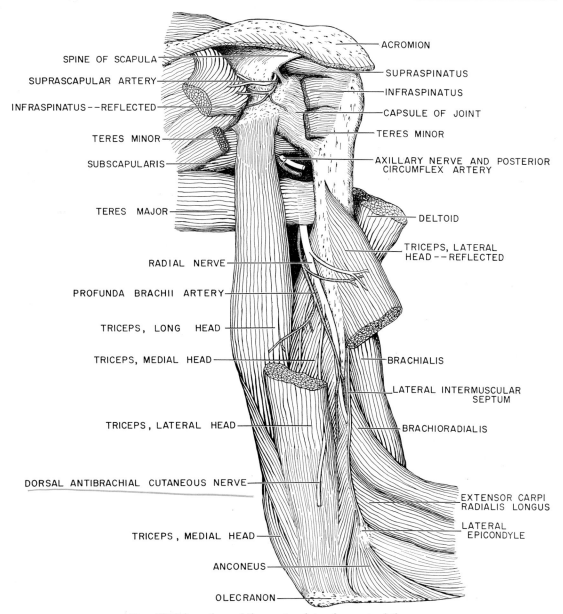

SPINE OF SCAPULA

SUPRASCAPULAR ARTERY

INFRASPINATUS--REFLECTED

TERES MINOR

SUBSCAPULARIS

TERES MAJOR

RADIAL NERVE

PROFUNDA BRACHII ARTERY

TRICEPS, LONG HEAD

TRICEPS, MEDIAL HEAD

TRICEPS, LATERAL HEAD

DORSAL ANTIBRACHIAL CUTANEOUS NERVE

TRICEPS, MEDIAL HEAD

ANCONEUS

OLECRANON

ACROMION

SUPRASPINATUS

INFRASPINATUS

CAPSULE OF JOINT

TERES MINOR

AXILLARY NERVE AND POSTERIOR CIRCUMFLEX ARTERY

DELTOID

TRICEPS, LATERAL HEAD--REFLECTED

BRACHIALIS

LATERAL INTERMUSCULAR SEPTUM

BRACHIORADIALIS

EXTENSOR CARPI RADIALIS LONGUS

LATERAL EPICONDYLE

FIG. 80. Dissection of the posterolateral aspect of the arm.

of the medial head close to the ulnar nerve for some distance before finally entering the substance of the muscle (Fig. 76).

In the **radial groove,** the **radial nerve** passes laterally and distad **between** the **medial** and **lateral heads of** the **triceps.** At the distal end of the radial groove, it pierces the lateral inter-

muscular septum to enter the anterior compartment of the arm, where its further course has been seen. In the radial groove, it gives rise to a **branch to** the **lateral head,** a second branch to the **medial head,** and to the **dorsal antibrachial cutaneous nerve.** The latter nerve passes through the substance of the triceps to reach the posterolateral surface of the arm, from which point it has been traced (Fig. 80).

The **profunda brachii** is a branch of the **brachial artery**. It accompanies the **radial nerve** into the radial groove. It is distributed principally to the **triceps**. One branch, however, known as the **radial collateral artery,** accompanies the nerve into the anterior compartment to anastomose with the **radial recurrent artery.** Another **branch** usually ascends deep to the deltoid to anastomose with the **posterior humeral circumflex.**

Extensor Region of Forearm and Hand

Remove any superficial fascia which may remain on the dorsum (posterior) of the forearm and hand. Observe that the **deep fascia on** the **posterior aspect of** the **forearm** is more **dense** than the deep fascia on the anterior aspect. Proximad, it forms an aponeurotic sheet from the deep surface of which the superficial extensor muscles take partial origin. At the distal end of the forearm, it is strengthened by a strong transverse fibrous band known as the dorsal carpal ligament, whose limits should now be defined. Laterally, the **dorsal (extensor) carpal ligament** is attached to the **lateral border** of the distal end of the **radius;** medially, it is bound to the **styloid process of** the **ulna** and the **triangular** and **pisiform bones.** In addition to its lateral and medial attachments, the extensor carpal ligament is firmly attached to a series of bony ridges on the **posterior aspect** of the distal ends of the **radius** and **ulna.** There are thus formed, deep to the ligament, **six osteofibrous canals,** or compartments, through which the **extensor tendons** pass to the dorsum of the hand. Identify those various compartments and the tendons which traverse them (Fig. 81).

The **most lateral first compartment** is in relation to the lateral surface of the styloid process of the radius; through it pass the tendons of the **abductor pollicis longus** and the **extensor pollicis brevis.** Just medial to this is a broad **second** compartment for the tendons of the **extensor carpi radialis longus** and the **extensor carpi radialis brevis.** The **third** compartment is a narrow one for the slender tendon of the **extensor pollicis longus.** Medial to this is a much wider **fourth** compartment through which pass the four tendons of the **extensor digitorum communis** and the tendon of the **extensor indicis proprius.** The **fifth** compartment lies over the groove between the radius and the ulna and transmits the tendon of the **extensor digiti quinti (minimi) proprius.** The **sixth** compartment is in relation to the dorsal surface of the ulna, just lateral to the styloid process, and transmits the tendon of the **extensor carpi ulnaris.**

Explore with a blunt probe the limits of the **mucous sheaths** which surround the tendons as they pass deep to the dorsal carpal ligament. Each tendon has its own mucous sheath, with the exception that a single sheath encloses the four tendons of the extensor digitorum communis and the tendon of the extensor indicis proprius. The mucous sheaths begin proximad at or near the proximal border of the dorsal carpal ligament and extend distad to about the middle of the dorsum of the hand.

Clean the **anconeus.** This small triangular muscle arises from the back of the **lateral epicondyle of** the **humerus** and spreads distad and medially to be inserted on the **lateral border of** the **olecranon.** It is usually more or less continuous superiorly with the medial head of the triceps; its nerve of supply is derived from one of the branches of the **radial nerve** which supplies the medial head of the triceps.

Retaining the dorsal carpal ligament, clean the **muscles of** the **superficial layer** on the dorsal aspect of the forearm. Of these, the **extensor carpi radialis longus** is the most lateral. It arises from the distal portion of the lateral **supracondylar ridge of** the **humerus** and is partially overlapped near its origin by the brachioradialis. The **remaining muscles** of the superficial layer arise by a **common tendon** from the **lateral epicondyle** and from the **deep fascia** which covers them; they spread distad and medially over the dorsal aspect of the forearm.

of the deeper dorsal muscles, the abductor pollicis longus and the extensor pollicis brevis. The tendons of the two radial extensors pass deep to the dorsal carpal ligament as previously noted. Just distal to the ligament, they

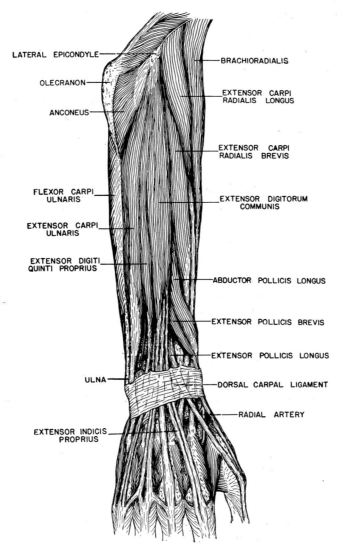

LATERAL EPICONDYLE

OLECRANON

ANCONEUS

FLEXOR CARPI ULNARIS

EXTENSOR CARPI ULNARIS

EXTENSOR DIGITI QUINTI PROPRIUS

ULNA

EXTENSOR INDICIS PROPRIUS

BRACHIORADIALIS

EXTENSOR CARPI RADIALIS LONGUS

EXTENSOR CARPI RADIALIS BREVIS

EXTENSOR DIGITORUM COMMUNIS

ABDUCTOR POLLICIS LONGUS

EXTENSOR POLLICIS BREVIS

EXTENSOR POLLICIS LONGUS

DORSAL CARPAL LIGAMENT

RADIAL ARTERY

FIG. 81. Superficial dissection of the dorsum of the forearm and hand.

The **extensor carpi radialis longus** and **brevis** descend along the lateral side of the forearm, the tendon of the former partially covering that of the latter. Just proximal to the dorsal carpal ligament they are crossed superficially by two

are crossed superficially by the tendon of the extensor pollicis longus. The **extensor carpi radialis longus** is inserted into the dorsal aspect of the **base of** the **second metacarpal;** the **extensor carpi radialis brevis** into the adjacent portions of the **bases of** the **second** and **third metacarpals.** The two radial extensors are supplied by branches which arise from the **radial nerve** just proximal to its termination or from the deep radial before it enters the substance of the supinator.

The **extensor digitorum communis** gives rise, some distance above the wrist, to **four tendons,** which pass deep to the dorsal carpal ligament side by side and diverge on the dorsum of the hand toward the backs of the fingers. Opposite the metacarpophalangeal joint, each tendon gives off a fibrous expansion which is attached to the **base of** the **first phalanx.** On the dorsum of the first phalanx, each tendon divides into **three slips.** Of these, the **middle slip** is inserted on the base of the **second phalanx,** while the two **collateral slips** pass distally to be inserted together into the base of the **terminal phalanx.** The tendon of the **extensor digiti quinti proprius** passes deep to the dorsal carpal ligament in its own compartment and, at the back of the fifth metacarpophalangeal joint, joins the **fourth tendon of** the **extensor digitorum communis.** At about the middle of the first phalanx, each extensor tendon receives on its lateral side the tendon of **insertion of** a **lumbrical muscle.** It should be noted further that, while the main insertion of the interossei is directly into the bases of the first phalanges, each **interosseous muscle** gives a fibrous expansion to the corresponding **extensor tendon,** and that the **adjacent tendons** of the extensor digitorum communis are usually united by oblique **fibrous bands** on the dorsum of the hand.

The **extensor carpi ulnaris** has an accessory origin from the proximal part of the dorsal border of the **ulna.** Its tendon passes deep to the most medial part of the dorsal carpal ligament and is inserted on the base of the **fifth metacarpal.**

Free and elevate the tendons of the extensor digitorum communis, the extensor digiti quinti proprius, and the extensor carpi ulnaris. De-

tach the ulnar head of the extensor carpi ulnaris from its origin and retract the superficial group laterally to expose the deep muscles. As this is done, clean and preserve the nerve twigs which enter the deep surfaces of the muscles in the proximal part of the forearm. In the interval between the superficial and the deep extensors, the **dorsal interosseous artery and nerve** and their branches will be found. These should therefore be cleaned as the deep muscles are cleaned.

The supinator is partly covered by the anconeus, which may be removed. The **supinator** arises in part from the common tendon on the **lateral epicondyle** but has a more extensive **ulnar origin,** from the area just below the radial notch and from the supinator crest. Its fibers form a muscular sheet, which wraps laterally around the proximal part of the **radius** to be inserted on the anterior surface of that bone from the tuberosity to the insertion of the pronator teres. The **deep radial nerve** has been seen to enter the supinator in the cubital fossa. Its continuation may now be found emerging from the distal part of the muscle at the back of the forearm. As it passes through the supinator, the deep radial nerve supplies that muscle; distal to its point of emergence from the supinator, the nerve is known as the **dorsal interosseous nerve.**

The **abductor pollicis longus** arises from the proximal part of the middle third (dorsal surface) of both the **radius** and the **ulna** and the intervening portion of the **interosseous membrane.** Its tendon runs distad and laterally, in company with the tendon of the extensor pollicis brevis, to cross the tendons of the radial extensors of the wrist superficially and pass through the most lateral of the dorsal carpal compartments. It is inserted on the lateral side of the **base of** the **first metacarpal.** The **extensor pollicis brevis** arises from the distal part of the middle third (dorsal surface) of the **radius** and the adjacent part of the **interosse-**

ous membrane. It is inserted at the base of the first phalanx of the thumb.

The extensor pollicis longus arises from the distal part of the middle third (dorsal surface) of the ulna and the adjacent portion of the interosseous membrane. Its tendon passes deep to the dorsal carpal ligament in a compartment of its own and is inserted into the base of the second phalanx of the thumb.

The extensor indicis proprius takes origin from a small area on the dorsal surface of the ulna and the interosseous membrane, just distal to the origin of the extensor pollicis longus. Its tendon crosses the wrist in the same compartment with the tendons of the extensor digitorum communis. Both here and on the dorsum of the hand, it is covered by the first tendon of the latter muscle, which it joins at the back of the second metacarpophalangeal joint.

The dorsal interosseous artery has been seen to arise in the front of the forearm and pass backward above the interosseous membrane. It appears at the back of the forearm between the adjacent borders of the supinator and the abductor pollicis longus and descends between the deep and superficial muscles, to all of which it gives branches. Near the lower border of the supinator, it gives rise to the interosseous recurrent artery, which ascends under cover of the anconeus to anastomose behind the lateral epicondyle with a branch of the profunda brachii.

The dorsal interosseous nerve emerges from the supinator near its distal border and descends between the deep and superficial muscles. Its branches supply all of the extensor muscles with the exception of the two radial extensors of the wrist. A slender continuation of the nerve descends on the dorsal surface of the interosseous membrane, deep to the extensors pollicis longus and indicis proprius, and, passing deep to the tendons of the extensor digitorum communis, reaches the back of the wrist, where it is distributed to the carpal joints. To expose this nerve and the posterior branch of the anterior interosseous artery, the dorsal carpal ligament should be divided over the tendons of the extensor digitorum communis. The posterior branch of the anterior interosseous artery pierces the interosseous membrane some distance proximal to the wrist and descends in company with the dorsal interosseous nerve to the back of the carpus.

The course of the radial artery in the forearm and palm has already been studied. The small intervening segment of its course at the lateral side of the wrist should now be cleaned. As it winds laterally and dorsally around the wrist, the radial artery passes deep to the tendons of the abductor pollicis longus and the extensors pollicis longus and brevis. At the base of the first interosseous space, it turns forward into the palm as the deep palmar arch. From this part of its course, the radial artery gives two branches, the dorsal radial carpal and the first dorsal metacarpal. The dorsal carpal branch runs medially across the back of the carpus to anastomose with the dorsal carpal branch of the ulnar artery and with terminal twigs of the posterior branch of the anterior interosseous. From it arise the second, third, and fourth dorsal metacarpal arteries. The dorsal metacarpals descend in the interosseous spaces; each divides into two small dorsal digital branches for the adjacent sides of two fingers.

Scapular Region

Define and clean the infraspinatus, teres minor, and teres major muscles and the upper part of the long head of the triceps brachii, all of which were partially covered by the posterior part of the deltoid (Fig. 82).

The infraspinatus occupies the infraspinous fossa of the scapula. It arises from the medial part of this fossa and, to some extent, from the layer of deep fascia which covers its outer surface. Its fibers converge laterally to join a strong flat tendon which is closely attached to the posterior part of the capsule of the shoulder joint and is inserted on the **middle facet** on the **greater tuberosity of** the **humerus.** The **teres minor** is a small muscle, which is often fused to a greater or lesser extent with the infraspinatus, immediately below which it lies. It arises from the middle portion of the **axillary border of** the **infraspinous fossa;** its fibers ex-

head of the triceps to reach the anterior aspect of the humerus, where it is inserted into the **medial lip of** the **intertubercular sulcus,** under cover of the coracobrachialis muscle and the tendon of insertion of the latissimus dorsi. The supraspinatus and subscapularis muscles and the remaining dissection of the infraspinatus and teres muscles are described in their relationship to the shoulder joint.

The **axillary nerve** has already been seen to arise as a branch of the **posterior cord of** the

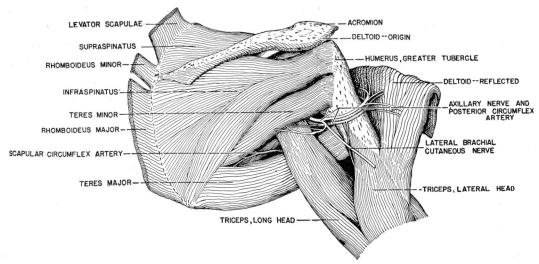

FIG. 82. Posterior aspect of the shoulder region after reflection of the deltoid.

tend laterally to join a tendon which crosses the lower posterior part of the capsule of the shoulder joint to be inserted on the **lowest facet** of the **greater tuberosity of** the **humerus.** The origin of the **long head of the triceps** is covered posteriorly by the teres minor. It arises from the **infraglenoid tuberosity** at the lateral end of the axillary border of the scapula and descends in front of the teres minor and behind the teres major to reach the back of the arm. The **teres major** is a rounded fleshy muscle which arises from the medial part of the **axillary border of** the **infraspinous fossa** and extends laterally, passing in front of the long

brachial plexus within the axilla, which it leaves by passing between the adjacent borders of the subscapularis and teres major muscles in company with the **posterior humeral circumflex branch of** the **axillary artery.** The nerve and artery may now be found reaching the back of the shoulder region by passing through a small **quadrangular space** bounded by the lower border of the **teres minor,** the upper border of the **teres major,** the lateral margin of the **long head of** the **triceps,** and the medial aspect of the **surgical neck of** the **humerus.** It should be noted that the teres minor lies immediately behind the lower part of the subscapularis. Clean and study the further course of the axillary nerve and the posterior humeral circumflex artery (Fig. 82).

The **axillary nerve,** soon after it reaches the back of the shoulder, divides into a superior and an inferior division. The **superior division** is distributed entirely to the **deltoid muscle** by numerous large twigs which enter the deep surface of the muscle. The **inferior division** gives rise to a branch which supplies the **teres minor** and ends as the **lateral brachial cutaneous nerve,** which winds around the posterior border of the deltoid to reach the skin, as previously noted. It may also give a few additional twigs of supply to the deltoid. The largest branches of the **posterior humeral circumflex artery** accompany the branches of the superior division of the axillary nerve into the **deltoid.** A small branch winds anteriorly around the lateral side of the neck of the humerus to anastomose with the **anterior humeral circumflex artery.**

The origin of the **scapular circumflex artery** as a branch of the subscapular in the axilla has already been seen. It leaves the axilla by passing between the adjacent borders of the subscapularis and the teres major. Its continuation may now be seen between the teres minor and the teres major medial to the long head of the triceps. It is distributed to the muscles near the axillary border of the scapula.

Joints

The dissection of the joints should be done only in one extremity; the other should be saved for a review of the entire dissected limb and for the relationships of the various structures to the joints. While dissecting the muscles and other structures away in preparation for the actual dissection of the joints, the opportunity should be utilized to follow the course of the anastomotic, **collateral vessels,** and the **nerves to** the **joints,** which could not

be dissected adequately in the preceding dissection of the upper extremity.

Scapuloclavicular Joint

The clavicle is joined to the scapula by means of a diarthrodial joint between the **lateral end of** the **clavicle** and the **acromion process** (acromioclavicular articulation) and a ligamentous union between the inferior surface of the flattened lateral part of the clavicle and the **coracoid process** (coracoclavicular articulation). These should now be studied. Push the clavicle upward from in front and clean the conoid and trapezoid ligaments; these are the two portions of the **coracoclavicular ligament.** The **conoid ligament** is the **more medial;** it is a strong fibrous cord which passes upward and laterally from the medial side of the root of the **coracoid process** to the **conoid tubercle** on the inferior surface **of** the **clavicle.** The **trapezoid ligament** is a flat fibrous band; it is attached below to a rough ridge on the medial border of the **coracoid process** and above to an oblique line on the **inferior surface of** the **clavicle,** which runs forward and laterally from the conoid tubercle (Fig. 75). The **acromioclavicular joint** is a simple diarthrodial joint surrounded by a fibrous capsule which is attached to the margins of the opposing articular surfaces of the two bones. Open this capsule and observe the articular surfaces of the two bones. Divide the conoid and trapezoid ligaments and disarticulate the clavicle.

Clean the **coracoacromial ligament.** This is a flat, strong fibrous band which arches above the shoulder joint from the lateral border of the **coracoid process** to the tip of the **acromion;** it is wider at its coracoid than at its acromial attachment. Open the **subacromial bursa.** This is a large mucous bursa which lies below the acromion and the coracoacromial ligament, between these structures and the muscles which cover the upper part of the shoulder joint.

Then clean the supraspinatus muscle (Figs. 80 and 82).

The **supraspinatus** occupies the **supraspinous fossa,** from the medial two-thirds of which its fibers take origin. Extending laterally to pass below the acromion and the coracoacromial ligament, the muscle fibers join a strong flat tendon, which is closely bound to the highest part of the capsule of the shoulder joint and is inserted into the **highest facet** on the **greater tuberosity of** the **humerus.** Draw the superior border of the supraspinatus backward to expose the superior border of the scapula. Clean the **superior transverse ligament** of the scapula. This is a strong fibrous band by which the notch in the superior border of the scapula is converted into a foramen. Observe that the **suprascapular nerve,** whose origin from the upper trunk of the brachial plexus in the posterior triangle of the neck has already been seen, passes through this foramen to enter the supraspinous fossa. The **suprascapular artery** passes above the ligament to enter the supraspinous fossa close to the nerve (Fig. 75).

Divide the supraspinatus by an incision at right angles to the direction of its fibers; this incision should be made slightly lateral to the scapular notch. Then reflect the medial segment of the muscle backward and medially and follow the course of the suprascapular nerve. Observe that it runs inferiorly through the supraspinous fossa close to the bone, giving twigs of supply to the supraspinatus, and then passes through the great scapular notch to enter the infraspinous fossa. Attempt to define the **inferior transverse ligament.** This is a fibrous band, not so well defined as is the superior ligament, which converts the medial part of the great scapular notch into a foramen through which both the **suprascapular nerve** and the **suprascapular artery** pass from the supraspinous to the infraspinous fossa (Fig. 80).

Divide the infraspinatus about 1½ in.

medial to its insertion and reflect the medial segment backward and medially from the bony surface of the infraspinous fossa. Observe that the **suprascapular nerve** terminates in twigs of supply to the **infraspinatus.** The **suprascapular** artery is also distributed to the **supraspinatus** and **infraspinatus.** It will be apparent that it enters into anastomoses near the axillary border of the scapula with terminal branches of the **scapular circumflex artery.** The teres minor should also be dissected free from the adjacent structures and elevated to expose the origin of the **long head of** the **triceps,** then transected. Observe that at its origin the long head lies between the teres minor and the lower part of the subscapularis.

Turn to the anterior aspect of the shoulder region and clean the **subscapularis.** This is a wide, thick muscle which fills the entire **subscapular fossa,** from whose bony surface it takes origin. Stretching laterally across the front of the shoulder joint, the muscle narrows toward its insertion, which is on the **lesser tuberosity of** the **humerus.** Its tendon of insertion passes below the coracoid process and behind the common origin of the coracobrachialis and the short head of the biceps. The subscapularis is supplied by the **upper subscapular nerve** and by twigs from the **lower subscapular nerve.** Observe that the latter nerve is distributed principally to the **teres major.** Draw the upper border of the subscapularis forward and downward and open the **subscapular bursa.** This is a large synovial bursa which lies between the deep surface of the **subscapularis** and the inner surface of the **scapula** near the glenoid border; it communicates laterally with the cavity of the shoulder joint.

Clean the anterior surface of the teres major and the tendon of insertion of the latissimus dorsi, if this has not already been done, and examine the manner of insertion of these muscles. Observe that the tendon of the **latissimus dorsi** winds upward over the anterior surface of the teres major to be inserted into the **depth of** the **intertubercular sulcus,** while the **teres major** is inserted into the **medial lip of** this **sulcus.** Both insertions lie behind the coracobrachialis and the biceps. The tendon of insertion of the **pectoralis major** should also be cleaned at this time. This tendon crosses in front of the coracobrachialis and the biceps to be inserted into the **lateral lip of** the **intertubercular sulcus** under cover of the anterior border of the deltoid (Fig. 76).

Shoulder Joint

The **shoulder joint** should be studied next. Cleaning of its **articular capsule** will be facilitated if the following procedure is followed. Divide the coracoacromial ligament along its line of attachment to the coracoid. Then saw through the acromion at its junction with the scapular spine and remove the acromion and the coracoacromial ligament. The **fibrous capsule** of the shoulder joint is attached medially to the **margin of** the **glenoid fossa** and laterally to the **anatomical neck of** the **humerus.** It is almost entirely surrounded by the muscles which pass from the scapula to the tuberosities of the humerus. The **supraspinatus, infraspinatus,** and **teres minor** have already been divided; reflect the lateral segments of these muscles laterally and posteriorly toward their insertions and observe how closely they are bound to the articular capsule. Anteriorly, the capsule is covered by the **subscapularis.** Divide this muscle about 2 in. medial to the lesser tuberosity and reflect its lateral segment forward and laterally. As this is done, the opening in the fibrous capsule by which the **articular cavity communicates with** the **subscapular bursa** will be exposed.

Clean the **coracohumeral ligament.** This ligament is a strong band which stretches from the lateral border of the **coracoid** downward and laterally to the upper part of the **greater tuberosity.** Only at its medial end is it distinctly separable from the fibrous capsule. The **transverse ligament of** the **humerus** is a fibrous band, closely connected with the capsule, which extends **between** the **two tuberosities,** roofing over the proximal portion of the intertubercular sulcus. The **glenohumeral ligaments** are thickenings in the anterior part of the capsule, which may best be seen from the inside. Divide the posterior part of the capsule vertically and turn the head of the humerus laterally and posteriorly, so that the internal surface of the anterior part of the capsule may be seen. The **superior glenohumeral ligament** stretches from the **glenoid border** at the root of the coracoid downward and laterally to the summit of the **lesser tuberosity.** The **middle** and **inferior glenohumeral ligaments** are less distinct thickenings in the lower anterior part of the capsule. The **opening into** the **subscapular bursa** lies between the superior and the middle glenohumeral ligaments.

Observe that the tendon of the **long head of** the **biceps** arises from the **supraglenoid tubercle of** the **scapula** and passes through the articular cavity to reach the **intertubercular sulcus.** Divide this tendon and the anterior part of the capsule and separate the humerus from the scapula. Observe the **glenoid lip.** This is a narrow fibrocartilaginous ring which surmounts the edge of the glenoid cavity and slightly deepens it.

Elbow Joint

Clean the **capsule of** the **elbow joint.** Anteriorly, the lower part of the **brachialis** is closely applied to the capsule; posteriorly, it is covered by the **triceps** and the **anconeus.** These muscles must therefore be removed in cleaning the capsule. The origins of the superficial flexors and extensors should also be cut away from the medial and lateral epicondyles. The **elbow joint** (articulatio cubiti) is the joint at which the distal end of the **humerus** meets the proximal articular surfaces of the **radius** and the

ulna. Enclosed in the same capsule, however, and with a common articular cavity, is the proximal **radioulnar joint** (also a diarthrodial joint). The **fibrous capsule** is attached above to the **humerus** and below to the margins of the **articular surfaces** of the **ulna** and the **neck of** the radius. The **ligaments of** the **elbow joint** are all merely thickenings of the fibrous capsule. The strongest of these are the radial and ulnar collateral ligaments. The **ulnar collateral ligament** extends from the **medial epicondyle** and spreads distad, to be attached to a ridge on the medial borders of the **coronoid** and **olecranon processes of** the **ulna.** The **radial collateral ligament** arises from the lateral **epicondyle.** Its fibers pass distad, and most of them end by joining the lateral part of the **anular ligament;** some fibers, however, are prolonged as far as the neck of the radius. The **anular ligament** is the proper ligament of the proximal radioulnar joint. It is a strong fibrous band whose two ends are attached to the anterior and posterior margins of the **radial notch of** the **ulna.** It encircles the **head of** the **radius** and holds the latter in place as it rotates against the radial notch in the actions of **pronation and supination.** The anular ligament may be seen to better advantage if the joint capsule is opened by a transverse incision across its anterior portion. Observe that the bony articular surfaces are covered by a layer of **cartilage** and that the **articular cavity** is elsewhere lined by the **synovial membrane.**

Wrist Joint

Clean the fibrous capsules of the distal radioulnar joint and the wrist joint. At the **distal radioulnar joint,** the distal end of the **ulna** articulates with the **ulnar notch on** the **radius** and with the proximal surface of the **radial articular disc.** Its external ligaments are the **palmar** and **dorsal radioulnar ligaments,** which connect the distal ends of the two bones. At the **wrist joint** (radiocarpal articulation), the

distal surfaces of the **radius** and of the **radial articular disc** articulate with the proximal surfaces of the navicular (scaphoid) and lunate. Its external ligaments are the radial and ulnar collateral ligaments of the wrist and the palmar and dorsal radiocarpal ligaments. The **ulnar collateral ligament** is a strong fibrous cord which descends from the **styloid process of** the **ulna** to the **pisiform** and **triangular bones.** The **radial collateral ligament** consists of fibers which radiate from the tip of the **styloid process of** the **radius** to the **navicular (scaphoid)** and **greater multangular (trapezium) bones.** The **dorsal** and **palmar radiocarpal ligaments** are thickened parts of the capsule, which spread distad from the lateral part of the distal end of the **radius** to the dorsal and **palmar** surfaces of the **carpal bones.** Open the joint by a transverse incision across the anterior part of the capsule and study the articular surfaces. The **articular disc** is a **plate of fibrocartilage** which is attached laterally to the medial border of the **radial articular surface** and medially to the **styloid process of** the **ulna.** It articulates distad with the **triangular bone** and separates the cavity of the wrist joint from that of the distal radioulnar joint.

Carpal and Metacarpal Joints

The carpal bones are joined to one another by dorsal, palmar, and interosseous ligaments. **Four separate articular cavities,** in addition to that of the wrist joint, are found in connection with the carpal bones. These may be investigated by dividing the ligaments which bind the dorsal surfaces of the bones together and spreading the bones apart to expose the articular surfaces. The **first,** a single large cavity, includes the articulations of the **scaphoid, lunate,** and **triangular** with each other and with the four **bones of** the **distal row.** It is further prolonged along both sides of the lesser multangular to include the articulations between the **second** and **third metacarpals** and the **capitate** and **trapezium.** A **second** articular cavity is found at the junction of the **trapezoid** and the **first metacarpal.** A **third** cavity is for the

articulation of the **fourth** and **fifth metacarpals** with the **hamate.** The **fourth** is a small cavity between the **pisiform** and the **triangular.**

Inferior Extremity ·

Surface Anatomy

The order of dissection followed in this chapter presupposes that the abdomen and pelvis have already been dissected and that one-half of the pelvis has been separated from the vertebral column. If it is desired to dissect the extremity while the abdomen is still intact, it is advisable to make a slight rearrangement to avoid the necessity of turning the body too frequently. This can be accomplished by dissecting the anterior part of the thigh, leg, and foot while the body is in the supine position. Then turn the body over and dissect the gluteal region, posterior part of the thigh, popliteal fossa, and flexor surfaces of the leg and foot as indicated in the subsequent dissection procedure.

Before the skin is reflected from the inferior extremity, attention should be directed to the surface anatomy. Anteriorly, the **thigh** is marked off from the **anterior abdominal wall** by a depressed line running from the anterior superior iliac spine to the pubic tubercle and corresponding to the line of the **inguinal ligament.** The **gluteal region** or buttock, which forms the upper lateral and posterior portion of the inferior extremity, is bounded above by the **iliac crest;** the prominence of the buttock is caused principally by the **gluteus maximus muscle.** Medially, the thigh is separated from the perineum by the border of the **ischiopubic rami.** The head and shaft of the femur are for the most part deeply placed and covered by

thick layers of muscle. These give the thigh its rounded contour. The lateral surface of the **greater trochanter,** however, is subcutaneous. It lies 2 or 3 in. below the anterior superior iliac spine and usually projects slightly farther laterally than the most lateral portion of the iliac crest. At the front of the knee, the anterior surface of the **patella** is subcutaneous. At the lateral side of the knee, the **lateral condyle of the femur** may be palpated; immediately below it is the **lateral condyle of the tibia** and the **head of the fibula.** At the medial side of the knee, locate the **medial condyle of the femur and** the medial condyle of the **tibia.**

The surface landmarks of the **leg** and **foot** should be identified. Observe that the broad, flat, medial surface of the **tibia is subcutaneous** through its length and is continuous below with the **medial malleolus,** which is also subcutaneous. The shaft of the fibula is, for the most part, covered by muscles. The **head of the fibula,** however, may be palpated just below the posterior part of the lateral condyle of the tibia. At the lateral side of the ankle, the **lateral malleolus of the fibula** is subcutaneous and is continuous above with a narrow triangular subcutaneous surface which is interposed between the anterior and lateral surfaces of the fibula in its distal portion. The individual tarsal bones cannot all be recognized. However, the **tuberosity of the calcaneus** forming the prominence of the heel and the **tendon of Achilles** (tendo calcaneus) attaching to it posteriorly are easily recognizable. On the medial border of the foot, slightly below and in front of the medial malleolus, the **tuberosity of** the **navicular bone** should be identified. Somewhat farther anteriorly, on the lateral margin of the foot, the **tuberosity of** the **fifth metatarsal** forms a prominent bony projection.

The skin should be reflected from the entire extremity. Make a longitudinal incision through the skin downward along the medial aspect of the **thigh** from the lower border of the pubic symphysis to the medial condyle of the tibia. From the lower end of this incision, carry a transverse incision across the front of the leg, about 1 in. below the patella, to the head of the fibula. Starting at the upper end of the longitudinal incision, reflect the skin laterally from the entire anterior aspect of the thigh; then continue the reflection of skin posteriorly and downward from the buttock and the posterior aspect of the thigh. The skin over the **gluteal region** should be reflected laterally from the sides of the incisions over the sacrum and coccyx made during the dissection of the back.

The **skin** is now to be reflected from the **entire leg** and the **dorsum of** the **foot.** First remove the large skin flap previously reflected from the thigh, cutting it away along the line where it still remains attached to the upper back part of the leg. Then make a longitudinal incision through the skin of the leg along the middle of the medial surface of the tibia as far as the lower tip of the medial malleolus. From the lower end of this incision, make another incision which completely encircles the posterior part of the foot. This incision must go transversely across the front of the ankle, downward and backward below the lateral malleolus, then across the lower back part of the heel, and upward and forward below the medial malleolus, to reach its point of beginning. This will mark out one large skin flap which should now be reflected and completely removed from

the entire circumference of the leg. Then make a transverse incision across the dorsum of the foot at the level of the bases of the toes and a longitudinal incision running backward along the dorsum from the middle of this transverse incision to the front of the ankle. This will mark out two flaps of skin on the dorsum of the foot which should now be reflected to the lateral and medial borders of the foot respectively.

Make a transverse incision through the **skin** across the **sole of** the **foot** at the bases of the toes. From the middle of this incision, carry a longitudinal incision backward to the heel. Then reflect the two skin flaps thus marked out to each side. The skin should also be reflected from the plantar aspect of the toes. This may be done by means of a longitudinal incision along the middle of each toe. Observe that the **plantar skin** is very **thick** and is closely bound to the superficial fascia by means of fibrous strands which extend through the superficial fascia from the plantar aponeurosis to reach the skin.

Cutaneous Veins and Nerves

The **superficial fascia** of the thigh is usually moderately thick and exhibits the typical characteristics of the panniculus adiposus. Within it are numerous **superficial veins.** The largest and most constant of these is the **great saphenous vein,** which should now be cleaned. This vein begins from the **dorsal venous arch of** the **foot.** Ascending on the **medial side of** the leg, it will be found behind the medial side of the knee. It passes upward along the **medial side of** the **thigh,** inclining somewhat forward, and joins the **femoral vein** about 1 in. below the inguinal ligament by passing through the **saphenous hiatus.** This is an oval opening in the deep fascia (fascia lata) of the thigh, which lies immediately in front of the femoral vein, below the medial part of the inguinal ligament.

Observe the **superficial inguinal lymph**

Ing. Lig.

nodes. These are from 10 to 20 in number and often of considerable size. They lie in the superficial fascia below the inguinal ligament in the region of the saphenous hiatus. In many cases, the fine **lymphatic vessels** which communicate with them may be made out.

Attention should next be directed to the **cutaneous nerves of** the **thigh.** The main trunks or branches of these nerves pierce the fascia lata at variable distances below the inguinal ligament or the iliac crest and descend along the deep surface of the superficial fascia. As they are displayed, the superficial fascia should be removed.

The **lateral femoral cutaneous nerve is** a **branch of** the **lumbar plexus.** It enters the thigh by passing behind the lateral end of the inguinal ligament. Below the inguinal ligament, it divides into an anterior and a posterior branch, which will be found piercing the fascia lata separately. The **posterior branch** supplies the skin on the upper lateral part of the thigh. The **anterior branch** becomes superficial somewhat lower and more anteriorly and supplies the skin of the lower lateral part of the thigh.

The **lumboinguinal nerve** is one of the terminal branches of the **genitofemoral nerve.** It emerges through the saphenous hiatus or may pierce the fascia lata near that opening. It supplies a variable area of skin below the inguinal ligament on the upper anterior aspect of the thigh.

The **intermediate femoral cutaneous nerve** and the **medial femoral cutaneous nerve** are the anterior cutaneous branches of the **femoral nerve.** Their origin from the femoral nerve will be seen in the dissection of the femoral triangle. At present, their terminal branches should be found piercing the fascia lata and traced downward on the thigh. Each usually divides into two branches before piercing the fascia lata. The **medial** and **lateral branches of** the **intermediate nerve** will be found piercing the fascia lata close together, at the middle of the an-

terior aspect of the thigh about a third of the distance between the inguinal ligament and the knee. The **branches of** the **medial cutaneous nerve** usually appear close to the great saphenous vein. Small branches of this nerve may be found piercing the fascia lata at any point along the course of the vein; its larger terminal anterior and posterior branches become cutaneous in the lower part of the thigh, the former lying in front of the vein and the latter behind it.

The **infrapatellar branch of** the **saphenous nerve is** a cutaneous nerve which becomes superficial at the medial side of the knee, from which point it takes a curved course downward and forward below the patella.

The **cutaneous nerves of** the **gluteal region** include the lateral cutaneous **branch of** the **iliohypogastric nerve** and a group of small nerves known as the **cluneal nerves.** They are small and usually difficult to demonstrate, but an attempt at their identification should be made as the superficial fascia is removed from the region below the iliac crest.

The **lateral cutaneous branch of** the **iliohypogastric nerve** runs downward over the iliac crest at about the junction of its anterior and middle thirds and is distributed to the skin over the outer surface of the anterior part of the ilium. The **superior cluneal nerves** are the lateral branches of the **posterior** primary **divisions** of the first three **lumbar nerves.** They cross the iliac crest in series behind the lateral cutaneous branch of the iliohypogastric nerve and are distributed to the skin of the gluteal region. The **middle cluneal nerves** are small nerves derived from the lateral branches of the **posterior** primary **divisions** of the first three **sacral nerves.** They pierce the gluteus maximus in a line running from the posterior superior iliac spine to the tip of the coccyx to supply the skin over the medial part of the gluteus maximus. The **inferior cluneal nerves** are branches of the **posterior femoral cutaneous** nerve, which supplies the skin on the posterior aspect of the thigh. They may be most easily identified when the gluteus maximus is cleaned.

The **cutaneous nerves of** the **leg** and **foot** should now be investigated. Some variation occurs in the distribution of these nerves, but most commonly they will be found to follow approximately the description given here. The **medial** and **lateral sural cutaneous nerves** arise from the **tibial** and **common peroneal nerves,** respectively, in or near the popliteal fossa. Their distributions should now be followed. The **lateral sural cutaneous nerve** is distributed to the skin on the upper lateral and antero-lateral part of the leg; it gives rise to a branch known as the **peroneal anastomotic nerve,** which passes downward and backward across the calf and joins the medial sural cutaneous nerve to form the sural nerve. The peroneal anastomotic nerve sometimes arises independently from the common peroneal. The **medial sural cutaneous nerve** accompanies the **small saphenous vein** down the back of the calf. Below its junction with the peroneal anastomotic, it is known as the sural nerve. The **sural nerve** supplies the lower lateral part of the leg and turns forward below the lateral malleolus to supply the lateral margin of the foot, where it is known as the **lateral dorsal cutaneous nerve,** and may be traced as far forward as the lateral side of the fifth toe.

The **saphenous nerve** becomes superficial, emerging between the sartorius and the gracilis. It descends in company with the **great saphenous vein** and supplies the skin on the medial and anteromedial part of the leg as far down as the medial malleolus; branches of the saphenous nerve can often be followed for a considerable distance along the medial margin of the foot.

The **superficial peroneal nerve** is one of the terminal branches of the **common peroneal.** It may be found piercing the deep fascia on the anterolateral aspect of the leg about halfway between the knee and the ankle, or a little

lower. Traced distad, it divides almost at once into a medial and a lateral branch. The **medial branch** passes downward in front of the ankle and divides into **two trunks;** of these, the more **medial** passes forward to the skin along the medial side of the great toe, while the more **lateral** reaches the cleft between the second and third toes and divides into two dorsal digital branches which supply the skin on the adjacent sides of these toes. The **lateral branch of** the **superficial peroneal** also gives rise to **two trunks,** from which **dorsal digital nerves** arise to supply the adjacent sides of the third and fourth and fourth and fifth toes. The **terminal part of** the **deep peroneal nerve** will be found emerging in the cleft between the bases of the great and second toes. It gives rise to two **dorsal digital branches** which supply the adjacent sides of these two toes.

Thigh

The **superficial fascia** should now be entirely removed from the anterior and lateral aspects of the thigh to expose the **deep fascia.** Retain the **medial** and **intermediate femoral cutaneous nerves** so that their origin from the femoral nerve may later be recognized. The deep fascia which invests the thigh is known as the **fascia lata.** Superiorly, it is attached to the inguinal ligament and the iliac crest. Toward the medial aspect of the thigh, the fascia lata is relatively thin and does not differ appreciably from the deep fascia which is ordinarily found investing muscles. Along the lateral aspect of the thigh, however, it is resolved into a very dense apo-neurotic band known as the **iliotibial tract,** which should now be investigated. Superiorly, it is attached to the **anterior part of** the **iliac crest** through the fascia covering the gluteus medius muscle. Inferiorly, it extends over the lateral side of the knee joint to be attached to the **lateral condyle of** the **tibia.** The iliotibial tract receives the insertions of the **tensor muscle of** the **fascia lata** and most of the fibers of the **gluteus maximus.** The external surfaces of these two muscles should now be cleaned to demonstrate their relation to the fascia lata.

The **tensor fasciae latae** is a flat quadrilateral muscle which arises from the anterior portion ciculi. It arises from the most **posterior part of the iliac crest** and the **dorsum of the ilium** behind the posterior gluteal line, from the lateral part of the posterior surface of the **sacrum** and **coccyx,** and from the **sacrotuberous**

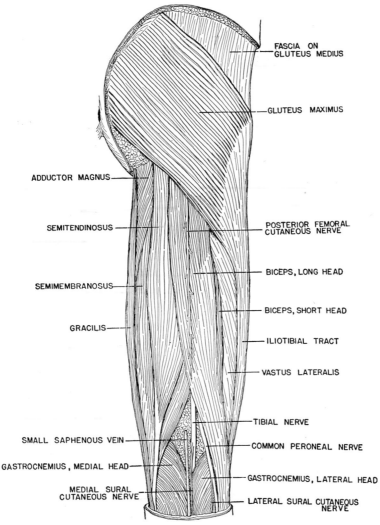

FASCIA ON
GLUTEUS MEDIUS

GLUTEUS MAXIMUS

ADDUCTOR MAGNUS

SEMITENDINOSUS

SEMIMEMBRANOSUS

GRACILIS

POSTERIOR FEMORAL
CUTANEOUS NERVE

BICEPS, LONG HEAD

BICEPS, SHORT HEAD

ILIOTIBIAL TRACT

VASTUS LATERALIS

TIBIAL NERVE

SMALL SAPHENOUS VEIN

COMMON PERONEAL NERVE

GASTROCNEMIUS, MEDIAL HEAD

MEDIAL SURAL
CUTANEOUS NERVE

GASTROCNEMIUS, LATERAL HEAD

LATERAL SURAL CUTANEOUS
NERVE

Fig. 83. Superficial dissection of the posterior aspect of the thigh.

of the **external lip of** the **iliac crest** and the **anterior superior iliac spine.** Its fibers run downward and somewhat laterally to join the **iliotibial tract** about one-third of the distance down the thigh.

The **gluteus maximus** is a large, thick quadrangular muscle, made up of very coarse fas-

ligament. Its fibers pass downward and laterally across the buttock, and the greater portion of them are inserted into the **iliotibial tract** of the fascia lata.

The two borders of the **gluteus maximus** should be carefully defined. Stretching across a roughly triangular area bounded by the superior border of the gluteus maximus, the posterior border of the tensor fasciae, and the iliac crest, the fascia lata covers the external surface of the gluteus medius. This portion of the fascia lata is usually covered by a relatively thick layer of superficial fascia, all of which should be removed (Fig. 83).

As the inferior border of the gluteus maximus is cleaned, the **inferior cluneal branches of** the **posterior femoral cutaneous nerve** will be found turning upward around this border. The **trunk of** the **posterior femoral cutaneous nerve** will be found emerging from behind the middle of the lower border of the gluteus maximus to run downward on the posterior aspect of the thigh.

The **iliotibial tract** is merely a greatly **thickened portion of** the **fascia lata** and is continuous with the thinner portion of the fascia stretching medially across the anterior aspect of the thigh. Since the fascia covering the anterior thigh muscles must be removed in cleaning the muscles and since it is desirable for the present to retain the iliotibial tract, an artificial anterior border for the iliotibial tract may be made by dissection. To do this, make a longitudinal incision through the fascia lata, running downward from the lower end of the anterior border of the tensor fasciae latae to the lateral condyle of the tibia. The thick portion of the fascia lata behind this incision is the iliotibial tract; the continuation of the fascia lata across the thigh in front of this incision may be removed as the anterior thigh muscles are cleaned. In the preliminary cleaning of the superficial muscles of the thigh, which is to be the next step in the dissection, care should be taken to avoid displacing the muscles. Clean only their external surfaces and keep their relative positions undisturbed.

Extensor Region of Thigh

Clean first the **sartorius.** This is a long, narrow straplike muscle which crosses the anterior aspect of the thigh obliquely. Arising from the **anterior superior spine of** the **ilium,** its fibers run downward and medially to the medial side of the knee; from here, the muscle is continued downward as a flat tendon which is inserted into the upper part of the **medial surface of** the **tibia.** This insertion will be seen later in the dissection.

The anterior and lateral portions of the thigh, below and lateral to the sartorius, are occupied by the four muscles which make up the **quadriceps femoris;** these are the **rectus femoris** and the **vastus medialis,** vastus **intermedius,** and vastus **lateralis.**

The uppermost portion of the **rectus femoris** is overlapped by the sartorius medially and the tensor fasciae latae laterally. It arises from the **coxal (hip) bone** by two separate short tendons, which will be seen to better advantage somewhat later. The **straight tendon** arises from the **anterior inferior iliac spine,** the **reflected tendon** from the upper surface of the **rim of** the **acetabulum.** The two tendons unite to form an aponeurotic expansion, whose anterior surface may now be seen in the interval between the upper part of the sartorius and the tensor fasciae. Observe that muscle fibers spread downward from this aponeurosis to form a thick spindle-shaped muscle on the front of the thigh, which is inserted by a strong flat tendon into the **upper border of** the **patella.**

Lateral to the rectus femoris, clean the exposed portion of the **vastus lateralis.** Draw the iliotibial tract laterally and observe that it lies immediately external to the broad lateral surface of the vastus lateralis. Pass the hand posteriorly on the internal surface of the fascia lata, in the interval between the fascia and the vastus lateralis, and observe that a short fascial septum extends inward from the deep surface of the posterolateral portion of the fascia lata to the lateral lip of the linea aspera and the lateral supracondylar ridge. This is the **lateral intermuscular septum of** the **thigh, which sep-**

arates the **anterior** or **extensor group** of muscles from the **posterior flexor** or hamstring **muscles.**

Turn next to the medial aspect of the thigh and clean the external surface of the **gracilis.**

the thigh, it becomes narrower and thicker, finally giving rise to a rounded tendon which descends behind the medial condyle of the femur. Its insertion on the **medial surface of**

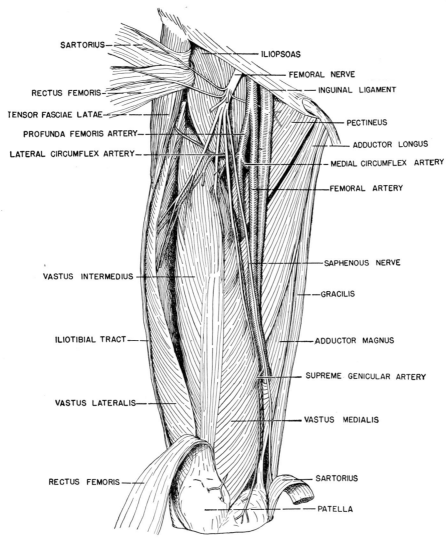

FIG. 84. Dissection of the anterior aspect of the thigh. The sartorius and rectus femoris have been reflected and the vastus lateralis and iliotibial tract displaced laterally.

This muscle arises by a flat tendon from the margin of the **inferior ramus of** the **pubis** and the adjacent part of the **inferior ramus of the ischium.** Its upper portion is flat and relatively broad. As it descends on the medial aspect of

the **tibia** will be seen later. In the lower half of the thigh, the gracilis lies immediately posterior to the sartorius (Fig. 84). The interval on the upper anterior part of the thigh, between the medial border of the sartorius and the anterior border of the gracilis, from which the deep fascia has not yet been removed is occupied by the muscles of the **adductor group.**

Attention should first be directed to the **femoral triangle.** This space is bounded **above** by the **inguinal ligament, laterally** by the medial border of the upper part of the **sartorius,** and **medially** by the medial border of the **adductor longus.** Its **roof,** or superficial boundary, is formed by the **fascia lata,** which is here relatively thin. Its **floor,** or deep boundary, is formed by the anterior surfaces of the **adductor longus, pectineus,** and **iliopsoas muscles.** Within the femoral triangle are the upper portions of the **femoral vessels** and the terminal part of the **femoral nerve.** Remove the fascia lata from the roof of the femoral triangle, define the medial border of the adductor longus, and study the femoral vessels and the femoral sheath.

The **adductor longus** arises by a narrow flat tendon from the **superior ramus of the pubis** near the pubic tubercle. The fibers pass downward and laterally from this origin as the muscle widens toward its insertion on the middle third of the **linea aspera.** Its medial border, particularly near the origin, is usually adjacent to the anterior border of the gracilis (Fig. 84).

The **femoral artery** begins behind the inguinal ligament as a direct continuation of the **external iliac artery.** It descends in the femoral triangle, which it leaves a short distance above the apex of the triangle, by passing behind the sartorius. At its beginning, the femoral artery is lateral to the femoral vein; lower down it comes to lie in front of the vein. In the uppermost part of the femoral triangle, both the artery and the vein are enclosed within the femoral sheath, which should now be investigated.

The **femoral sheath** is a funnel-shaped fascial sheath which represents a prolongation behind the inguinal ligament into the thigh of portions of the **transversalis fascia and** the **iliac fascia.**

Its **anterior wall** is continuous above the inguinal ligament with the transversalis fascia; its **posterior wall** is continuous with the portion of the iliac fascia which lies behind the external iliac vessels. The **lateral boundary** of the femoral sheath is formed by the blending of these two layers of fascia around the lateral side of the femoral artery. The femoral sheath can be traced as a distinct structure for only about 1 in. below the inguinal ligament; lower than this, it joins the general fascial covering of the vessels. Its chief importance lies in the fact that its anterior and posterior walls do not blend immediately on the medial side of the femoral vein but are prolonged farther medially to enclose a loosely filled compartment of the sheath known as the **femoral canal,** which lies along the medial side of the uppermost part of the femoral vein and may be the seat of a **femoral hernia.**

The upper or **abdominal end of** the **femoral canal** is known as the **femoral ring.** It is here that a femoral hernia leaves the abdominal cavity. The femoral ring lies behind the medial part of the **inguinal ligament.** It is bounded laterally by the **femoral vein,** medially by the free margin of the **lacunar ligament,** and posteriorly by the **pecten of** the **pubis.** It is loosely filled by fat and a few small lymph glands and consequently forms a weak spot in the abdominal wall. Identify the aperture into the femoral canal and restudy the boundaries of this canal by the procedure described in the chapter on the abdominal wall (inguinal region).

Clear away the femoral sheath and, without injury to the femoral artery, the femoral nerve, and their branches, define the borders of the muscles which form the **floor of** the **femoral triangle.** The **adductor longus** has already been seen to form the lower medial portion of the floor. The upper lateral portion of the floor of the femoral triangle is formed by the **iliopsoas.** This muscle, which here consists of the psoas tendon and the lower fibers of the iliacus, enters the thigh by passing behind the lateral part of the inguinal ligament. Its insertion on the **lesser trochanter of** the **femur** is at present hidden by the sartorius. Between the iliopsoas and the adductor longus, the floor of the femoral triangle is formed by the anterior surface of the **pectineus.** This flat muscle has a fleshy origin from the **outer surface of** the **pubis** below the pecten; its fibers pass downward and laterally to be inserted in the **pectineal** line behind and below the lesser trochanter **of** the **femur.**

Identify the three large branches which arise from the **femoral artery** within the femoral triangle. These are the profunda femoris and the medial and lateral femoral circumflex arteries. The **profunda** arises from the posterior aspect of the femoral about $1\frac{1}{2}$ in. below the inguinal ligament and runs downward through the triangle behind and slightly lateral to the femoral. The femoral circumflex arteries are somewhat variable in origin. In many cases, they appear as branches of the profunda. It is very common, however, to find one or both of them arising as direct branches of the femoral a short distance below the origin of the profunda. The **medial femoral circumflex artery** passes medially and posteriorly to leave the femoral triangle between the adjacent borders of the psoas and pectineus muscles, first giving rise to a **superficial branch to** the muscles of the **adductor group.** The **lateral femoral circumflex artery** passes laterally behind the sartorius and rectus muscles.

The **femoral nerve** enters the femoral triangle by passing downward behind the inguinal ligament lateral to the psoas tendon. It ends in the upper part of the triangle by dividing into two groups of terminal branches, an **anterior** or **superficial** and a **posterior** or **deep group.** The **superficial group** should now be studied. It includes the **nerve to** the **pectineus,** the **nerve to** the **sartorius,** and the **medial** and **intermediate femoral cutaneous nerves.** The

nerve to the pectineus passes medially and downward behind the femoral vessels to reach the anterior surface of the pectineus. The nerve to the sartorius often arises in common with the intermediate cutaneous branch, from which it separates before entering the upper part of the sartorius. The distribution of the cutaneous branches has already been studied; the intermediate cutaneous nerve frequently pierces the sartorius before becoming superficial.

As the **femoral artery** leaves the femoral triangle, it enters a space known as the **adductor canal.** To open this canal for study, it will be necessary to reflect the sartorius. Divide this muscle at about its middle by an incision at right angles to the direction of its fibers, and reflect the two segments toward the origin and the insertion of the muscle. The adductor canal is triangular in section, possessing a lateral, a posterior, and an anteromedial wall. The **lateral wall** is formed by the external surface of the **vastus medialis muscle.** The **posterior wall** is formed by portions of the anterior surfaces of the **adductor longus** and **adductor magnus muscles.** The canal is covered **anteromedially** by the **sartorius,** but its anteromedial wall is further reinforced by an **aponeurotic septum** which bridges across from the adductors to the vastus medialis under cover of the sartorius. Make a longitudinal incision through this aponeurosis to expose the femoral vessels and the saphenous nerve within the canal.

Observe that within the adductor canal the **femoral vein** lies **behind** the **femoral artery.** Posteriorly, the vessels rest against the adductor longus in the upper part of the canal and, below the medial border of the adductor longus, against the adductor magnus. Observe the **tendinous opening in** the **adductor magnus** at the side of the medial supracondylar ridge of the femur. As it passes through this opening, the **femoral artery** terminates by becoming the **popliteal artery;** the **femoral vein** begins here as a direct continuation of the **popliteal vein.**

In the adductor canal, the femoral artery is crossed anteriorly by the **saphenous nerve.** Trace this nerve proximad and observe that it is one of the deep terminal branches of the **femoral nerve.** Traced distad, it does not accompany the femoral vessels through the adductor magnus but continues downward under cover of the sartorius to become superficial at the medial side of the knee between the tendons of the sartorius and the gracilis. Its distribution as a cutaneous nerve of the leg will be seen later.

Clean the course of the **supreme (descending) genicular artery.** This artery arises from the **femoral** just above the tendinous opening in the adductor magnus and almost immediately divides into a saphenous and a musculoarticular branch. The two branches frequently arise separately from the femoral. The **saphenous branch** accompanies the saphenous nerve; the **musculoarticular branch** enters the vastus medialis, giving twigs to that muscle and taking part in the general arterial anastomosis around the knee joint.

Now return to the **deep branches of** the **femoral nerve.** These are the **saphenous nerve,** which has already been traced, and the **nerves to** the **rectus femoris,** the **vastus lateralis,** the vastus **intermedius,** and the vastus **medialis.** Secure first the nerve to the rectus femoris and trace it into the deep surface of that muscle. Then divide the rectus femoris transversely at about its middle and reflect the cut segments toward the origin and the insertion. The reflection of the rectus femoris will expose a portion of the vastus intermedius and will also facilitate the study of the distribution of the lateral femoral circumflex artery and the nerves to the vasti.

The **lateral femoral circumflex artery** ends behind the upper part of the rectus femoris by dividing into ascending and descending branches. These should now be cleaned. The

ascending branch runs upward and laterally under cover of the rectus and sartorius, to both of which it gives branches, and ends under cover of the tensor fasciae latae, where it anastomoses with the **gluteal arteries.** The **descending branches** run downward and laterally and provide the main supply of the vastus intermedius and vastus lateralis. The most lateral of these branches, which accompanies the nerve to the vastus lateralis, will serve as a guide to the anterior border of that muscle (Fig. 84).

Define the anterior border of the vastus lateralis, raise it from the subjacent vastus intermedius, and study the origins of these two muscles. The **lower fibers** of the **vastus lateralis** arise from the lateral lip of the **linea aspera** and the **lateral intermuscular septum.** Observe that its **upper fibers** arise from the anteroinferior margin of the **great trochanter** and, below this, from a **line** curving downward and laterally **around** the **femur** to join the lateral lip of the linea aspera. Its nerve passes under the anterior border of the muscle to reach its deep surface. The **vastus intermedius** has a broad origin from the lateral and anterior surfaces of the upper two-thirds of the **shaft of** the **femur.** Its fibers pass downward and forward to join an aponeurosis which lies on the anterior surface of the muscle and is inserted, in common with the rectus tendon and fibers of the other two vasti, into the **proximal border of** the **patella.** The nerve to the vastus intermedius enters the upper part of its anteromedial surface.

The **vastus medialis** arises from the entire length of the medial lip of the **linea aspera.** It is intimately associated above with the vastus intermedius. Distad, its upper fibers join a flat tendon which overlies the medial margin of the tendon of the vastus intermedius and is difficult to separate from it. If the proper separation is made, however, and the vastus medialis pushed medially, it will be seen that the broad medial surface of the femur is bare of muscle attachments and is simply overlain by the deep surface of the vastus medialis (Figs. 84 and 95).

Adductor Region of Thigh

Attention should now be directed to the **adductor group of muscles** and the nerves and vessels which supply them. If the anterior surfaces of the adductor longus and pectineus the adductor longus. Elevate the **adductor longus.** At the same time, secure and preserve the nerve which enters its deep surface; this is a **branch of the obturator nerve.** The elevation of the adductor longus will expose the lower part of the adductor brevis muscle, which lies behind the lower part of the pectineus and the upper part of the adductor longus. Define the lower (medial) border of this muscle and then

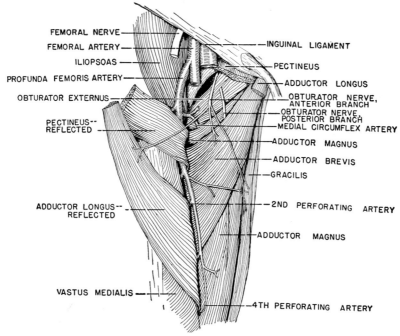

FEMORAL NERVE

FEMORAL ARTERY

ILIOPSOAS

PROFUNDA FEMORIS ARTERY

OBTURATOR EXTERNUS

PECTINEUS-- REFLECTED

ADDUCTOR LONGUS-- REFLECTED

VASTUS MEDIALIS

INGUINAL LIGAMENT

PECTINEUS

ADDUCTOR LONGUS

OBTURATOR NERVE, ANTERIOR BRANCH

OBTURATOR NERVE, POSTERIOR BRANCH

MEDIAL CIRCUMFLEX ARTERY

ADDUCTOR MAGNUS

ADDUCTOR BREVIS

GRACILIS

2ND PERFORATING ARTERY

ADDUCTOR MAGNUS

4TH PERFORATING ARTERY

FIG. 85. Dissection of the upper medial portion of the thigh to display the adductor muscles and the obturator nerve.

have not been completely cleaned, this should be done now. At the same time, clean the insertion of the iliopsoas. Observe that most of the fibers of the **iliacus** join the **psoas tendon,** which is inserted into the **lesser trochanter,** but that a few of the lowest fibers of the iliacus are inserted directly into the **femur** in a line extending for a short distance below the lesser trochanter.

Trace the **profunda femoris artery** distad and observe that it passes downward behind clean and study the full course of the **profunda femoris artery** (Fig. 85).

From its posterior aspect, the **profunda** gives rise to a series of **perforating arteries,** which pass posteriorly through the adductor muscles to reach the back of the thigh. The **first perforating artery** arises at about the level of the upper border of the adductor longus and pierces both the adductor brevis and the adductor magnus. The **second perforating artery** arises somewhat lower and also pierces both of these muscles. The **third perforating artery** passes below the adductor brevis, piercing only the magnus. The **fourth perforating artery** is the termination of the profunda itself. From the medial aspect of the profunda, one or two small branches are given to the adductor muscles.

Detach the pectineus from its origin and reflect it anteriorly and laterally to its insertion. Then, by tracing proximad the nerve to the adductor longus previously identified, find the **anterior division of the obturator nerve.** This nerve descends under cover of the pectineus, where it divides into three branches which may now be traced into the **adductor longus,** the **adductor brevis,** and the **gracilis.**

Clean the anterior surface of the **adductor brevis.** This muscle has a narrow origin from the outer surface of the **inferior ramus of** the **pubis** under cover of the origins of the pectineus and adductor longus. The fibers diverge laterally to form a flat triangular muscle which is inserted into the upper part of the **linea aspera** immediately lateral to the insertions of the pectineus and adductor longus. Define clearly the upper border of the adductor brevis and observe that the uppermost portion of the adductor magnus is exposed above it. Running downward on the anterior surface of the adductor magnus to disappear behind the adductor brevis is the **posterior division of** the **obturator nerve.** Above the upper border of the adductor magnus, the upper part of the external surface of the **obturator externus muscle,** which covers the obturator foramen and obturator membrane, is exposed. The two divisions of the **obturator nerve** usually emerge separately into the upper medial part of the thigh—the **anterior division** running downward over the upper border of the obturator externus, and the **posterior division** piercing that muscle slightly below its superior border (Fig. 85).

Retract the adductor brevis anteriorly and

laterally. Then study the anterior surface of the **adductor magnus.** This muscle has a long origin, beginning on the **inferior ramus of** the **pubis** and running backward along the **outer surface of** the **ischium** to the tuberosity. It has a very extensive linear insertion on the entire length of the **linea aspera** and the **medial supracondylar ridge.** This insertion is broken at the tendinous opening already observed, through which the femoral vessels leave the front of the thigh. The most distal part of the insertion of the **adductor magnus** is by means of a strong rounded **tendon** which joins the **adductor tubercle.**

Running downward on the anterior surface of the **adductor magnus** and supplying it is the **posterior division of** the **obturator nerve.** This nerve also gives rise to a long, slender twig which pierces the lower part of the adductor magnus to reach the **knee joint.**

The medial femoral circumflex artery has already been seen to leave the femoral triangle by passing between the psoas and the pectineus. It may now be seen to proceed farther toward the back of the thigh above the upper border of the adductor magnus, between that muscle and the obturator externus.

Gluteal Region

The external surface of the **gluteus maximus** muscle has already been cleaned. Clearly define the entire length of both the upper and lower borders of the gluteus maximus if this was not previously done. Then make an incision through the entire thickness of the muscle, taking care to avoid injury to underlying structures. This incision should start at about the middle of the upper border and run vertically downward to the lower border. Then reflect the lateral cut segment of the muscle to its insertion. Observe that while the muscle is for the most part inserted into the **iliotibial tract,** the deeper fibers of its inferior portion are inserted directly into the **gluteal tuberosity of** the **femur.** Between the deep surface of the muscle and the greater trochanter, a closed **mucous bursa,** sometimes very large, is usually found. Next reflect the medial segment of the muscle to its origin. As this is done, clean and preserve the **inferior gluteal nerve** and the branches of the **superior and inferior gluteal arteries,** which ramify on the deep surface of the gluteus maximus and supply it. Observe

pelvic cavity is put into communication with the **gluteal region,** are covered externally by the gluteus maximus. Attention should next be given to the various structures which emerge from the pelvis through the greater sciatic foramen.

Clean first the **piriformis.** This small muscle arises within the pelvis from the **lateral part of** the **sacrum** and also, to some extent, from

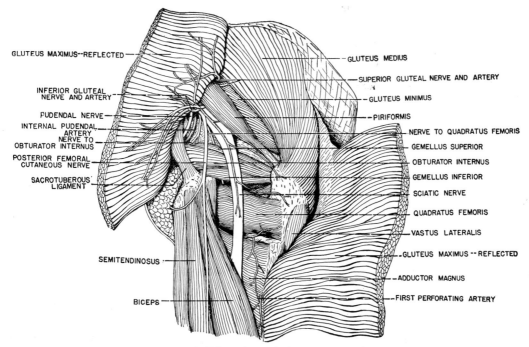

GLUTEUS MAXIMUS--REFLECTED
INFERIOR GLUTEAL NERVE AND ARTERY
PUDENDAL NERVE
INTERNAL PUDENDAL ARTERY
NERVE TO OBTURATOR INTERNUS
POSTERIOR FEMORAL CUTANEOUS NERVE
SACROTUBEROUS LIGAMENT
SEMITENDINOSUS
BICEPS

GLUTEUS MEDIUS
SUPERIOR GLUTEAL NERVE AND ARTERY
GLUTEUS MINIMUS
PIRIFORMIS
NERVE TO QUADRATUS FEMORIS
GEMELLUS SUPERIOR
OBTURATOR INTERNUS
GEMELLUS INFERIOR
SCIATIC NERVE
QUADRATUS FEMORIS
VASTUS LATERALIS
GLUTEUS MAXIMUS -- REFLECTED
ADDUCTOR MAGNUS
FIRST PERFORATING ARTERY

FIG. 86. Dissection of the gluteal region.

that some of the lower fibers of the muscle take origin from the outer surface of the **sacrotuberous ligament;** these fibers should be detached and the ligament cleaned (Fig. 86).

The **sacrotuberous ligament,** which runs downward and laterally from the **sacrum** and **coccyx** to the **ischial tuberosity,** forms the inferomedial boundary of the **lesser sciatic foramen,** the passage by which the **gluteal region** communicates **with** the ischiorectal fossa of the **perineum.** Both this foramen and the **greater sciatic foramen** above it, by which the

the upper border of the **greater sciatic notch.** Emerging from the **greater sciatic foramen,** its fibers run downward and laterally, narrowing to a round tendon which is inserted upon the highest part of the **great trochanter of** the **femur.** In some cases, the fleshy belly of the muscle is divided by the passage through it of the **common peroneal (fibular) nerve.** This nerve, which is normally one of the terminal branches of the **schiadic (sciatic) nerve,** does not in most cases appear in the gluteal region at all. Fairly frequently, however, the ischiadic nerve as a whole is lacking, its two terminal branches, the **tibial** and **common peroneal (fibular) nerves,** arising directly from the sacral plexus. In such cases, the common peroneal nerve usually pierces the piriformis, the tibial nerve passing below it.

The **superior gluteal nerve and artery** emerge through the **greater sciatic foramen** immediately **above** the **piriformis.** Only a small segment of the superior gluteal nerve may be seen at present, since it disappears almost at once under cover of the posterior border of the gluteus medius. The superior gluteal artery lies above the nerve. It gives several large branches to the upper part of the **gluteus maximus** and then accompanies the nerve under cover of the gluteus medius.

The **inferior gluteal nerve and vessels** emerge immediately **below the piriformis.** The **inferior gluteal nerve** is distributed entirely to the **gluteus maximus.** The **inferior gluteal artery** breaks up into numerous branches, the **largest** of which enter the **gluteus maximus.** Others pass downward and laterally to take part in the general arterial anastomosis around the greater trochanter, while one long, slender branch accompanies the ischiadic nerve downward into the thigh.

The **ischiadic nerve** is the largest nerve in the body. It appears **below** the **piriformis** and runs somewhat laterally and downward into the thigh, to pass from view under cover of the long head of the biceps femoris. No branches arise from it in the gluteal region. Occasionally, as noted above, it is represented by two nerves, the tibial and the common fibular; of these, the common fibular is the more lateral.

The **posterior femoral cutaneous nerve** emerges from the greater sciatic foramen **below** the **piriformis** and passes downward, lying at first under cover of the gluteus maximus in close relation to the ischiadic nerve. The remaining structures which pass through the greater

sciatic foramen will also be found below the piriformis. Before exposing them, however, it is advisable to identify and clean the tendon of the obturator internus, the gemelli muscles, and the quadratus femoris.

The **obturator internus** has a wide origin on the **internal wall of** the **pelvis minor** from the inner surface of the **coxal bone** and the **obturator membrane.** Its fibers converge toward the lesser sciatic notch to join a flat tendon which curves laterally across the notch and extends laterally and upward in front of the ischiadic nerve to be inserted into the medial surface of the **greater trochanter of** the **femur.** This tendon is overlapped above by the gemellus superior and below by the gemellus inferior.

The **gemelli** are two small muscles which are inserted together with the **obturator internus** and intimately connected with its **tendon** throughout. The **gemellus superior** arises from the outer surface of the **spine of** the **ischium.** The **gemellus inferior** arises from the upper part of the **ischial tuberosity and** the **sacrotuberous ligament** near the tuberosity.

The **quadratus femoris** lies below the gemellus inferior. It arises from the **outer border of** the **ischial tuberosity.** Its fibers pass almost directly laterally to be inserted into a vertical ridge on the **femur** immediately below the posterior border of the greater trochanter (Fig. 86).

The **nerve to** the **quadratus femoris,** the nerve to the **obturator internus,** the **internal pudendal vessels,** and the **pudendal nerve,** all of which emerge from the pelvis through the **greater sciatic foramen below** the **piriformis,** will be found running downward across the outer surface of the ischium in the roughly triangular space bounded by the sacrotuberous ligament, the gemellus superior, and the ischiadic nerve. Most medial is the **pudendal nerve.** This nerve runs downward and somewhat medially across the outer surface of the **ischial spine** and passes through the **lesser sciatic foramen** to enter **Alcock's canal** on the lateral wall of the ischiorectal fossa. Immediately lateral to it is the **internal pudendal artery,** which follows a similar course. In some cases, the **inferior rectal nerve,** which is usually a branch of the pudendal, arises separately from the sacral plexus and so will also be found accompanying the pudendal. The **nerve to** the **obturator internus** crosses the ischium lateral to the internal pudendal artery. It gives a branch of supply to the **gemellus superior** and then passes through the lesser sciatic foramen to enter the deep surface of the **obturator internus.** The **nerve to** the **quadratus femoris** is still farther lateral and often overlapped externally by the ischiadic nerve. It passes downward, anterior to the obturator tendon and the gemelli, gives a branch of supply to the **gemellus inferior,** and enters the deep (anterior) surface of the **quadratus femoris.**

Clean and study the **gluteus medius.** This muscle, which is only partly covered by the gluteus maximus, arises from the **outer lip of** the **iliac crest,** the **external surface of** the **ilium** between the anterior and posterior gluteal lines, and the deep surface of the portion of the **fascia lata** which covers it externally above the gluteus maximus. Its fibers converge downward to a broad flat tendon which is inserted on the external surface of the **greater trochanter** in a diagonal line running from the posterosuperior to the anteroinferior angle of the trochanter. At its insertion, this tendon is usually more or less intimately connected with the tendon of origin of the uppermost part of the vastus lateralis. Carefully define the posterior border of the **gluteus medius** and observe that, while the **gluteus minimus** lies for the most part under cover of the gluteus medius, a small portion of it is exposed behind and below the posterior border of the medius. To expose the gluteus minimus, the gluteus medius should now be carefully detached from its origin and turned downward and laterally to its insertion. As this is done, observe the twigs of supply

which enter its deep surface from the **superior gluteal nerve.**

Clean and study the gluteus minimus; the superior gluteal nerve and artery should be cleaned at the same time. The **gluteus minimus** arises from the **outer surface of** the **ilium** between the anterior and inferior gluteal lines; at the upper anterior part, it is often partially blended with the gluteus medius. Its fibers converge downward and laterally to a tendon which is inserted on the **anterior border of** the **greater trochanter** (Fig. 94).

The **superior gluteal nerve** has already been seen to emerge from the greater sciatic foramen and pass laterally under cover of the gluteus medius. Here it divides almost immediately into a superior and an inferior branch. The **superior branch** goes forward along the upper border of the gluteus minimus and is distributed entirely to the **gluteus medius;** the **inferior branch** crosses the middle of the gluteus minimus, gives twigs of supply to both the **medius and** the **minimus,** and ends anteriorly in the deep surface of the **tensor fasciae latae,** which it also supplies. The **superficial branches of** the **superior gluteal artery** enter the gluteus maximus; its **deeper continuation** divides into **two branches** which are distributed with the two branches of the superior gluteal nerve. The **inferior branch** anastomoses with the ascending branch of the **lateral femoral circumflex artery,** under cover of the tensor fasciae latae.

Now turn to the interior of the pelvis and study the **sacral plexus.** This plexus, part of which is often separately described as the pudendal plexus, lies in front of the lateral part of the sacrum and the origin of the piriformis and external to the parietal pelvic fascia, which must be removed for its display. The **roots of** the **plexus** are the **lumbosacral trunk** and the **anterior divisions of the first four sacral nerves.** The **lumbosacral trunk** is formed by the junction of a branch of the **fourth lumbar** with the entire anterior division of the **fifth lumbar nerve.** The **trunk** descends behind the common iliac artery into the pelvis and unites with the **first sacral** to form a **loop** through which the superior gluteal artery usually passes. This loop joins with the **anterior divisions** of the **second** and **third** and part of the **fourth sacrals** to form a flattened nervous mass which is the **sacral plexus.** Passing downward in front of the origin of the piriformis muscle, the plexus becomes resolved into two bands, a very large upper and lateral ischiadic band and a much smaller lower and medial pudendal band. Passing between the adjacent borders of the coccygeus and piriformis muscles and outward through the greater sciatic foramen, these bands are continued as the ischiadic and pudendal nerves. The **ischiadic band** is derived from the lumbosacral trunk and the first three sacral nerves, the **pudendal band** from the second, third, and fourth sacrals. The branches of the second, third, and fourth sacral nerves, which were found going to the pelvic viscera, should now be traced back to the main trunks of these nerves. These visceral branches are known by many names: pelvic parasympathetics, nervus erigens, pelvic nerve, etc.

Of the remaining **branches of** the **plexus,** some arise from its anterior and some from its posterior aspect. Those arising **anteriorly** are the **nerves to** the **quadratus femoris and** the **obturator internus,** both of which leave the pelvis below the piriformis. From the **posterior aspect** of the plexus arise the **superior gluteal nerve,** which accompanies the superior gluteal vessels above the piriformis and through the upper part of the greater sciatic foramen, and the **inferior gluteal** and **posterior femoral cutaneous nerves,** which pass below the piriformis. Twigs of supply to the **piriformis** are usually derived directly from the **first and second sacral nerves.**

Attempt to display the **sacral portions of** the **sympathetic trunks** and the **rami communi-**

cantes by which they are connected with the sacral nerves. The trunks lie in front of the sacrum immediately medial to the anterior sacral foramina. At their terminations in front of the first piece of the coccyx, the trunks of the two sides communicate freely with each other.

Flexor Region of Thigh

Turn to the back of the thigh and clean the exposed surfaces of the **flexor** or **hamstring muscles.** These three muscles are the **biceps femoris, semitendinosus,** and **semimembranosus.**

The thick, fleshy belly of the **long head of** the **biceps** will be found below the lateral part of the lower border of the gluteus maximus. Its fibers run downward and somewhat laterally to join a thick flat tendon which passes downward along the lateral side of the back of the knee. The medial border of this tendon forms the superolateral boundary of the popliteal fossa, the fat-filled space at the back of the knee. On its lateral side, this tendon is joined by the fibers of the **short head,** which arise from the distal part of the **linea aspera** near its lateral lip, from the lateral **supracondylar ridge,** and from the posterior surface of the **lateral intermuscular septum.** Observe that the short head of the biceps is separated from the vastus lateralis only by the intermuscular septum.

Medial to the biceps and partly overlapped by it laterally is the **semitendinosus.** Its flat belly begins to contract at about the middle of the thigh toward a thick rounded tendon, which passes downward behind the medial condyle of the femur. The **semimembranosus** lies immediately in front of the semitendinosus and, consequently, is partially hidden by the latter. In the lower part of the thigh, however, it is considerably wider than the semitendinosus, so that its posterior surface is exposed both medial and lateral to the latter. The medial portion of the semimembranosus lies immediately behind the gracilis; the lower part of its lateral border forms the superomedial boundary of the popliteal fossa. The flat tendon of insertion of the **semimembranosus,** whose insertion on the **medial condyle of** the tibia will be demonstrated later, is covered externally by the tendons of the gracilis and the semitendinosus.

Observe that the **long head of** the **biceps and** the **semitendinosus** arise by a **common tendon** from the medial part of the back of the **ischial tuberosity** and separate from each other a short distance below this origin. The broad flat tendon of origin of the semimembranosus lies in front of the upper part of the semitendinosus; it arises from the lateral part of the back of the ischial tuberosity. Clean the **branches** which the **ischiadic nerve** gives to the **long head of** the **biceps, semitendinosus,** and **semimembranosus.** These usually arise from the ischiadic nerve under cover of the biceps but may appear at a higher level. Somewhat lower will be found the **branch of** the **ischiadic nerve** which supplies the **short head of** the **biceps.**

Elevate the semimembranosus and semitendinosus muscles. By this means, the posterior surface of the adductor magnus will be exposed and should be cleaned. The **adductor magnus** has already been seen to receive its main **nerve supply** from the **posterior division of** the **obturator nerve;** it should now be noted that it receives an additional branch from the **ischiadic nerve.** The terminal portions of the medial femoral circumflex and the four perforating arteries may now be observed. **The medial circumflex** will be found reaching the back of the thigh above the adductor magnus, between that muscle and the lower border of the quadratus femoris. The **perforating arteries** pierce the adductor magnus in longitudinal series close to the linea aspera (Fig. 94).

Before completing the dissection of the hip region and the back of the thigh, it is advisable to dissect the **popliteal fossa** while the hamstring muscles, which form a part of its boundaries, are still in place. If these muscles have been partially displaced, they should be restored to their normal position.

Popliteal Fossa

The **popliteal fossa** is the diamond-shaped space which lies at the back of the knee. Its highest point or **apex** is the point at which the **biceps** and **semimembranosus muscles** separate from each other. Its **superolateral** boundary is formed by the medial border of the **biceps,** its **superomedial** boundary by the lateral border of the **semimembranosus.** Its **inferolateral** and **inferomedial boundaries** are formed by the lateral and medial **heads of** the **gastrocnemius** muscle, which arise from the lateral and medial condyles of the femur under cover of the biceps and semimembranosus respectively. The **roof** or superficial boundary of the fossa is formed merely by **skin and fascia**; its **floor** or deep boundary is formed from above downward by the popliteal surface of the **femur,** the **oblique popliteal ligament** at the back of the knee joint, and the **fascia covering the popliteus muscle.** The fossa itself is filled with fatty areolar tissue, which must be removed as the dissection proceeds, to expose the other structures contained (Figs. 83 and 87).

Clean first the terminal part of the **small saphenous vein.** This vein ascends in the superficial fascia on the middle of the calf to enter the popliteal fossa at about its middle and terminate in the **popliteal vein.** Just lateral to it, but on a slightly deeper plane, is the **medial sural cutaneous nerve,** which arises from the **tibial nerve** in the upper part of the popliteal fossa and descends on the external surface of the gastrocnemius.

Identify the **common fibular nerve.** This nerve and the tibial nerve are the two terminal branches of the **ischiadic nerve.** They arise from the ischiadic, usually under cover of the biceps, but occasionally not until the apex of the popliteal fossa is reached. The common peroneal is, at its origin, lateral to the tibial. It passes downward and laterally, close to the medial margin of the biceps, and leaves the popliteal fossa by crossing the external surface of the lateral head of the gastrocnemius, still closely following the border of the biceps. It gives rise to one or two small **articular branches,** which pass deeply into the fossa to

sels, which it crosses obliquely downward from the lateral to the medial side. It is crossed by the plantaris muscle or its tendon. In the lower part of the fossa, sometimes under cover of the gastrocnemius, the tibial nerve gives rise to a group of **muscular branches.** If the **two heads of** the **gastrocnemius** are spread apart, one of these branches may be followed into the deep surface of each head. A small branch is given to the **plantaris.** The remaining branches will be seen later to supply the **soleus** and **popliteus**

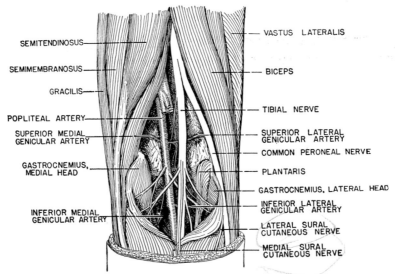

FIG. 87. Dissection of the popliteal fossa; its boundaries have been somewhat spread apart, the better to expose the structures within.

reach the **knee joint** and the **lateral sural cutaneous nerve,** which descends on the lateral head of the gastrocnemius. Now clean the upper portions of the two heads of the gastrocnemius muscle, which have been exposed, so that the boundaries of the fossa may be clearly defined. Then proceed to the display of the more important structures contained in the fossa.

The **tibial nerve** enters the popliteal fossa at its apex and descends through it almost vertically, but inclining somewhat medially. It lies superficial (posterior) to the popliteal ves-

muscles. In addition to these muscular and cutaneous branches, the tibial nerve gives rise to two or three minute **articular branches to the knee joint.**

Clean the **plantaris.** This is a somewhat variable muscle whose small, fleshy belly is partially overlapped by the lateral head of the gastrocnemius. It arises from the **lateral part of the femur** immediately above the lateral condyle. Its fibers run downward and medially in the popliteal fossa to converge to a long, slender tendon which descends deep to the gastrocnemius.

The **popliteal artery** begins at the tendinous opening in the adductor magnus and descends through the popliteal fossa to the lower border of the popliteus muscle, where it ends by dividing into the **anterior** and **posterior tibial arteries.** It is the most deeply placed of the structures in the fossa, being in contact with the floor (anterior wall) of the fossa throughout. Posteriorly, it is covered above by the semimembranosus and below by the gastrocnemius and plantaris. The vein lies behind or medial to the artery; it may be removed, if desired, in cleaning the artery and its branches.

The constant, named branches of the **popliteal artery** are its five **genicular branches.** Its largest branches, however, are usually the somewhat variable muscular branches which are given to the hamstring muscles and the gastrocnemius, soleus, and plantaris. The two superior genicular arteries arise from each side of the popliteal and wind around the femur immediately above the condyles. The **medial superior genicular** runs medially in front of the semitendinosus and semimembranosus above the medial head of the gastrocnemius and turns forward deep to the tendon of the adductor magnus. The **lateral superior genicular** runs laterally above the lateral condyle and in front of the biceps. The **middle genicular** is a small vessel which pierces the oblique popliteal ligament to enter the knee joint; it may arise by a common stem with one of the superior geniculars. The two inferior genicular arteries arise from the lower part of the popliteal under cover of the upper part of the gastrocnemius. The **medial inferior genicular** runs downward and medially to pass forward below the medial condyle of the tibia. The **lateral inferior genicular** runs straight laterally across the lateral condyle of the tibia and above the head of the fibula and turns forward to reach the front of the knee joint. All of these vessels take part in the **arterial anastomosis around** the **knee joint.**

Posterior Crural Region

Turn now to the **posterior crural region.** The **muscles** of this region are arranged in **three layers** from without inward. The muscles of the **superficial layer** are the **gastrocnemius, plantaris,** and **soleus** and constitute the fleshy prominence known as the calf. The upper part of the gastrocnemius has already been seen in connection with the popliteal fossa. The entire external surface of this muscle should now be cleaned.

The **gastrocnemius** arises by **two heads** which take origin from the upper posterior parts of the **lateral** and **medial condyles of** the **femur** and join below the popliteal fossa. The muscle is fleshy above and tendinous below. It is inserted into the **tuberosity of** the **calcaneus** through the **tendon of Achilles** (tendo calcaneus), which is **common to** the **gastrocnemius, plantaris,** and **soleus.** Before reflecting the gastrocnemius, clean and study the tendon of insertion of the **semimembranosus.** This muscle is inserted into a facet on the posterior surface of the **medial condyle of** the **tibia,** medial to the medial head of the gastrocnemius and partially overlapped by it. A **mucous bursa** is usually found to intervene between the **semimembranosus** tendon and the **medial head of** the **gastrocnemius.** Divide the two heads of the gastrocnemius $\frac{1}{2}$ in. below their attachments to the femur and reflect the entire muscle downward and backward to its junction with the tendon of Achilles. As this is being done, observe the branches which it receives from the **tibial nerve** and the **popliteal artery.** When these have been seen, they may be cut so that the muscle may be completely reflected.

Observe now that the tendon of the **plantaris muscle** passes downward and medially behind the popliteal artery and the tibial nerve and descends between the gastrocnemius and soleus to join the **tendon of Achilles.** It also is supplied by a twig from the **tibial nerve.** Divide the plantaris just below its origin and turn it downward. Then clean and study the popliteus and soleus muscles (Fig. 88).

The **popliteus** is a flat triangular muscle which lies in front of the lower part of the popliteal artery in relation to the popliteal surface of the tibia; it is covered by a fairly dense layer of fascia. Its tendon of origin arises within the cavity of the knee joint from

The **soleus** is a thick fleshy muscle whose long linear origin has roughly the outline of an inverted V. It arises from the middle third of the **medial border of** the **tibia,** from the **soleus line** on the back **of** the **tibia,** from a strong **fibrous band** which bridges across the interval between the upper end of the popliteal line and the head of the fibula, from the posterior

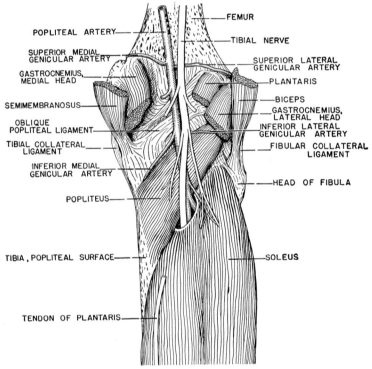

FIG. 88. The back of the knee and the upper part of the calf after removal of the gastrocnemius.

the lower lateral part of the **lateral condyle of** the **femur.** It may now be found emerging from the lateral side of the posterior aspect of the joint capsule. From this tendon, muscle fibers diverge downward and medially to cover the **popliteal surface of** the **tibia,** upon which they are inserted. The popliteus is supplied by a branch of the **tibial nerve,** which arises in the popliteal fossa and usually winds around the lower border of the muscle to reach its deep surface.

surface of the **head of** the **fibula,** and from the upper third of the **posterior surface of** the **fibula.** It is inserted, together with the plantaris and the gastrocnemius, into the **tuberosity of** the **calcaneus** by means of the **tendon of Achilles.** Find and clean the nerve of supply which arises from the **tibial nerve** in the popliteal fossa and enters the proximal part of the external surface of the soleus.

The terminal part of the popliteal artery may now be seen to better advantage than was possible when the popliteal fossa was dissected. The **popliteal artery** ends, usually opposite the lower border of the popliteus, by dividing into the **anterior** and **posterior tibial arteries.** Observe that these two vessels and the tibial nerve descend into the leg by passing in front of the fibrous band between the tibia and fibula, from which the soleus takes partial origin.

Detach the **soleus** entirely from its origin and reflect it downward and backward toward the calcaneus. As this is being done, observe that its deep surface receives an additional nerve of supply which arises from the **tibial nerve in** the **leg** and several branches from the **posterior tibial artery.** When these have been cleaned, they should be cut so that the muscle may be completely reflected. Observe that in front of the tendon of Achilles, between it and the posterior aspect of the ankle joint, is a considerable amount of fatty areolar tissue.

The **second layer** in the posterior crural compartment consists of two muscles, the **flexor hallucis longus** and the **flexor digitorum longus.** Before cleaning these, clean and define the **laciniate ligament (flexor retinaculum),** a thickened portion of the deep fascia at the medial side of the heel. It is a strong fascial band which stretches downward and backward from the **medial malleolus** to the prominence on the posterior part of the **medial surface of** the **calcaneus** and serves to retain in position against the talus and the calcaneus the tendons of the tibialis posterior, the flexor digitorum longus, and the flexor hallucis longus and the terminal portions of the tibial nerve and the posterior tibial artery. Piercing it will be found some small medial **calcaneal branches of** the **tibial nerve** which supply the skin on the medial side of the heel; they are accompanied by the medial **calcaneal branches of** the **posterior tibial artery.** Retaining the laciniate ligament, proceed to clean and study the flexor digitorum longus and the flexor hallucis longus. The posterior tibial artery will be found to descend through the posterior crural compartment, in company with the tibial nerve, in the groove between the adjacent borders of these two muscles (Fig. 89).

The **flexor digitorum longus** arises from the distal part of the **popliteal line** and the middle half of the medial side of the **posterior surface of** the **tibia;** its fibers pass obliquely downward to join a tendon which passes behind the medial malleolus and deep to the laciniate ligament. The **flexor hallucis longus** arises from the distal two-thirds of the **posterior surface of** the **fibula.** Its tendon also passes deep to the laciniate ligament, lying a short distance behind the tendon of the flexor digitorum longus.

The **third layer** of the posterior crural compartment is represented by a single muscle, the **tibialis posterior.** Except for its most proximal portion, this muscle is covered posteriorly by the two muscles of the second layer. It can, therefore, be studied to better advantage if the flexor hallucis longus and the flexor digitorum longus are spread laterally and medially respectively. First, however, it is advisable to clean the posterior tibial artery and the tibial nerve.

The **posterior tibial artery** begins at the lower border of the popliteus and descends in front of the soleus and between the flexor digitorum longus and the flexor hallucis longus. It is in relation anteriorly, successively from above downward, with the tibialis posterior, the posterior surface of the tibia, and the capsule of the ankle joint. Its largest branch is the **peroneal artery;** this vessel arises about 1 in. below the origin of the posterior tibial and runs laterally and distad across the tibialis posterior to pass from view at present under cover of the flexor hallucis longus. The **posterior tibial** gives **muscular branches** to the soleus and the deeper posterior crural muscles, several small **medial calcaneal branches,** and a **posterior medial malleolar branch,** which runs forward across the medial malleolus to anasto-mose with the anterior medial malleolar branch of the anterior tibial. It ends under cover of the laciniate ligament by dividing into the **medial and lateral plantar arteries.**

which supply the **flexor digitorum longus,** the **flexor hallucis longus,** and the **tibialis posterior.** It terminates under cover of the laciniate ligament by dividing into the **medial** and **lateral plantar nerves.** Just proximal to its termina-

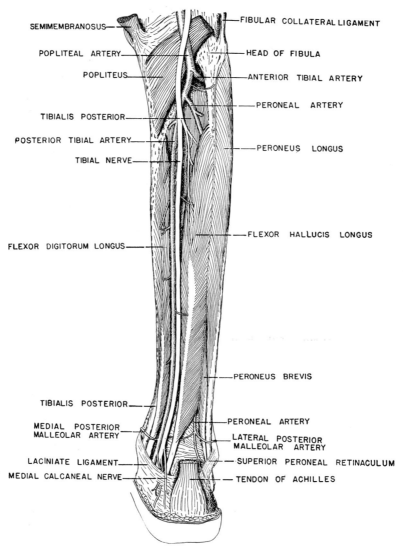

SEMIMEMBRANOSUS—

POPLITEAL ARTERY—

POPLITEUS—

TIBIALIS POSTERIOR—

POSTERIOR TIBIAL ARTERY—

TIBIAL NERVE—

FLEXOR DIGITORUM LONGUS—

TIBIALIS POSTERIOR—

MEDIAL POSTERIOR MALLEOLAR ARTERY

LACINIATE LIGAMENT—

MEDIAL CALCANEAL NERVE—

—FIBULAR COLLATERAL LIGAMENT

—HEAD OF FIBULA

—ANTERIOR TIBIAL ARTERY

—PERONEAL ARTERY

—PERONEUS LONGUS

—FLEXOR HALLUCIS LONGUS

—PERONEUS BREVIS

—PERONEAL ARTERY

—LATERAL POSTERIOR MALLEOLAR ARTERY

—SUPERIOR PERONEAL RETINACULUM

—TENDON OF ACHILLES

FIG. 89. The posterior aspect of the leg, after removal of the gastrocnemius and soleus.

The **tibial nerve** is at first medial to the posterior tibial artery but soon crosses behind it and for the rest of its course lies on the lateral side of the artery. It gives a **branch to** the deep surface of the **soleus** and **branches**

tion, it gives a **small articular** twig **to** the **ankle joint** and the **medial calcaneal cutaneous** branches.

The **tibialis posterior** should now be cleaned. It arises from the upper two-thirds of the

Post. Lat. malleolar of Common peroneal A.
"   Med.   "   of Post. t.b. A.

Inferior Extremity   225

lateral part of the **posterior surface of** the **tibia** below the popliteal line, from the entire **medial surface of** the **fibula,** and from the posterior surface of the upper two-thirds of the **interosseous membrane.** Its tendon passes distad and medially deep to the flexor digitorum longus behind the medial malleolus and deep to the laciniate ligament, where it lies immediately in front of the tendon of the flexor digitorum longus.

Displace the flexor hallucis longus laterally and trace the further course of the **peroneal (fibular) artery.** This vessel descends in close relation to the fibula, between the **tibialis posterior** and the **flexor hallucis longus,** giving branches to those muscles and to the **peronei longus and brevis.** In the distal part of the leg, it lies on the interosseous membrane and here gives rise to the **perforating branch** on the front of the leg. Behind the lateral malleolus, it gives rise to a **posterior lateral malleolar** branch which passes forward across the lateral malleolus to anastomose with the anterior lateral malleolar. The peroneal artery terminates in some small **lateral calcaneal branches** which ramify on the lateral side of the heel.

The course of the **anterior tibial artery** in the posterior crural region is very short. From its origin, it runs downward and forward to pierce the proximal part of the interosseous membrane above the tibialis posterior. Before piercing the membrane, however, it gives rise to a **posterior tibial recurrent branch,** which ascends, deep to the popliteus muscle, to reach the knee joint.

The laciniate ligament (flexor retinaculum) should now be reflected, to expose the terminations of the tibial nerve and the posterior tibial artery and the relative positions of these structures and the three flexor tendons. Observe that, under cover of the **laciniate ligament (flexor retinaculum),** these structures are arranged in the following order from before backward (or, as sometimes described, from

medial to lateral): the **tendon of** the **tibialis posterior,** the tendon of the **flexor digitorum longus,** the **posterior tibial artery,** the **tibial nerve,** and the **tendon of** the **flexor hallucis longus.** The three tendons and the medial and lateral plantar nerves and arteries, which arise here, all pass distad into the sole of the foot.

Anterior Crural Region

The **muscles of the leg** are arranged in **three groups,** each of which occupies a **separate osteofascial compartment.** Superficially, each compartment is limited by the deep fascia which encircles the leg; the deep boundaries of the various compartments are formed by the bones and the fascial septa of the leg. The muscles of the **anterior group,** which **dorsiflex** the **foot** and **extend** the **toes,** are in relation to the anterior surfaces of the fibula and the interosseus membrane and the lateral surface of the tibia. The muscles of the **posterior group,** which **plantarflex** the **foot** and **flex** the **toes,** are in relation to the posterior and medial surfaces of the fibula and the posterior surfaces of the interosseus membrane and the tibia. The **lateral group,** which are primarily **evertors of the foot,** occupy a narrow compartment which is limited deeply by the lateral surface of the fibula and separated anteriorly and posteriorly from the lateral parts of the anterior and posterior compartments by short fascial intermuscular septa. Medially, the subcutaneous medial surface of the tibia intervenes between the muscles of the anterior and posterior groups. The deep fascia covering this surface of the tibia is intimately blended with the periosteum. The anterior compartment should be examined next. Before doing this, however, it is advisable to clean and study the patellar ligament and the insertions of the sartorius, gracilis, and semitendinosus muscles (Fig. 90).

The **patellar ligament** is a strong, flat fibrous band which extends from the **distal border of** the **patella** to the **tuberosity of** the **tibia** and represents the actual insertion of the four parts of the **quadriceps femoris.** It is an integral part of the capsule of the knee joint, as will be apparent when the joint is dissected. The **sartorius, gracilis,** and **semitendinosus** are all inserted close together on the upper part of the **medial surface of** the **tibia.** Observe that the flat tendon of insertion of the sartorius covers the other two tendons externally and that the gracilis lies at its insertion immediately above the semitendinosus and partially overlaps it.

Before cleaning the individual muscles of the anterior crural compartment, attempt to define the transverse and cruciate ligaments. These ligaments are merely thickened portions of the deep fascia of the leg. The **transverse crural ligament (superior extensor retinaculum)** stretches across the front of the leg just proximal to the malleoli; laterally, it blends with the periosteum of the triangular subcutaneous surface of the **fibula;** medially, with the **tibia.** The **cruciate crural ligament (inferior extensor retinaculum)** is somewhat lower. Laterally, it is a single band which stretches medially across the front of the ankle joint from the **anterior part of** the **calcaneus;** in front of the middle of the joint, it divides into two limbs, one of which passes proximad to reach the **medial malleolus,** while the other passes distad and turns around the medial margin of the foot to join the **plantar aponeurosis.**

The muscles in the anterior compartment should now be cleaned. Further, it will be found that the deep fascia covering these muscles in the upper part of the leg cannot all be satisfactorily removed, since the muscles take origin partially from its deep surface. This compartment also contains the anterior tibial artery and its accompanying veins and the deep peroneal nerve.

The **tibialis anterior** arises from the proximal half of the **lateral surface** of the **tibia,** the medial side of the anterior surface of the

interosseus membrane, and the **deep fascia** which covers it. Its fibers converge distad to a strong tendon which passes over the front of the ankle joint, onto the dorsum of the foot, and deep to the transverse and cruciate ligaments. It is inserted into the medial part of the **first cuneiform bone** and the adjoining part of the **base of the first metatarsal.**

The **extensor digitorum longus** arises from the anterior part of the **head of** the **fibula** and the proximal two-thirds of the anterior surface of the **shaft,** from the anterior surface of the **intermuscular septum** separating it from the lateral crural compartment, and from the **deep fascia** covering it. Its tendon descends in front of the ankle joint and on the dorsum of the foot divides into **four slips** which reach the dorsal surfaces of the **four lateral toes.** The skin should be reflected from the dorsum of the toes and the manner of insertion of these slips investigated. Observe that each slip expands on the dorsal aspect of the first phalanx and then divides into a **central** and **two collateral parts.** The **central part** is inserted into the **base of** the **second phalanx;** the **collateral parts** are prolonged distad to be inserted together into the **base of** the **terminal phalanx.**

The **peroneus (fibular) tertius,** while described as a separate muscle, usually has more the appearance of an additional **slip of** the **extensor digitorum longus.** It is continuous at its origin, which is from the distal part of the anterior surface of the fibula, with the latter muscle. Its slender tendon is inserted into the dorsal side of the **base of** the **fifth metatarsal.**

The **extensor hallucis longus** lies between the tibialis anterior and the extensor digitorum longus but does not reach so high a level as do these two muscles. Its proximal portion is covered by these muscles, which must be separated to expose it. It arises from the middle half of the **anterior surface of** the **fibula,** medial to the attachment of the extensor digitorum longus, and from the anterior surface of the adjacent part of the **interosseous membrane.** Its tendon crosses the front of the ankle joint just lateral to the tibialis anterior and passes proximally on the dorsum of the foot front of the ankle and on the dorsum of the foot. They cannot usually be very satisfactorily demonstrated in the ordinary dissecting room part, but an attempt should be made to inflate

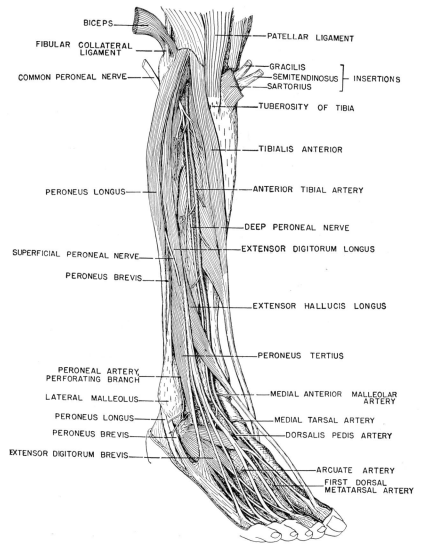

FIG. 90. Dissection of the anterior compartment of the leg and the dorsum of the foot. The muscles of the anterior compartment have been somewhat displaced to expose the anterior tibial artery and the deep peroneal nerve.

to be inserted into the **terminal phalanx of the great toe.**

Three closed **mucous sheaths** are found in relation to the tendons of these muscles in them with air by means of a blowpipe or to explore their limits with a blunt, flexible probe. The most **medial sheath** encircles the tendon of the **tibialis anterior** and extends from about the proximal border of the superior extensor retinaculum to within a short distance of the insertion of the muscle. A **second sheath** encloses the tendon of the **extensor hallucis longus** and extends from about the distal border of the transverse ligament to the base of the first phalanx of the great toe. The **third sheath** is common to the tendons of the **extensor digitorum longus** and those of the **fibularis tertius;** it extends from the distal border of the transverse ligament to about the middle of the dorsum of the foot.

Cut the superior extensor retinaculum and displace the tibialis anterior medially and the remaining muscles of the anterior compartment laterally, and clean and study the anterior tibial artery and the deep fibular nerve. The **anterior tibial** is one of the terminal branches of the **popliteal artery.** It enters the anterior compartment by piercing the proximal part of the interosseus membrane close to the neck of the fibula. It descends in the **anterior compartment** on the **interosseous membrane,** lying first between the tibialis anterior and the extensor digitorum longus and then between the tibialis anterior and the extensor hallucis longus. In the distal part of the leg, it rests on the anterior surface of the tibia and is crossed anteriorly by the tendon of the extensor hallucis longus; it becomes superficial just proximal to the ankle, where it lies between the tendons of the last-named muscle and the extensor digitorum longus. It ends in front of the ankle joint, from which point its continuation is known as the **dorsal artery of** the **foot** (a. dorsalis pedis). In addition to numerous branches to the muscles of the anterior compartment, it gives rise to the anterior tibial recurrent and the medial and lateral anterior malleolar arteries. The **anterior tibial recurrent** arises from the **anterior tibial** in the proximal part of its course and ascends through the substance of the upper part of the tibialis anterior to reach the front of the knee joint. The **anterior malleolar arteries** are small vessels which arise from either side of the anterior tibial just proximal to the ankle. The **lateral anterior malleolar** runs laterally deep to the tendons of the extensor digitorum longus and fibularis tertius and turns posteriorly on the lateral surface of the lateral malleolus. The **medial anterior malleolar** crosses the distal portion of the tibia deep to the tendons of the extensor hallucis longus and the tibialis anterior.

The **perforating branch of** the **fibular artery** should in addition be exposed at this time. It enters the anterior compartment by piercing the interosseous membrane about $1\frac{1}{2}$ in. above the lateral malleolus to descend in front of the distal part of the fibula and anastomose with the **lateral anterior malleolar artery.** It is usually a small vessel but, in some cases, is greatly enlarged and continued onto the dorsum of the foot as the **dorsalis pedis artery;** in such cases, the anterior tibial, which normally gives rise to the dorsalis pedis, ends in small twigs to the ankle joint.

Finally, the **deep fibular nerve** is one of the terminal branches of the **common fibular nerve.** It will be found entering the anterior compartment by piercing the upper part of the extensor digitorum longus. It accompanies the anterior tibial artery distad to the front of the ankle joint, from which point it accompanies the dorsalis pedis artery onto the dorsum of the foot. It lies to the lateral side of the anterior tibial throughout, with the exception that in the middle third of the leg it may lie in front of the artery. It gives branches of supply to the four **muscles of** the **anterior compartment.**

Dorsal Region of Foot

The deeper structures are now to be displayed on the dorsum of the foot. To render them more accessible, it is advisable to cut the **cruciate ligament (inferior extensor retinaculum)** so that the tendons of the extensor digitorum longus and the fibularis tertius may be displaced laterally. Then clean the extensor digitorum brevis.

The **extensor digitorum brevis** arises from the lateral and superior surfaces of the **body of** the **calcaneus.** As its fibers pass distad, they divide into **four fleshy bellies,** each of which gives rise to a separate **small tendon.** The **most medial of** these muscular **bellies** is sometimes described as a separate muscle, the **extensor hallucis brevis.** Its tendon is inserted into the dorsum of the **first phalanx of** the **great toe.** The **remaining** three **tendons** are given to the **second, third,** and **fourth toes.** They are not, however, inserted directly upon the phalanges of these toes, but each joins the lateral side of the corresponding **tendon of** the **long extensor** near the base of the first phalanx (Fig. 90).

Clean the **dorsalis pedis artery** and its branches. The dorsalis pedis begins in front of the ankle joint as a continuation of the **anterior tibial** and extends to the base of the first interosseous space, where it ends by dividing into the **deep plantar** and **first dorsal metatarsal arteries.** Deeply, it rests successively on the talus, the navicular bone, the second cuneiform, and the base of the second metatarsal. As it crosses the tarsal bones, it gives rise to a lateral tarsal and (usually) two medial tarsal branches. The **lateral tarsal** courses laterally deep to the extensor digitorum brevis and supplies this muscle and the bones and articulations of the region. The **medial tarsals** are small twigs which supply the skin and the bones in the medial tarsal region. Near its termination, the dorsalis pedis gives rise to the **arcuate artery.** This vessel runs laterally across the bases of the metatarsal bones; from it arise the second, third, and fourth **dorsal metatarsal arteries.** Each dorsal metatarsal artery passes forward along the corresponding interosseous space and divides into two **dorsal digital branches** which are distributed to the adjacent

sides of two toes. The dorsal metatarsal artery of the first space is, as has been seen, one of the terminal branches of the dorsalis pedis; it gives rise usually to a branch which supplies the medial side of the great toe. The other terminal branch, the **deep plantar artery,** passes downward through the base of the first interosseous space into the sole of the foot, where, as will be seen later, it takes part in the formation of the **deep plantar arch.**

Finally, the **deep fibular nerve** lies lateral to the first part of the dorsalis pedis artery. A short distance distal to the ankle joint it terminates by dividing into a lateral and a medial branch. The **lateral branch** passes deep to the **extensor digitorum brevis** and supplies that muscle and the **tarsal joints.** The **medial branch** passes forward with the dorsalis pedis artery; its distribution to the **skin** on the adjacent sides of the first and second toes has already been seen.

Lateral Crural Region

The lateral crural region is next to be examined. First clean and study the insertion of the **biceps femoris.** This muscle is inserted into the highest part of the **head of** the **fibula** and also gives a tendinous expansion to the fascia covering the lateral part of the leg. Observe that its insertion is split into two parts just above its attachment to the fibula by the **fibular collateral ligament.** This is a strong, rounded cord which extends from the upper lateral part of the **lateral condyle of** the **femur** downward to the lateral surface of the **head of** the **fibula.** Its upper part is covered externally by the biceps, which it pierces just above the head of the fibula (Fig. 90).

The **lateral crural compartment** contains two muscles; these are the **fibularis longus** and **brevis.** Before cleaning these muscles, attempt to locate and define the **fibular retinacula.** They are similar to the transverse crural and cruciate ligaments and represent thickenings in the deep fascia which serve to hold the tendons of the fibular muscles in place against the calcaneus. Note that the **superior fibular retinaculum** passes from the posterior distal part of the **lateral malleolus** downward and backward to the upper **lateral part of** the **calcaneus.** Note also the **inferior fibular retinaculum** taking a similar direction from the upper **anterior part of** the **calcaneus,** where it is continuous with the lateral end of the cruciate ligament, to the **trochlear process of** the **calcaneus.** Retaining carefully the fibular retinacula for the present, clean the fibularis longus by removing the remaining portions of deep fascia as completely as possible from its outer surface.

The **fibularis longus** arises from the proximal half of the **lateral surface of** the **fibula,** from the anterior and posterior fibular **intermuscular septa,** and, to some extent, from the deep fascia which covers it externally. Its fibers converge to a strong tendon which passes distad, running lateral to the fibularis brevis, and then across the lateral surface of the calcaneus behind and below the lateral malleolus and on a groove in the **cuboid bone** into the **sole of** the **foot,** where its further course will be seen later. As it lies against the calcaneus, located deep to the fibular retinacula, this tendon is enclosed in a mucous sheath which is common to it and the fibularis brevis.

Draw the lower part of the fibularis longus laterally and posteriorly and expose and clean the **fibularis brevis** with care. The muscle arises from the distal half of the **lateral surface of** the **fibula** and from the fibular **intermuscular septa.** Its tendon is at first covered by the tendon of the fibularis longus; however, as it turns forward across the calcaneus, it appears immediately above the latter tendon. It is inserted into the **tuberosity** at the **base of** the **fifth metatarsal bone** (Fig. 90).

The **common fibular nerve** has been followed downward and laterally along the border of the biceps femoris to the head of the fibula. At the posterior border of the upper section of the fibularis longus, it now disappears from view by passing deep to that muscle, between it and the neck of the fibula. Now cut carefully down through the substance of the fibularis longus in order to expose the further course of the nerve. Observe that as it crosses the neck of the fibula, the common fibular nerve gives off a small **recurrent articular branch to** the **knee joint** and then divides into the deep and superficial fibular nerves. Note that the **deep fibular nerve** passes through the upper part of the extensor digitorum longus, from which point its further course has been traced. The **superficial fibular nerve** passes distad in order to reach the interval between the **fibularis longus** and **brevis** muscles, both of which it supplies; in the distal part of the leg, it pierces the deep fascia, from which point its distribution is as a cutaneous nerve of the leg and foot.

Sole of Foot

Remove the superficial fascia and clean the plantar aponeurosis. The **plantar aponeurosis** stretches forward from the **calcaneus,** to which it is firmly attached posteriorly, to cover the superficial muscles on the plantar aspect of the foot. It is subdivided into **narrow medial** and **lateral portions,** which are relatively thin, and a broad, **thick intermediate portion.** As it reaches forward from the calcaneus, this portion widens out and toward the bases of the toes divides into five **digital slips,** which end anteriorly by blending with the fibrous sheaths which bind the flexor tendons down to the plantar surfaces of the metatarsophalangeal joints and the phalanges.

The **superficial muscles of** the **sole** should now be cleaned. They are covered by the medial, intermediate, and lateral portions, respectively, of the **plantar aponeurosis.** This aponeurosis must, therefore, be removed in cleaning them; its posterior portion cannot, however, be successfully removed, since the muscles take origin in part from its deep surface. As the muscles are being cleaned, care must be taken to preserve the **medial plantar nerve,** which emerges between the abductor hallucis and the flexor digitorum brevis, and the superficial branch of the **lateral plantar**

join a tendon which is inserted into the lateral side of the **base of** the **first phalanx of** the **fifth toe;** it often exhibits a secondary slip of insertion into the tuberosity at the base of the fifth metatarsal.

The **flexor digitorum brevis** arises from the medial process of the **tuberosity of** the **calcaneus** and from the deep surface of the **plantar**

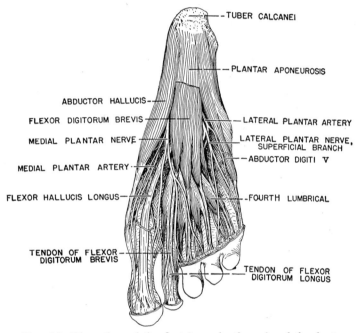

FIG. 91. Dissection of the first layer in the sole of the foot.

nerve, which appears at the lateral side of the flexor digitorum brevis.

The **abductor hallucis** arises from the medial process of the **tuberosity of** the **calcaneus** and from the portion of the **plantar aponeurosis** which covers it. Its fibers join a tendon which is inserted into the medial side of the **base of** the **first phalanx of** the **great toe;** as will be seen later, this insertion is common to the abductor hallucis and the medial belly of the flexor hallucis brevis. The **abductor digiti quinti** arises from the lateral process of the **tuberosity of** the **calcaneus.** Its fibers extend forward along the lateral side of the sole and

aponeurosis. As it passes distad, it divides into **four slips,** which give rise to four separate tendons which pass to the **second, third, fourth,** and **fifth toes;** the slip to the fifth toe is frequently lacking. The manner of insertion of these tendons will be examined later; for the present, they need be cleaned only as far forward as the heads of the metatarsal bones, where they enter the fibrous sheaths of the flexor tendons.

The **medial plantar nerve** will be found emerging between the abductor hallucis and the flexor digitorum brevis and running forward to divide into **four cutaneous branches.**

Of these, the **most medial passes** to the skin on the medial side of the plantar aspect of the great toe. The remaining **three,** which are known as **common plantar digital nerves,** each divide near the heads of the metatarsal bones into two proper plantar digital nerves which supply the adjacent sides of the first and sec-

the foot includes the tendons of the **flexor hallucis longus** and the **flexor digitorum longus,** the **quadratus plantae (accessory flexor),** and the four **lumbrical muscles.** At this same level will be found the trunks of the medial plantar nerve and artery, crossing deep to the abductor hallucis, and the lateral plantar nerve and

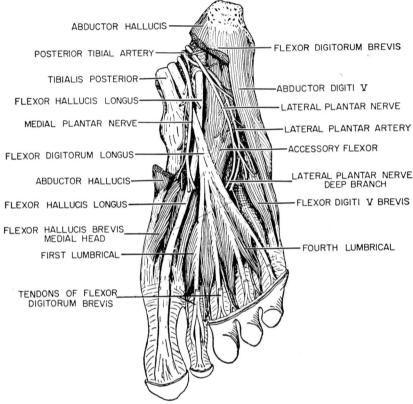

FIG. 92. The structures of the second layer in the sole of the foot as exposed by removal of the abductor hallucis and the flexor digitorum brevis.

ond, second and third, and third and fourth toes, respectively. The superficial branch of the **lateral plantar nerve** emerges from under cover of the lateral side of the flexor digitorum brevis and divides into **two branches;** the more **medial** of these gives rise to two proper digital branches which supply the adjacent sides of the fourth and fifth toes, and the more **lateral** supplies the lateral side of the fifth toe.

The **second layer of muscles** in the sole of

artery, which cross deep to both the abductor hallucis and the flexor digitorum brevis (Fig. 92).

Divide the **abductor hallucis** and the **flexor digitorum brevis** close to their origins and reflect them forward. As this is done, secure the nerves of supply which they receive from the **medial plantar nerve.** The beginnings of the medial plantar nerve and artery under cover of the laciniate ligament have already been seen.

1. Long Plantar Lig.
2. Calcaneo-Navicular Lig. (keeps boat Anchored) called spring Lig.
   helps stop Flat feet.
3. Deltoid Lig. (4 parts)

Inferior Extremity   233

Their full course may now be traced. In addition to the branches already described, the **medial plantar nerve** gives twigs of supply, usually from its two medial common digital branches, to the **flexor hallucis brevis** and the **first lumbrical muscle.** The **medial plantar artery** is usually much smaller than the lateral plantar. It accompanies the medial plantar nerve and gives rise to numerous small twigs which, for the most part, correspond to the branches of the nerve.

The **lateral plantar nerve** runs forward and laterally across the sole to about the base of the fourth interosseous space, where it ends by dividing into a deep and a superficial branch. From the **trunk of** the **nerve,** twigs of supply are given to the **abductor digiti quinti** and the **accessory flexor.** Near its beginning, the **superficial branch** supplies twigs to the **flexor digiti quinti brevis** and the **interosseous muscles of** the **fourth space;** its further course has been traced. The **deep branch** turns medially, deep to the accessory flexor, where it will be followed later. The **lateral plantar artery** accompanies the lateral plantar nerve to the base of the fourth interosseous space, at which it turns medially to pass deeply into the foot in company with the deep branch of the nerve. From the part of its course now visible, small twigs are given to the various neighboring muscles.

Trace the tendon of the **flexor digitorum longus** forward into the sole and observe that it divides into **four tendons** which pass into the fibrous sheaths on the plantar aspects of the **four lateral toes,** where they lie deep to the corresponding tendons of the flexor digitorum brevis. Clean the **accessory flexor.** This is a short flat muscle which arises by two heads from the lower parts of the **lateral** and **medial surfaces,** respectively, **of** the **calcaneus.** Its fibers pass forward to be inserted upon the **tendon of** the **flexor digitorum longus.** The lateral plantar nerve and artery rest directly on this muscle as they cross the sole. The **lumbrical muscles** are four small slips, which by their attachments make it possible to extend the interphalangeal joints of the four lateral toes at the same time that the metatarsophalangeal joints are flexed. The **first lumbrical** arises from the medial side of the first tendon of the flexor digitorum longus; the **remaining three** each arise from the adjacent sides of two tendons of the flexor longus. Each lumbrical gives rise to a slender tendon which passes around the medial side of its own digit to join the extensor expansion of that digit on the **dorsal side of** the **proximal phalanx.**

Now study the manner of insertion of the **flexor tendons** into the phalanges. First observe that these tendons are held in place on the plantar aspects of the phalanges by **fibrous bands,** which, with the plantar surfaces of the phalanges, form an **osteofibrous canal** in each digit, in which the flexor tendons lie. Within each of these canals, the tendons of the **flexor longus and** the **flexor brevis** are enclosed in a **common synovial sheath.** Open the fibrous sheath on the toes to see the insertions of the flexor tendons. Observe that the tendon of the **flexor longus** perforates the tendon of the flexor brevis and passes forward to be inserted at the **base of** the **terminal phalanx.** The **flexor brevis** tendon is inserted at the **base of** the **second phalanx.**

Trace the tendon of the **flexor hallucis longus** into the foot. Observe that as it enters the sole, it rests in a groove on the undersurface of the **sustentaculum tali,** to which it is bound by a strong fibrous band. It then passes forward, crossing deep to the tendon of the flexor digitorum longus, to which it gives a tendinous slip, to enter the fibrous sheath on the plantar aspect of the great toe. It is inserted into the **terminal phalanx.**

Divide the tendon of the flexor digitorum longus at the point where it enters the foot, detach the accessory flexor from its origin, and turn the divided portion of the tendon forward, together with the accessory flexor and the lumbrical muscles. As this is done, attempt to find the twigs which the **three lateral lumbricals** receive from the deep branch of the lateral **plantar nerve.**

Then clean and study the **muscles of** the **third layer.** These are the flexor hallucis brevis, the adductor hallucis, and the flexor digiti

is large and fleshy. It arises from the **tuberosity of** the **cuboid bone,** and its fibers pass forward and medially to join the tendon of insertion which is common to the adductor and the lateral belly of the flexor brevis. The **transverse head** is small and thin. It arises from the **capsules of** the third, fourth, and fifth **metatarsophalangeal joints,** its fibers passing medially to join the tendon of insertion. The **flexor**

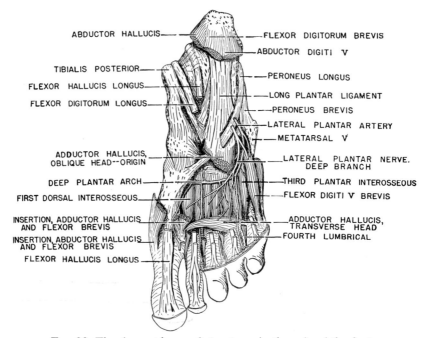

FIG. 93. The deepest layer of structures in the sole of the foot.

quinti brevis. The **flexor hallucis brevis** arises from the plantar surface of the **third cuneiform and** the **cuboid bone.** As its fibers pass forward, they become divided into two fleshy bellies which lie on each side of the tendon of the flexor hallucis longus. The **medial belly** is inserted in common with the abductor hallucis at the **medial side of** the **base of** the **first phalanx;** the **lateral belly** is inserted in common with the adductor hallucis into the **lateral side of** the **base of** the **first phalanx.** The **adductor hallucis** arises by two heads, an oblique and a transverse. The **oblique head**

digiti quinti brevis is a fleshy slip which arises on the **base of** the **fifth metatarsal** and runs straight forward to be inserted into the lateral side of the base of the **proximal phalanx of** the **little toe.**

The flexor hallucis brevis and the oblique head of the adductor hallucis should now be detached from their origins and turned forward, so that the deep plantar arch may be displayed. The **deep plantar arch** is formed by the medial continuation of the **lateral plantar artery,** deep to the accessory flexor and the adductor hallucis, and its junction with the deep plantar branch of the dorsalis pedis artery, which appears in the sole at the base of the first interosseous space. It rests upon the proximal ends of the second, third, and fourth metatarsal bones and gives rise to four **plantar metatarsal arteries.** These pass forward in the interosseous spaces, and each divides into two **plantar digital arteries** which supply the adjacent sides of two toes. The deep branch of the **lateral plantar nerve** accompanies the lateral part of the deep plantar arch. This nerve is distributed to the **adductor hallucis,** the **lateral three lumbrical muscles,** and the **interosseous muscles** of the first, second, and third spaces (Fig. 93).

To display the interosseous muscles, it is advisable to remove the transverse head of the adductor hallucis and to cut the transverse ligaments which bind the heads of the adjacent metatarsal bones together. The **interossei** occupy the **interosseous spaces.** They are arranged in two groups consisting of **three plantar** and **four dorsal interosseous muscles.** The **first, second, and third plantar interosseous muscles** arise from the proximal thirds of the medial plantar surfaces of the third, fourth, and fifth metatarsal bones, respectively. Their fibers pass obliquely forward to join three slender tendons which are inserted into the medial sides of the bases of the proximal phalanges of the third, fourth, and fifth toes. One dorsal interosseous muscle is found in each space. Each arises from the adjacent sides of the two metatarsal bones bounding the space in which it lies. The **first dorsal interosseous muscle** is inserted on the medial side of the base of the first phalanx of the second toe. The **second, third,** and **fourth** are inserted on the lateral side of the bases of the first phalanges of the second, third, and fourth toes.

The **tendon of** the **tibialis posterior** may now be traced to its insertion. Observe that while its principal attachment is to the **tuberosity of** the **navicular,** it gives off a secondary slip which spreads over the sole of the foot to gain attachment to the **second** and **third cuneiform,** the **cuboid,** and the **fourth metatarsal bones.** The **tendon of** the **fibularis longus** has been traced to the lateral border of the **cuboid bone;** follow it now across the sole to its insertion on the inferior surface of the **first cuneiform** and the adjacent part of the **first metatarsal.** Observe that as it crosses the cuboid bone it is partially ensheathed by the **long plantar ligament.** This ligament is a strong fibrous band which is attached posteriorly to the entire **inferior surface of** the **calcaneus** and passes forward to the **tuberosity of** the **cuboid,** from which its fibers spread out to reach the **bases of** the four lateral **metatarsal bones.** It is of considerable importance in preserving the **longitudinal arch of** the **foot.**

Joints

The dissection of the joints should be done only in one extremity; the other one should be saved for a review of the entire dissected limb and for the relationships of the various structures to the joints. As the muscles and other structures are being cleaned from the joints, the course of the **collateral vessels** and the **nerves to** the **joints** should be studied, since they could not be dissected adequately in the preceding dissection of the lower extremity.

Hip Joint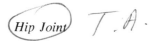

The posterior aspect of the **capsule of** the **hip joint** should next be cleaned. First, divide the ischiadic nerve about 1 in. below the greater sciatic foramen and turn the distal portion downward. Then sever the tendons of the piriformis, the obturator internus, and the gemelli about ¾ in. medial to their insertions and turn the cut ends of these muscles laterally and medially. Observe that as they approach their insertions all of these muscles lie immediately behind the joint capsule. Observe the

mucous bursa which intervenes between the deep surface of the **obturator internus** and the **lesser sciatic notch.** Detach the quadratus femoris from its insertion on the femur and

capsule to be inserted into the **trochanteric fossa.** The upper posterior part of the joint capsule is covered by the gluteus minimus. First, cut the tensor fasciae latae away from its

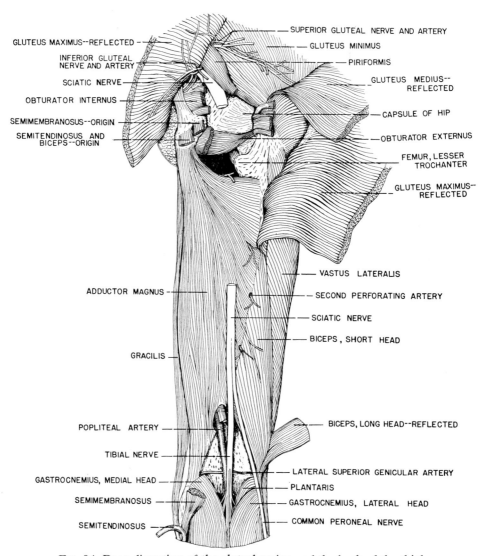

FIG. 94. Deep dissection of the gluteal region and the back of the thigh.

turn it medially. The removal of a little fatty areolar tissue in front of the quadratus will now expose the **tendon of** the **obturator externus,** which here winds laterally and superiorly across the lower posterior part of the joint

origin, if this has not already been done, and turn it downward; then detach the **gluteus minimus** from its origin and reflect it completely to its insertion. As this is being done, it should be noted that some of its deeper fibers arise from the **joint capsule;** these should be cut away and the posterior part of the capsule cleaned.

The **fibrous capsule** of the hip joint is attached posteriorly to the **ilium and the ischium** about ¼ in. medial to the acetabular rim; from here, it stretches laterally and downward to be attached to the posterior surface of the **neck of the femur.** Its thickened upper portion is known as the **ischiocapsular ligament;** this reaches as

Review the origins of the pectineus, gracilis, and adductor muscles. Sever the gracilis close to its origin and turn it downward. Then define clearly the upper border of the **adductor magnus,** taking care to distinguish between this muscle and the **obturator externus,** which lies behind it but reaches a higher level. Then divide the adductor magnus along the entire length of its origin and reflect the main mass of the muscle backward and laterally toward

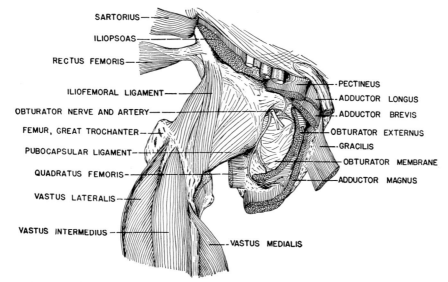

FIG. 95. Dissection to expose the anterior aspect of the capsule of the hip joint and the distribution of the obturator artery.

far laterally as the upper part of the great trochanter and is closely associated with the insertions of the piriformis, obturator internus, and gemelli.

Turn next to the front of the hip. A favorable opportunity is now offered to study the manner of origin of the **rectus femoris.** The **straight head** runs downward from the anterior inferior spine of the ilium; the **reflected head** arises from the posterosuperior surface of the border of the acetabulum in close relation to the capsule of the hip joint and goes forward under cover of the gluteus minimus and tensor fasciae to join the straight head (Fig. 95).

its insertion. The obturator externus is now exposed and should be cleaned.

The **obturator externus** arises, under cover of the origins of the adductors brevis and magnus, from the outer surface of the **ischiopubic rami** along the anterior margin of the obturator foramen and, to a slight extent, from the external surface of the **obturator membrane.** Its fibers converge laterally and posteriorly to join a tendon which winds around the lower part of the joint capsule, as already noted.

The anterior aspect of the capsule of the hip joint is covered by the **iliopsoas muscle.** Sever this muscle just above its insertion into the lesser trochanter and turn it upward to expose the anterior surface of the capsule. Observe the **large mucous bursa** which intervenes between the deep surface of the muscle and the anterior surface of the capsule; this bursa frequently communicates with the cavity of the joint. Study of the joint capsule will be facilitated if the lower reflected portion of the iliopsoas is completely removed by cutting through its entire thickness along the line of the inguinal ligament.

Anteriorly, the **articular capsule** is attached to the **ilium** and the **pubis** close to the rim of the acetabulum, from which it stretches downward and laterally to be attached to the **intertrochanteric line of** the **femur.** It exhibits two special thickened portions which are described as distinct ligaments. The stronger of these is the **iliofemoral ligament.** This is a very thick triangular portion of the capsule which is attached above to the **ilium** immediately below the anterior inferior spine and widens out inferiorly to reach the upper two-thirds of the **intertrochanteric line.** The **pubocapsular ligament** is a less marked thickening of capsule which stretches from the outer surface of the **pubis** near its junction with the ilium to the lower part of the **intertrochanteric line.** Superiorly, between these two ligaments, the capsule is often very thin; it is here that it may communicate with the **psoas bursa.**

Before the joint cavity is opened, the obturator externus should be reflected to expose the **obturator membrane** and the distribution of the **obturator artery.** Cut through the entire breadth of the obturator externus close to its origin and turn the cut portion of the muscle downward and backward toward its insertion. As this is being done, observe the twigs of supply which it receives from the **obturator nerve.** Then clean the outer surface of the obturator membrane. The **obturator artery** will be found emerging from the pelvis at the obturator canal, in company with the obturator nerve,

above the short upper free margin of the obturator membrane. It divides almost at once into an **anterior** and a **posterior branch,** which follow in their further course the anterior and posterior borders, respectively, of the obturator foramen. The **anterior branch** is usually smaller than the posterior; it is distributed to the **adductor muscles** near their origins and to the **obturator externus.** The **posterior branch** gives rise to an **acetabular branch** which pierces the joint capsule in the region of the acetabular notch to reach the **head of** the **femur** by way of the **ligamentum teres.** From the posterior branch, branches are also given to the various muscles which arise from the ischial ramus (inferior).

The **interior of** the **hip joint** should now be studied. Make an incision through the entire circumference of the articular capsule about ½ in. proximal to its attachment to the femur. As this is done, note the extreme thickness of the **iliofemoral ligament.** Then draw the head of the femur away from the acetabulum. Observe that the bones cannot be drawn entirely apart because of the presence of the **ligamentum teres (capitis femoris),** a strong fibrous band which stretches between the **head of** the **femur** and the **acetabular fossa.** Observe that the **head of** the **femur,** except at the attachment of the ligamentum capitis femoris, and the **articular surface of** the **acetabulum** are each covered with a layer of **cartilage.** All other portions of the internal surface of the **joint cavity** are covered by the **synovial stratum.**

The **internal ligaments of** the **hip joint** are the ligamentum capitis femoris, the transverse acetabular ligament, and the glenoid lip (labrum glenoidale). The **transverse acetabular ligament** is a fibrous band which bridges across the **acetabular notch** and converts it into a foramen, through which the acetabular branch of the obturator artery reaches the acetabular fossa. The **glenoid lip** is a **fibrocartilaginous** ring which surmounts the rim of the acetabulum and the transverse ligament and thus deepens the acetabulum.

Knee Joint

The **capsule of the knee joint** should now be cleaned. First, define clearly the inferior margins of the distal parts of the **vasti muscles;** observe that while these muscles for the most part are attached either directly or by means of the tendon of the quadriceps to the proximal border of the patella, tendinous expansions known as the **patellar retinacula** also pass distad from them to join the articular capsule. The capsule is covered on its lateral side by the **biceps femoris;** the short head of this muscle should now be detached from its origin on the femur and the entire muscle removed, except for the distal portion of its tendon of insertion, which may be left attached to the head of the fibula. The **semimembranosus** must also be removed from the capsule, except for about ½ in. proximal to its attachment to the tibia. With removal of the biceps, the full extent of the **fibular collateral ligament,** whose distal end was already seen piercing the tendon of the biceps, will be exposed and should be cleaned. This is the only one of the external ligaments of the knee joint which is not intimately blended with the articular capsule. Make a longitudinal incision through the middle of the **quadriceps tendon** a short distance above the patella to open the **suprapatellar bursa.** This bursa lies between the deep surface of the quadriceps tendon and the anterior surface of the distal part of the shaft of the femur; it is continuous distad with the articular cavity of the knee joint.

Attempt to demonstrate the **arterial anastomosis** which is found on the anterior aspect of the knee joint **encircling** the **patella.** The terminal portions of **six arteries,** the proximal parts of all of which have already been cleaned, take part in this anastomosis. They are the musculoarticular branches of the **supreme**

genicular from the femoral, the **medial and lateral superior and inferior genicular branches of** the **popliteal,** and the **anterior tibial recurrent** of the anterior tibial.

The **external ligaments of** the **knee joint,** with the exception of the fibular collateral ligament, are intimately blended with the fibrous capsule of the joint.

The fibular collateral and patellar ligaments have already been cleaned. The **tibial collateral ligament** is a strong flat band lying on the medial side of the joint under cover of the tendons of the sartorius, gracilis, and semitendinosus. It extends from the **medial condyle of** the **femur** to the uppermost portion of the **medial surface of** the **tibia,** below the medial condyle. The oblique and arcuate popliteal ligaments are thickenings in the posterior part of the capsule. The **oblique popliteal ligament** lies in front of the middle portion of the popliteal artery; it extends upward and laterally across the **back of** the **joint** from the posterior aspect of the medial condyle of the tibia. Observe that it receives a strong band of fibers from the tendon of insertion of the semimembranosus. The **arcuate popliteal ligament** lies at the posterolateral side of the knee, extending from the apex of the **head of** the **fibula** upward to the back of the **lateral condyle of** the **femur;** the tendon of the popliteus muscle emerges from the joint capsule at the medial border of this ligament.

Divide the entire thickness of the quadriceps femoris transversely about 2 in. above the patella and turn the distal segment of the muscle downward and forward. Then open the knee joint from the front by dividing the anterior part of the articular capsule close to its line of attachment to the distal portion of the anterior surface of the femur. Flex the knee completely, draw the distal portion of the quadriceps with the attached patella downward and forward, and study the **interior of** the **joint** (Fig. 96).

The bony **articular surfaces** of the knee joint include the **condyles** and the **patellar surface of** the **femur,** the superior **articular surface of** the **tibia,** and the **internal surface of** the **patella.** Observe that each of these surfaces is covered by a layer of **cartilage.** Elsewhere, the cavity of the joint is lined by the **synovial membrane,** between which and the fibrous capsule are numerous large depositions of fat. Observe the

these surfaces from the corresponding articular surfaces of the condyles of the femur. Their inner margins are sharp and free; their outer margins are thicker and attached to the fibrous capsule of the joint.

To expose the transverse and cruciate ligaments, it will be necessary to clear away the patellar synovial fold and the fat contained in it. The **transverse ligament** is a fibrous cord

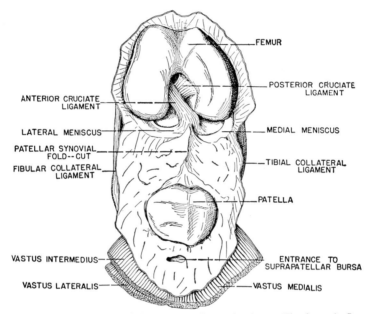

FIG. 96. The interior of the knee joint as seen from the front. The knee is flexed and the patella drawn downward. The femoral attachment of the patellar synovial fold has been cut away to expose the cruciate ligaments.

patellar synovial fold; this is a fat-filled fold of the synovial stratum, which runs from the lower border of the **patella** back **to the inter-condyloid fossa of** the **femur.**

The **internal ligaments** of the knee joint include the **medial** and **lateral menisci,** the **transverse ligament,** and the **anterior** and **posterior cruciate ligaments.** The **menisci** may be seen without dissection. They are **two** semilunar **fibrocartilaginous discs** which rest upon the outer portions of the **articular surfaces of** the **condyles of** the **tibia** and partially separate

which extends across the anterior margin of the upper surface of the tibia from the rounded anterior margin of the **lateral meniscus** to the sharp anterior extremity or cornu of the **medial meniscus.** The cruciate ligaments are strong fibrous bands which occupy the intercondyloid fossa of the femur. The **anterior cruciate ligament** extends upward, backward, and laterally from the **anterior intercondyloid fossa of** the **tibia** to the medial surface of the **lateral condyle of** the **femur.** The **posterior cruciate ligament** is partly covered anteriorly by the anterior ligament. It extends upward and medially from the **posterior intercondyloid fossa of** the **tibia** to the lateral surface of the **medial condyle of** the **femur.**

Extend the knee, divide the posterior portion of the capsule of the joint, and observe the origin of the popliteus muscle from the lower lateral part of the lateral condyle of the femur, within the cavity of the joint.

Ankle Joint *T.A.*

Clean the capsule of the **ankle joint.** At this joint, the **talus** articulates with the **distal end** and **medial malleolus** of the **tibia** and the **lateral malleolus of the fibula.** Its capsule is very thin anteriorly and posteriorly but is thickened on the lateral and medial sides. The thickened medial portion is known as the **deltoid ligament.** It is attached above to the **medial malleolus** and spreads out inferiorly to be attached, from before backward, to the **navicular,** the **talus,** the **sustentaculum tali of** the **calcaneus,** and the **posterior part of** the **talus.** The thickened lateral portion of the capsule consists of three distinct slips, the **anterior talofibular ligament,** the **calcaneofibular ligament,** and the **posterior talofibular ligament.**

Tarsal and Metatarsal Joints

The **articulations of** the **foot** include the **intertarsal, tarsometatarsal,** and **intermetatarsal** joints, the **metatarsophalangeal** joints, and the **interphalangeal** joints. The joints of the first groups are worthy of some attention; study of them should be accompanied by constant reference to the mounted skeleton of a foot or to a set of disarticulated bones.

The **tarsal** and **metatarsal bones** are arranged in the form of **two arches,** a **longitudinal** and a **transverse,** the concavities of both facing toward the sole. The **longitudinal arch** rests posteriorly on the tuberosity of the **calcaneus** and anteriorly on the **metatarsal** bones. It is supported principally by the **long plantar liga-**

ment (Fig. 93) and the **plantar calcaneonavicular ligament** (Fig. 97).

The **tarsal** and **metatarsal bones** are connected to one another by **dorsal, plantar,** and **interosseous ligaments.** There are **six** separate **articular cavities** for the various intertarsal, tarsometatarsal, and intermetatarsal articulations. The **talus,** through which the entire weight of the body is transmitted to the foot, takes part in **two of these,** an articulation at which a facet on the **body of** the **talus** meets the **posterior facet of** the **calcaneus** and an articulation at which the **head of** the **talus** meets the **navicular**

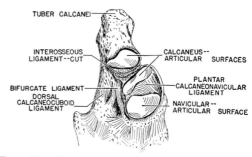

Fig. 97. The tarsal articulations of the talus, opened from above by removal of the talus.

and the **sustentaculum tali** of the calcaneus (Fig. 97).

Disarticulate the talus to open these two articular cavities. Observe that in order to disarticulate the talus, a very strong ligament which fills the tarsal canal (sinus tarsi) must be cut. This is the interosseus **talocalcaneal ligament,** which binds the **talus** and the **calcaneus** firmly together and separates the two articular cavities in which the talus takes part. Observe also that the articular surface of the head of the talus is not completely taken up by its articulations with the navicular and the calcaneus but rests also upon a strong ligament which stretches between the plantar surfaces of the two latter bones. This is the **plantar calcaneonavicular ligament;** it rests inferiorly on the tendon of the tibialis posterior.

Of the remaining four **articular cavities of the tarsus, one** is for the articulation between the **calcaneus** and the **cuboid. A second** single large articular **cavity** includes the articulations between the **navicular,** the three **cuneiforms,** the **cuboid,** and the **second** and **third metatarsals.** The **third cavity** includes the articulations between the **cuboid** and the **fourth** and **fifth metatarsals.** The **fourth cavity** is for the articulation of the **first cuneiform** with the **first metatarsal.** These cavities may be opened and the bones spread apart for observation of the articular surfaces by cutting through the dorsal ligaments.

Sacroiliac Joint

The sacroiliac joint is formed between the auricular surfaces of the sacrum and ilium. This joint is held together by the **anterior sacroiliac, posterior sacroiliac,** and **interosseous ligaments.** An attempt should be made to identify these ligaments since they are important in maintaining the sacrum between the two ilia.

Index ·

57
90
84
73
61

5⟌365⟌73
35
15

6⟌375
2
1
15

Mayberry
Rowry
Ashford